Atlas of Oral and Maxillofacial Anatomy

Joe Iwanaga • R. Shane Tubbs

Atlas of Oral and Maxillofacial Anatomy

Springer

Joe Iwanaga
Department of Neurosurgery
Clinical Neuroscience Research Center (CNRC)
Tulane University School of Medicine
New Orleans, LA
USA

R. Shane Tubbs
Department of Neurosurgery
Clinical Neuroscience Research Center (CNRC)
Tulane University School of Medicine
New Orleans, CA
USA

ISBN 978-3-030-78326-6 ISBN 978-3-030-78327-3 (eBook)
https://doi.org/10.1007/978-3-030-78327-3

This Springer imprint is published by the registered company Springer Nature Switzerland AG
The registered company address is: Gewerbestrasse 11, 6330 Cham, Switzerland

Preface

This atlas focuses on the oral and maxillofacial regions and is relevant in the disciplines of oral and maxillofacial surgery. The fine anatomy involved in oral and maxillofacial surgery has progressed greatly in recent years, and therefore knowledge of anatomical structures relevant to this field is now more important than ever. However, anatomical atlases that demonstrate the newest anatomical findings in the oral and maxillofacial regions in a comprehensive manner are scant. For oral and maxillofacial surgery, observing oral anatomy from the same view as seen in clinical practice is critical for a better understanding of various invasive procedures. However, to our knowledge, no other books have included high-resolution images of intraoral anatomical dissections, especially using fresh cadavers. For example, the lingual nerve is a structure that is always mentioned by mentors—"Be careful not to damage the lingual nerve as it runs next to the lingual cortical plate." Yes, we know that the lingual nerve is always at risk when we make an incision in the retromolar to molar areas of the mandible; however, how should we better minimize potential injury by an improved knowledge of this anatomy from an intraoral, surgical view? The answer to this question and others is found throughout this atlas via step-by-step fresh-cadaver dissections. We believe that this book will satisfy current needs in the discipline of oral and maxillofacial surgery and is timely.

New Orleans, LA, USA — Joe Iwanaga
New Orleans, CA, USA — R. Shane Tubbs

Contents

1 Anatomy of the Superficial Face

1.1 Superficial Face

Summary
The maxillofacial region has a rich blood and nerve supply. The former derived from the external carotid artery and terminal branches of the internal carotid artery. The mimetic muscles are innervated by the extracranial facial nerve branches, and the sensation of the skin is supplied by primarily, trigeminal nerve branches. Some of these nerve branches often communicate with adjacent nerves, e.g., marginal mandibular branch of the facial nerve and mental nerve, although the function of such connections is unclear. In this section, the superficial structures of the maxillofacial region will be demonstrated.

J. Iwanaga, R. S. Tubbs, *Atlas of Oral and Maxillofacial Anatomy*, https://doi.org/10.1007/978-3-030-78327-3_1

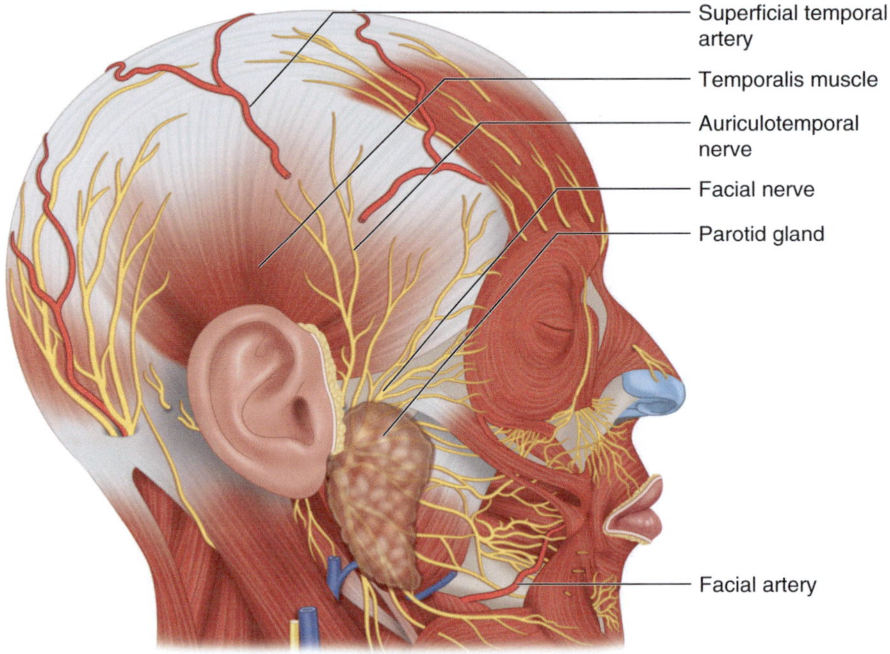

Fig. 1.1 Lateral view of the face

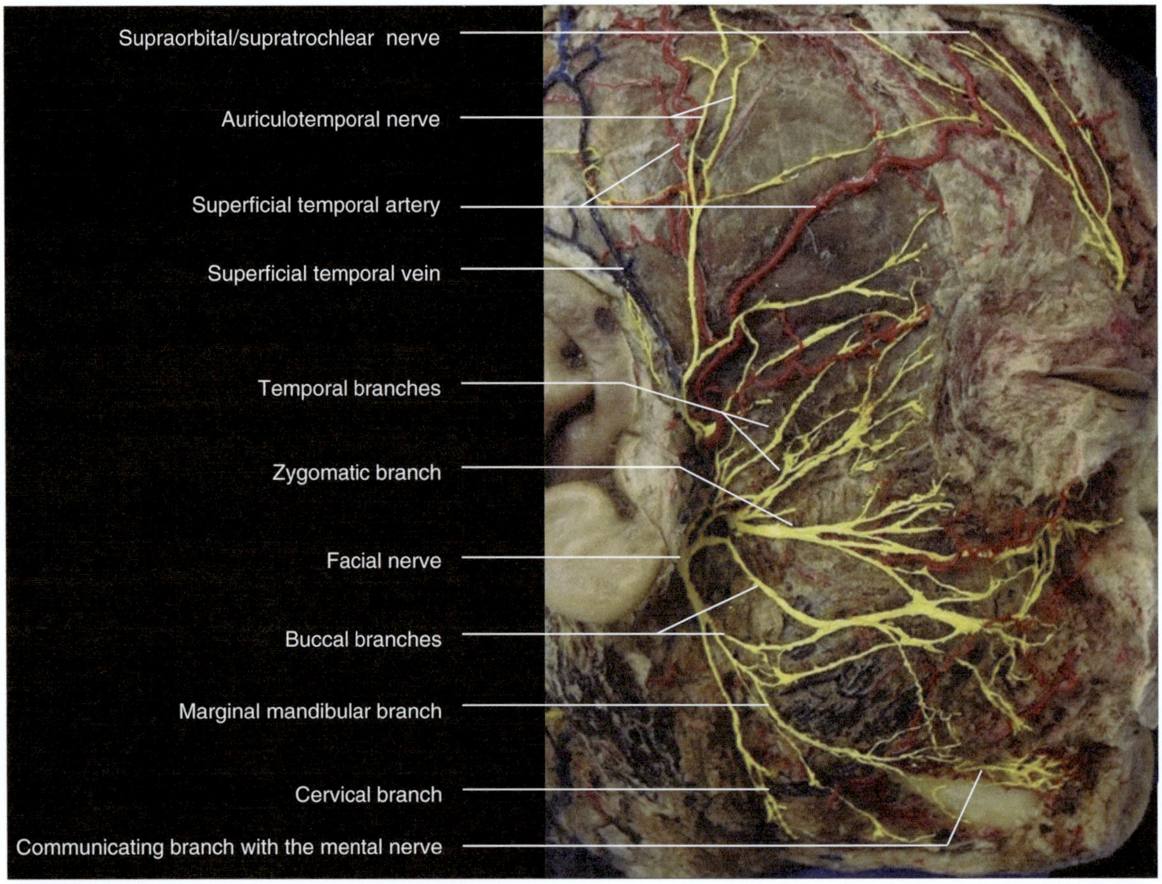

Fig. 1.2 Terminal branches of the facial nerve (lateral view)

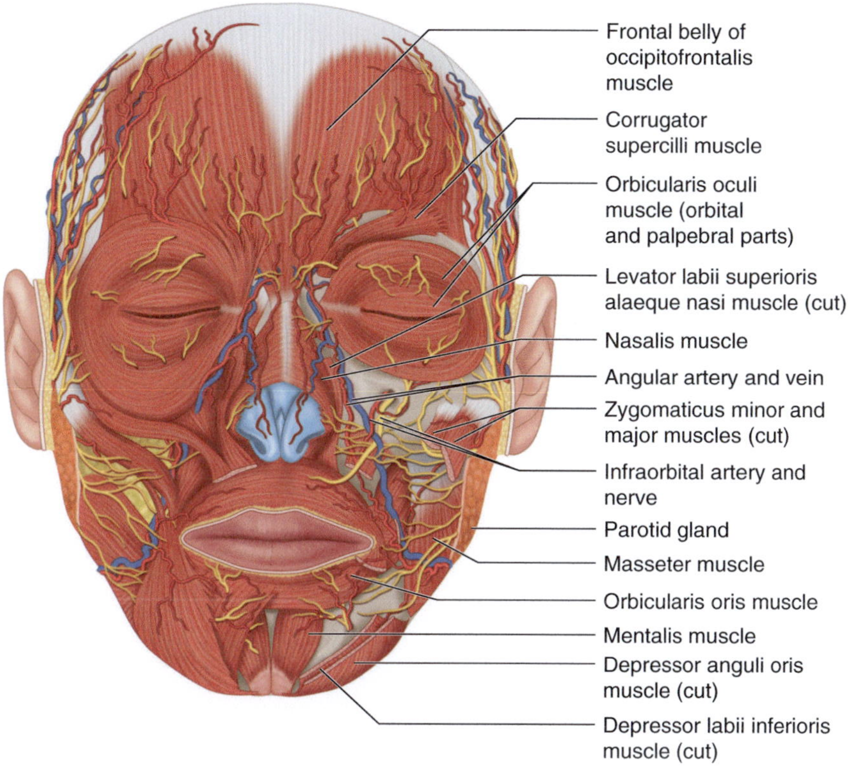

Fig. 1.3 Anterior view of the face

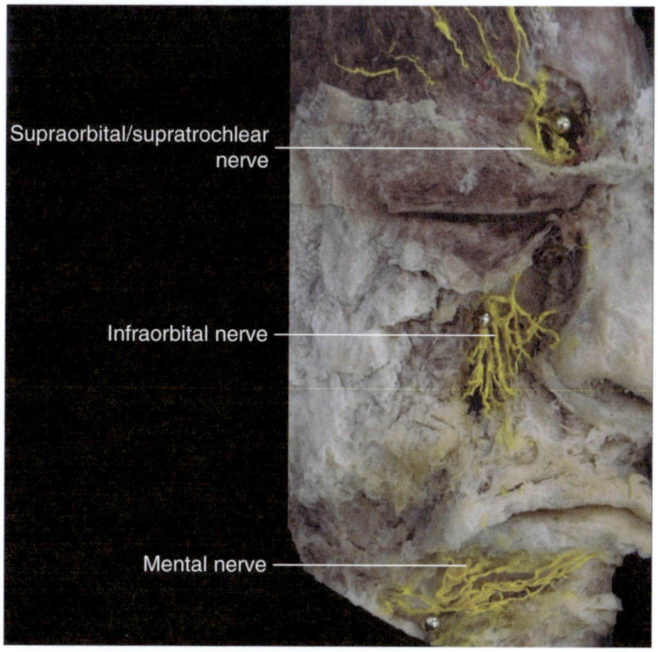

Fig. 1.4 Terminal cutaneous branches of the trigeminal nerve (anterior view)

Bones of the Head and Neck

2

2.1 Overview (Skull)

Summary
The skull consists of 23 bones including the hyoid bone: eight paired bones (temporal, zygomatic, parietal, maxillary, nasal, lacrimal and palatine bones, and the inferior nasal concha) and seven unpaired bones (occipital, frontal, sphenoid, ethmoid, hyoid, mandible, and vomer). The vomer and inferior nasal concha are within the nasal cavity. Three foramina (or notches) of the face, e.g., supraorbital, infraorbital, and mental foramina, are usually observed from an anterior view. A number of structures exist at the skull base as well as the cranial fossae, which allows vessels and nerves to leave and enter the skull and also act as the attachment of many skeletal muscles.

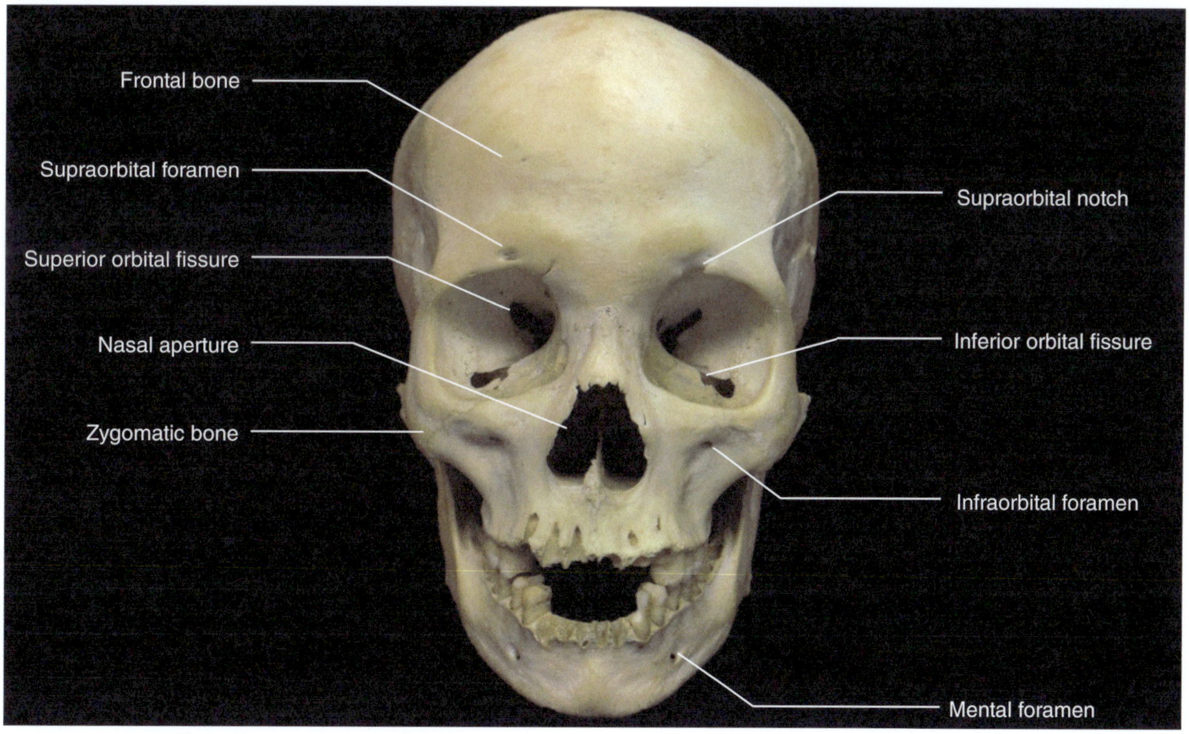

Fig. 2.1 Anterior view of the skull

J. Iwanaga, R. S. Tubbs, *Atlas of Oral and Maxillofacial Anatomy*, https://doi.org/10.1007/978-3-030-78327-3_2

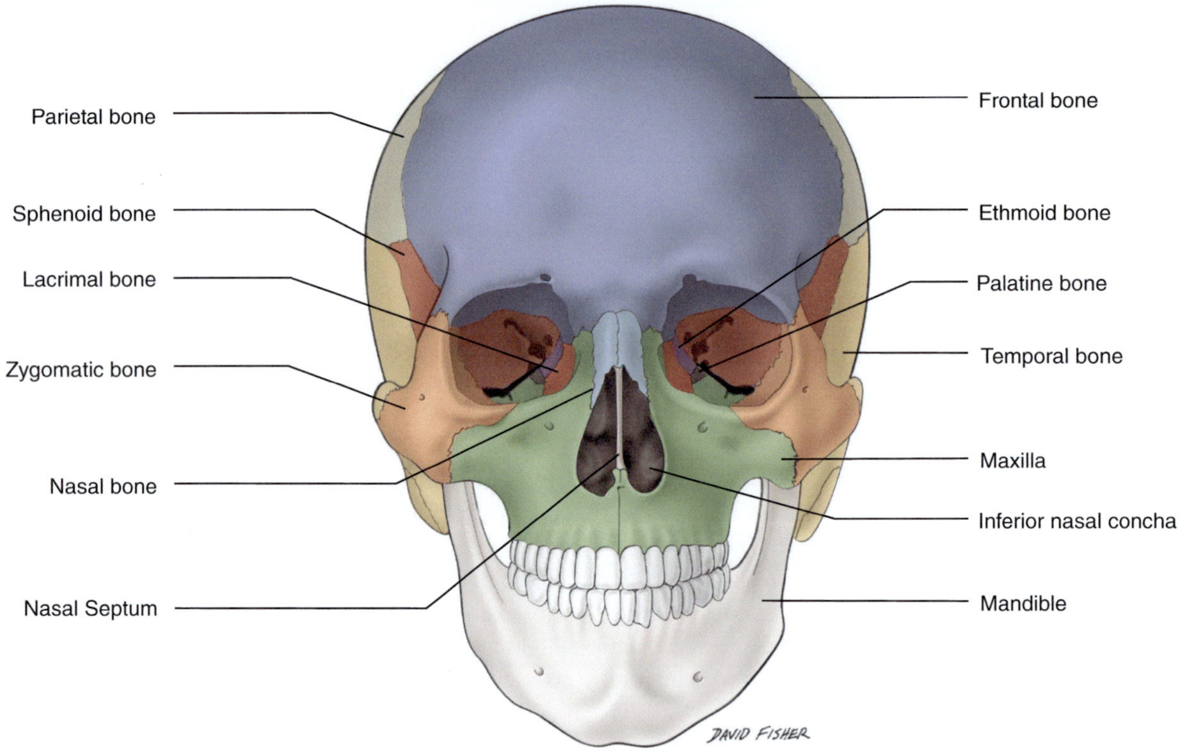

Fig. 2.2 Anterior view of the schematic skull.

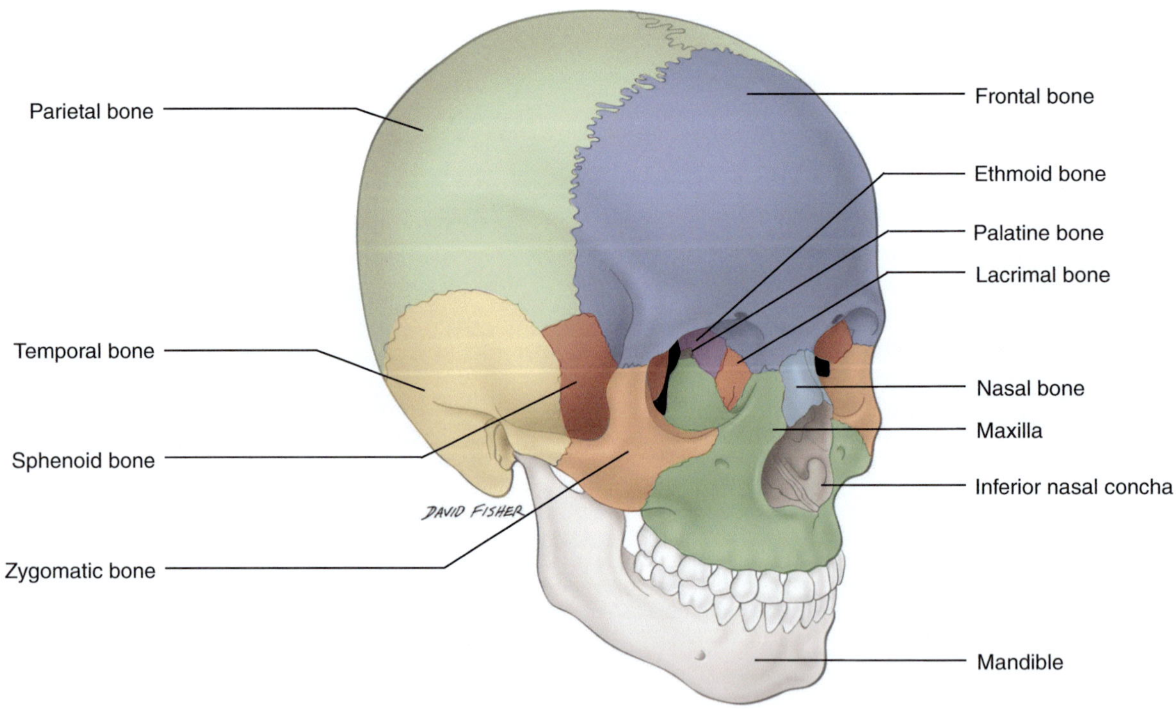

Fig. 2.3 Oblique view of the schematic skull.

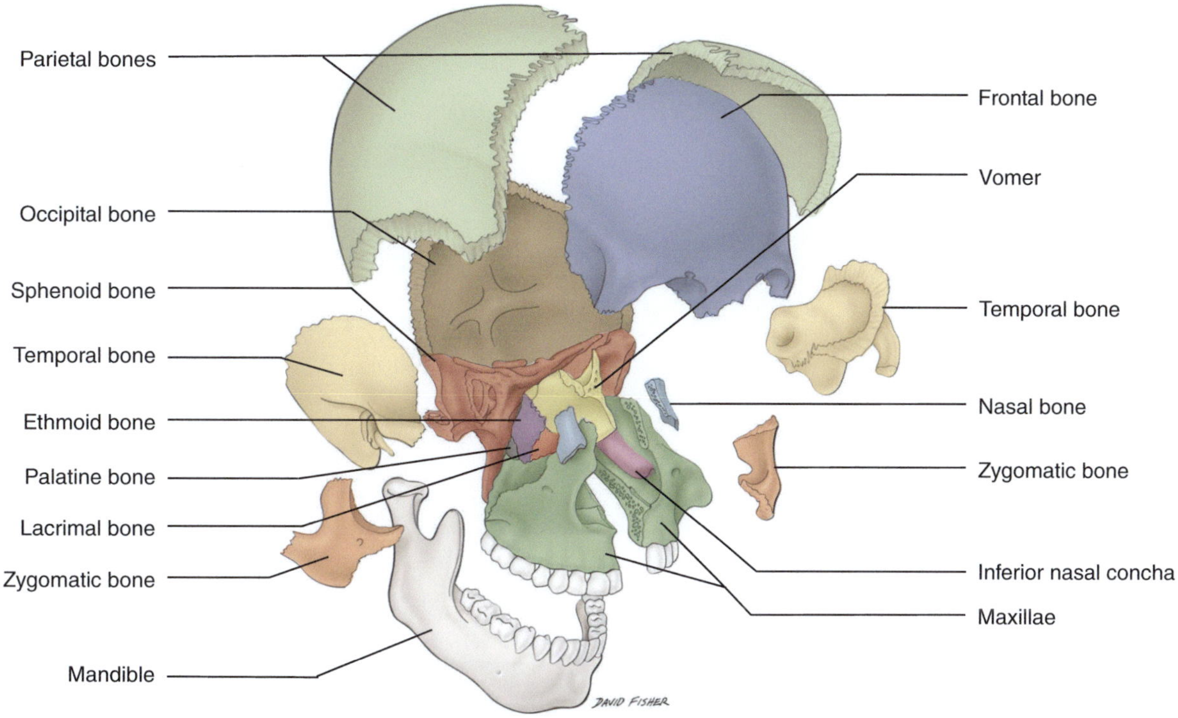

Fig. 2.4 Oblique view of the schematic exploded skull. © Fisher/Tubbs 2020. All Rights Reserved

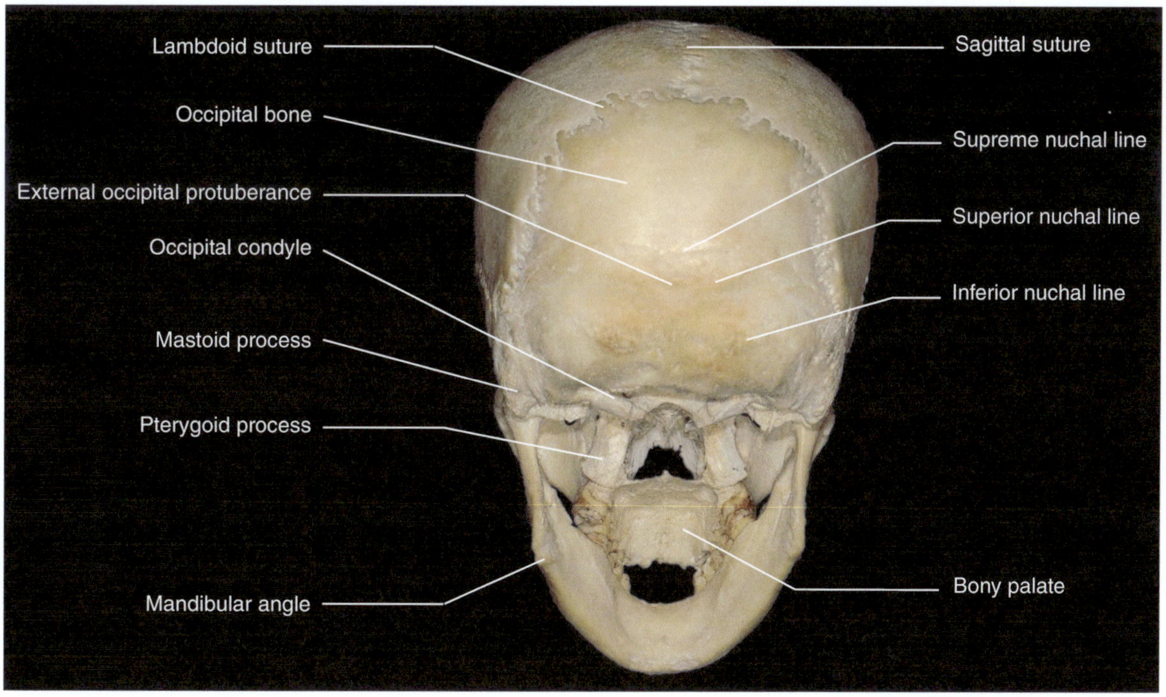

Fig. 2.5 Posterior view of the skull

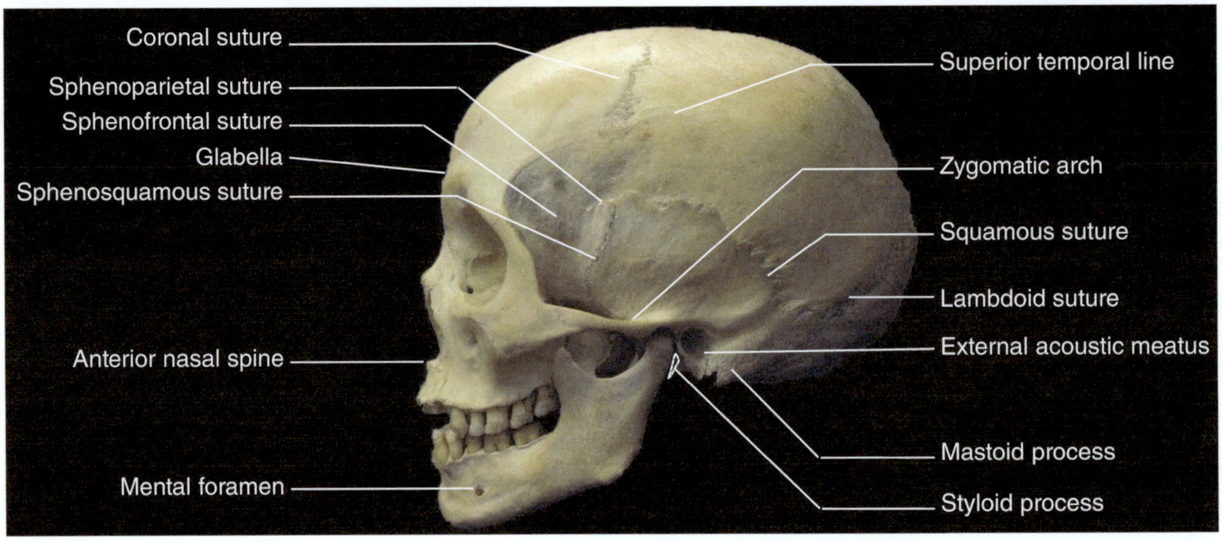

Fig. 2.6 Lateral view of the skull

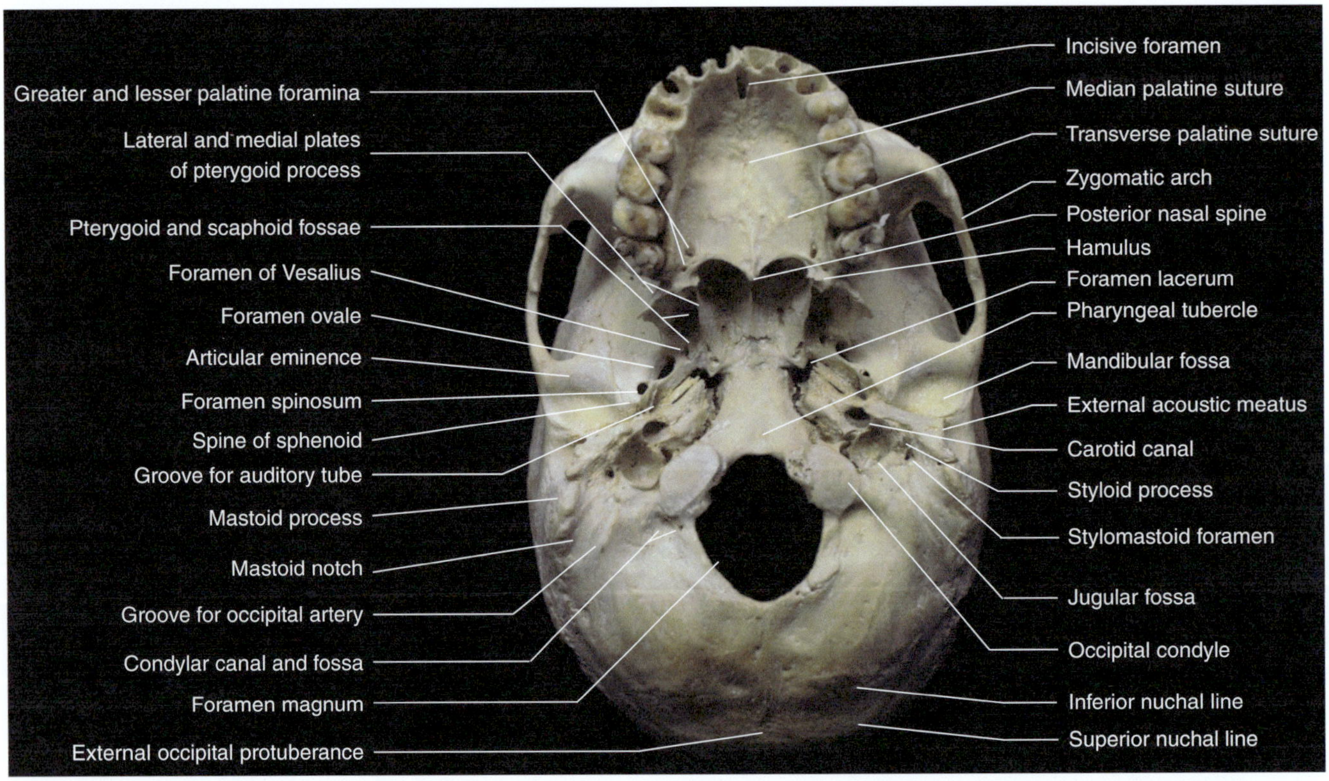

Fig. 2.7 Inferior view of the skull

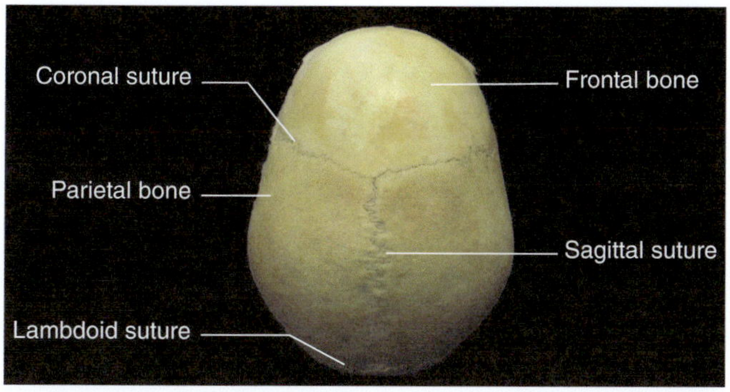

Fig. 2.8 Superior view of the skull

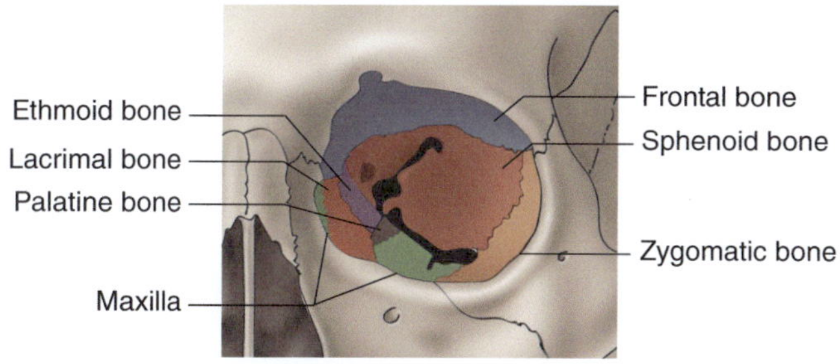

Fig. 2.10 Anterior view of the schematic orbit. The orbital wall consists of seven bones: frontal, sphenoid, zygomatic, ethmoid, lacrimal, palatine, and maxillary bones

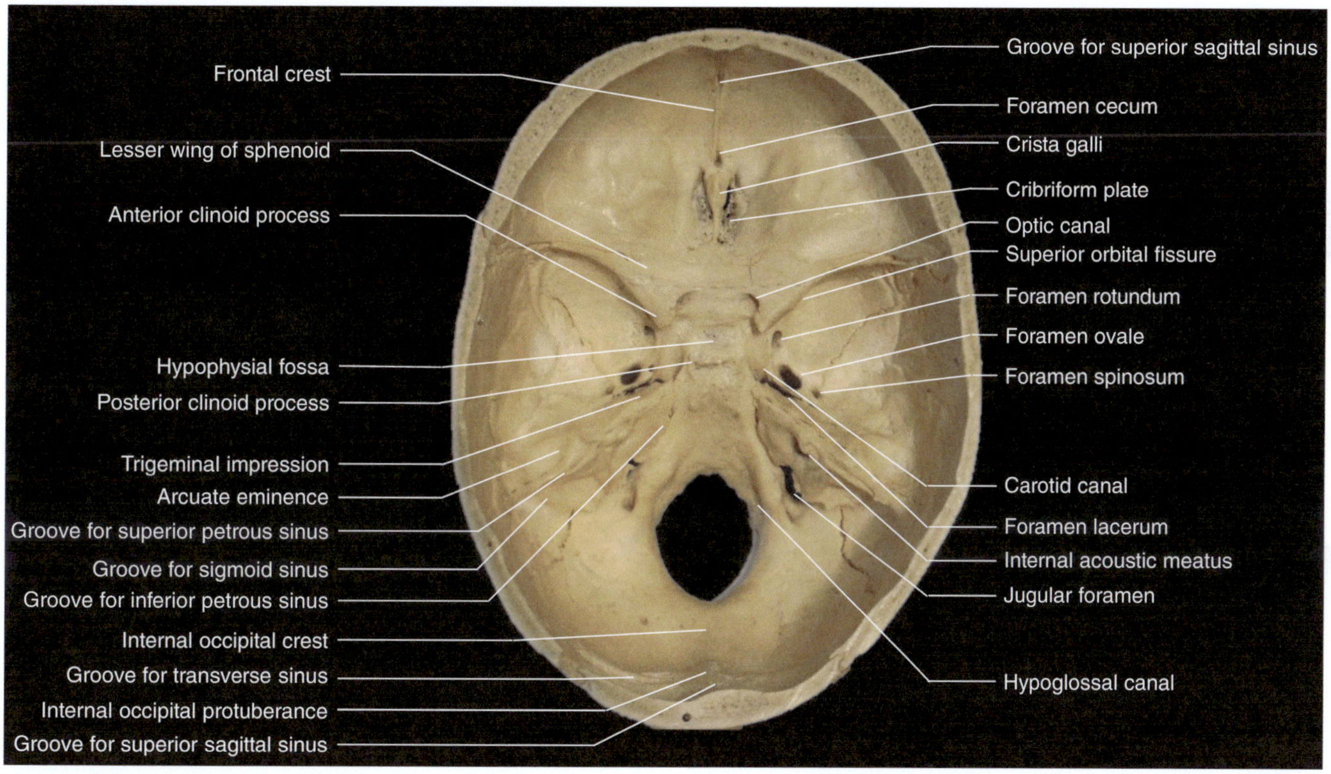

Fig. 2.9 Superior view of the cranial fossae

2.2 Sutures of the Skull

Summary
The sutures of the skull are mostly paired except for the sagittal, median palatine, intermaxillary, and internasal sutures. Many of these are still unfused at birth. For example, the metopic (frontal) suture usually closes at the age of 3 months to 2-years-old. Therefore, the metopic suture is usually not observed in adults. Also, the incisive suture is usually still open under the age of 12 years and is thus rarely visible in the adult. Usually, the anterior and posterior fontanelles close at the age of one and a half years old and three months old, respectively. The coronal, sagittal, and lambdoid sutures are still visible in the adult; however, some smaller sutures are often completely fused in adults. Knowledge of these sutures is vital to understanding clinical pathologies such as craniosynostosis, hydrocephalus, fractures, and rapid maxillary expansion.

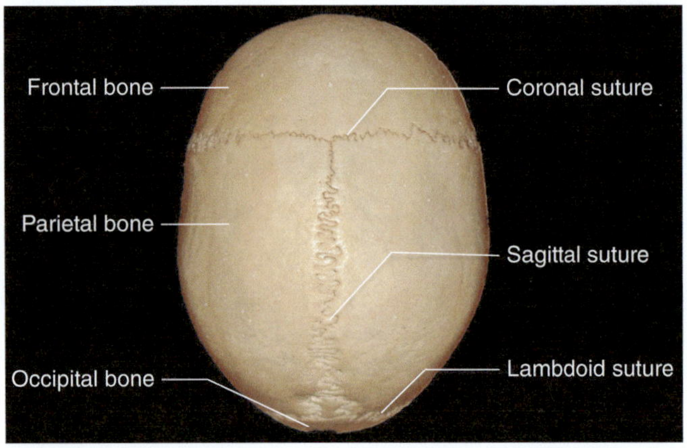

Fig. 2.11 Superior view showing the sutures of the calvaria

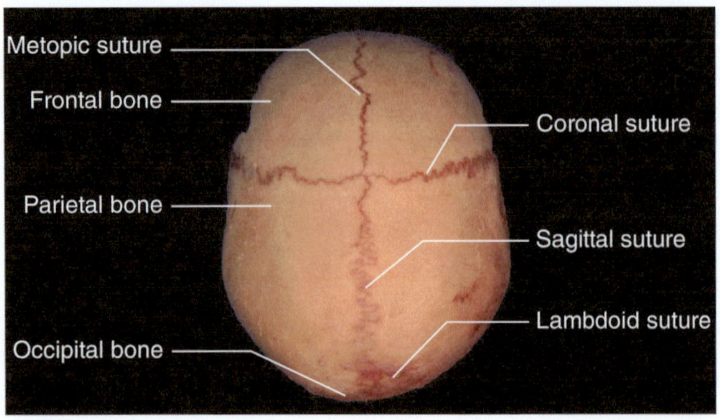

Fig. 2.12 Superior view of the calvaria with a metopic suture (also known as the frontal suture)

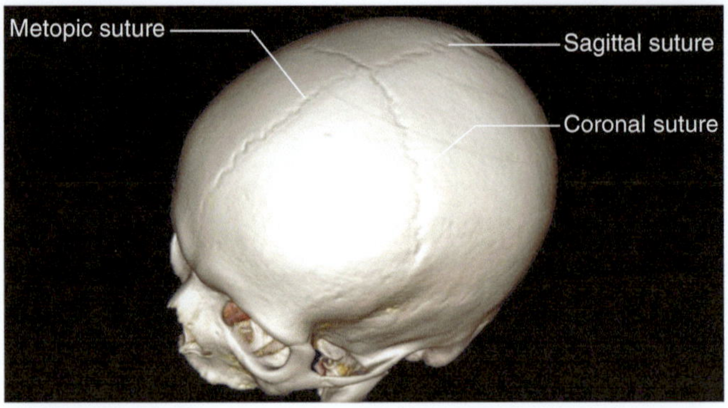

Fig. 2.13 Metopic suture on 3D reconstructed CT

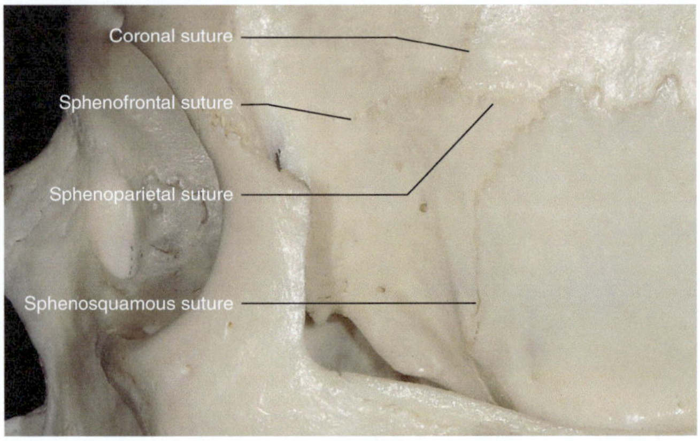

Fig. 2.14 Sutures in the temporal fossa

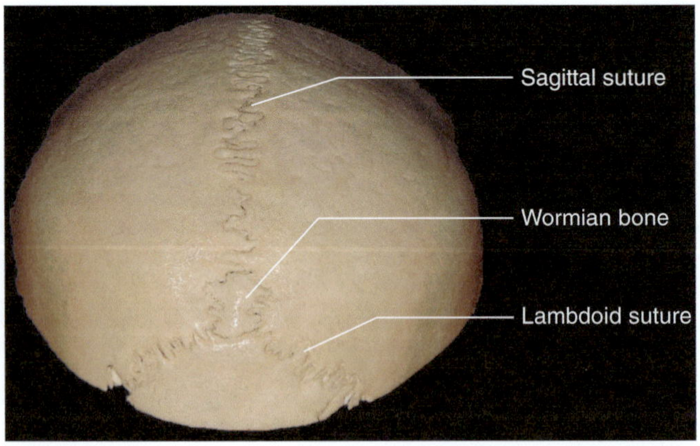

Fig. 2.15 Sutures of the posterior calvaria with a Wormian bone also known as an intrasutural or sutural bone

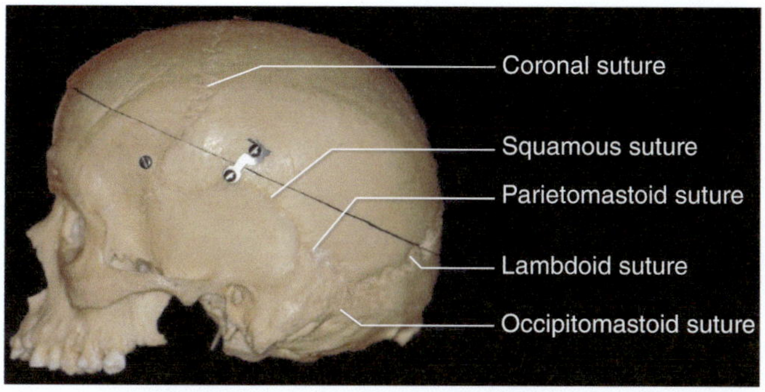

Fig. 2.16 Sutures of the lateral and posterior skull

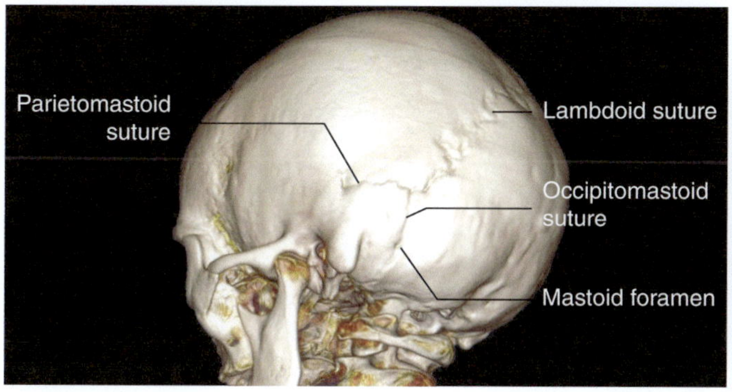

Fig. 2.17 Sutures and foramina around the mastoid process

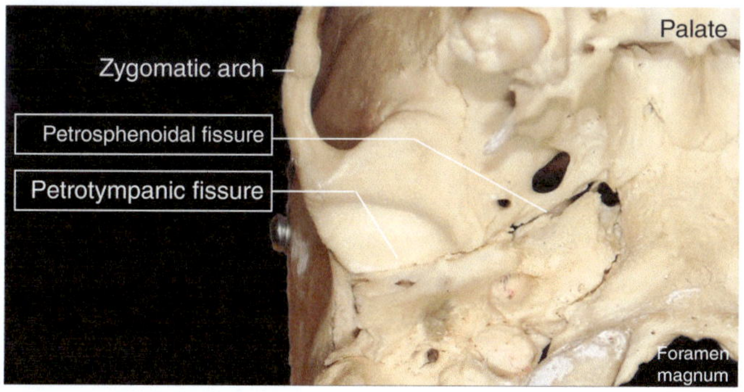

Fig. 2.18 Fissures of the inferior skull

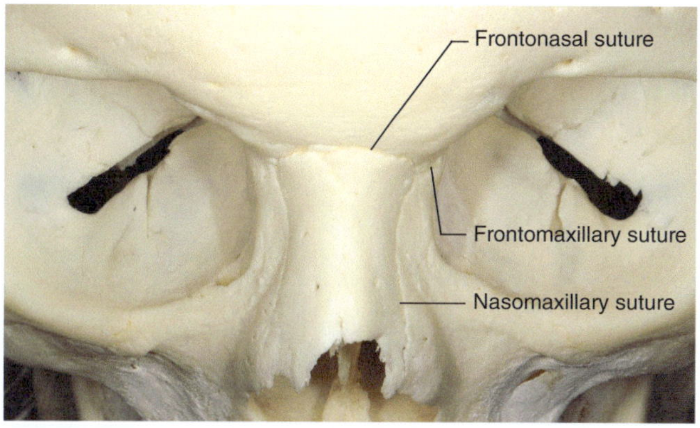

Fig. 2.19 Anterior view of the sutures around the nasal bones

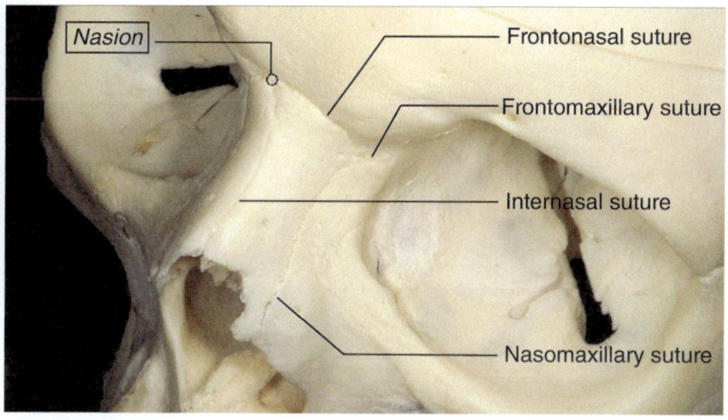

Fig. 2.20 Oblique view of the sutures related to the nasal bones

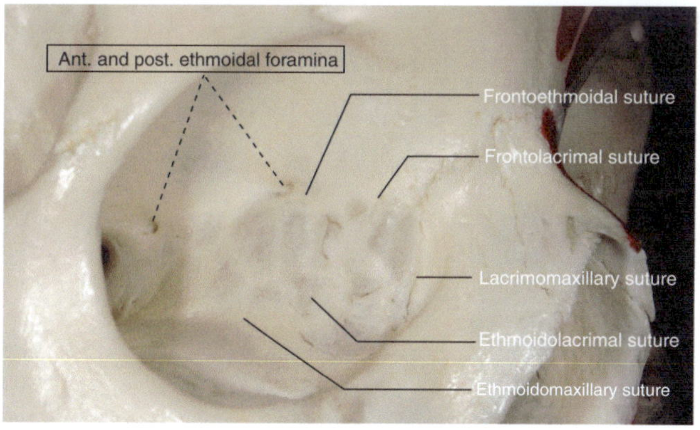

Fig. 2.21 Sutures of the medial wall of the orbit

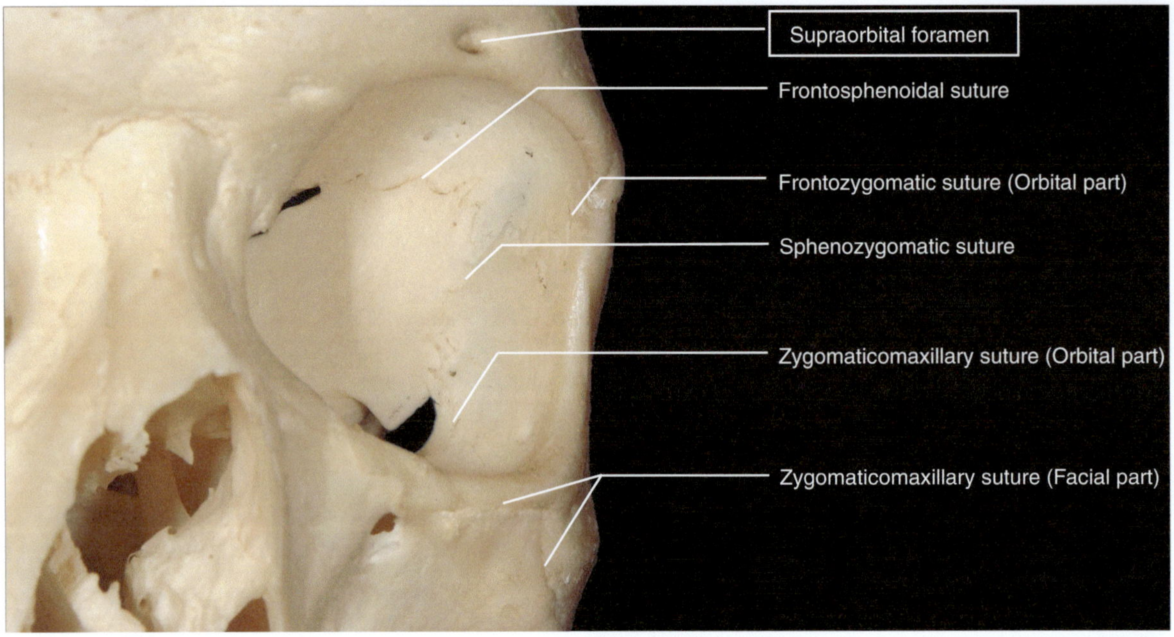

Fig. 2.22 Sutures of the lateral wall of the orbit

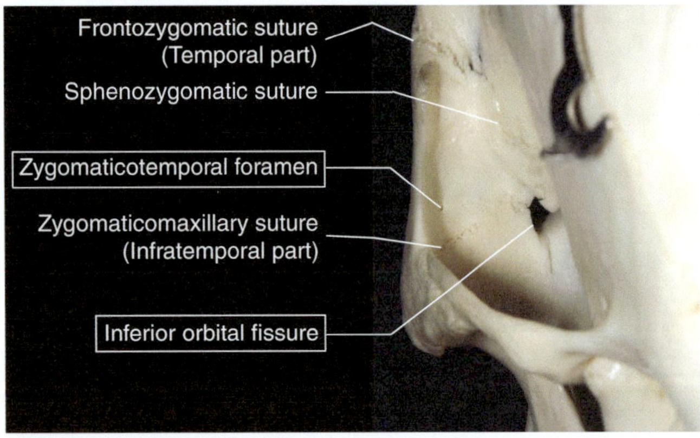

Fig. 2.23 Posterior view of the zygoma

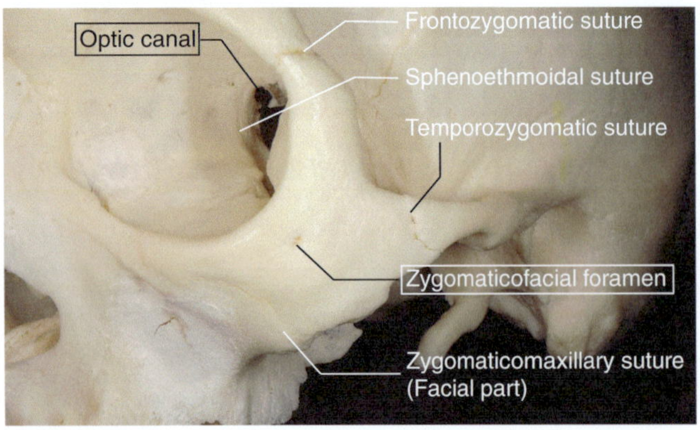

Fig. 2.24 Lateral view of the zygoma

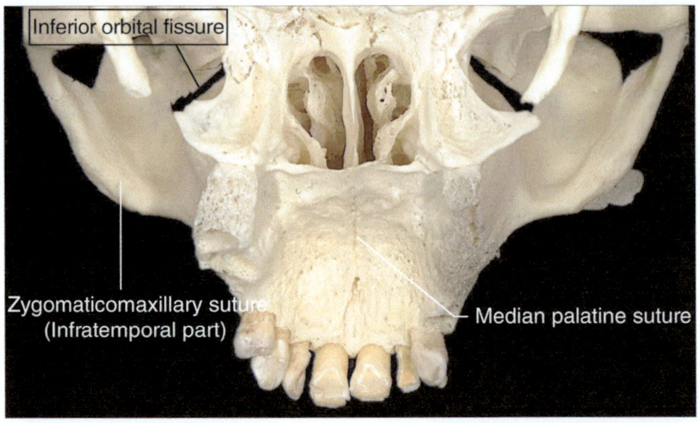

Fig. 2.25 Posteroinferior view

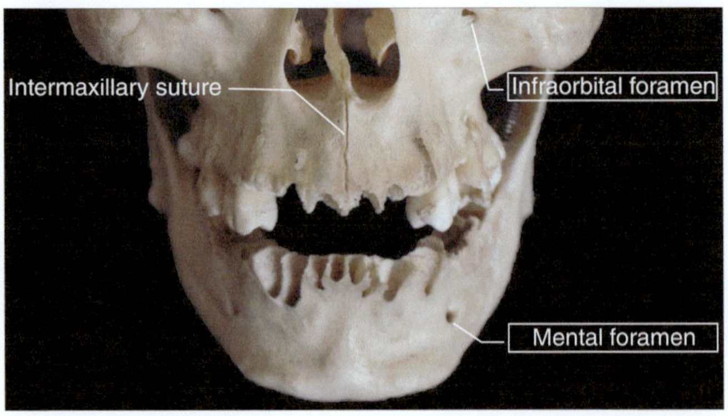

Fig. 2.26 Anterior view

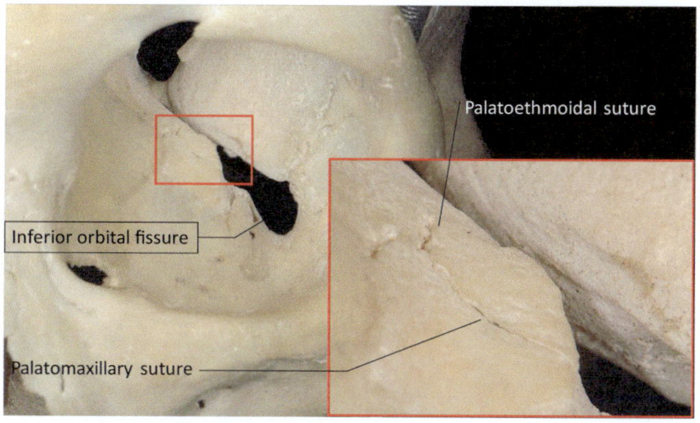

Fig. 2.27 Sutures in the posterior orbit

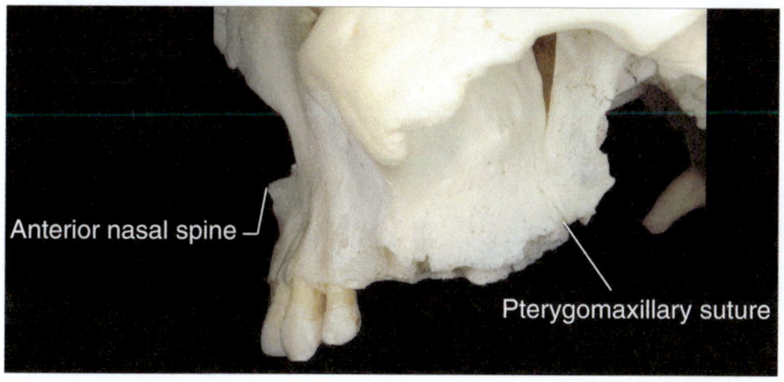

Fig. 2.28 Lateral view of the maxilla

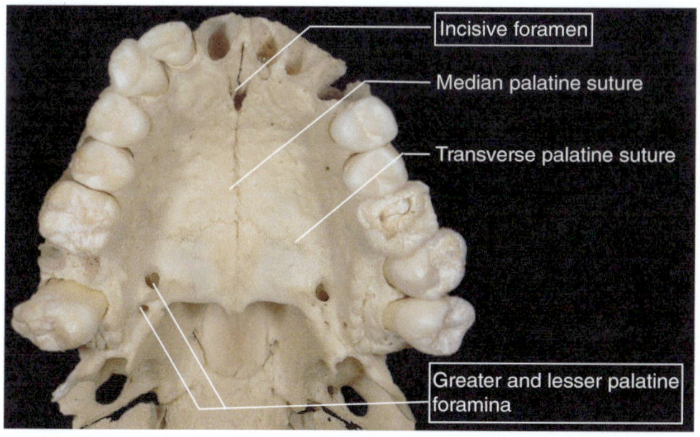

Fig. 2.29 Inferior view of the palate

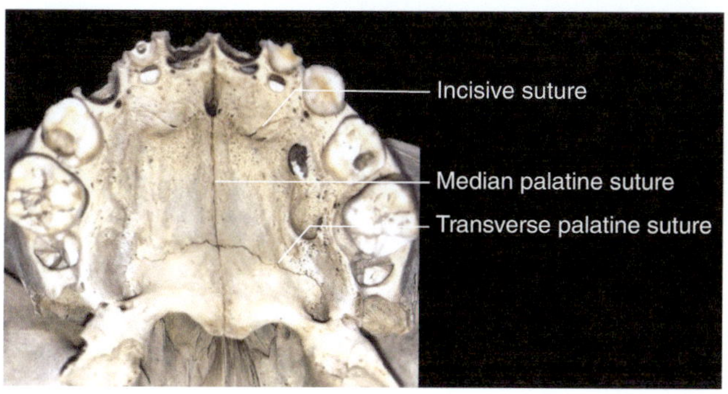

Fig. 2.30 Inferior view of the palate with an incisive suture

2.3 Separate Bones

Summary

In this chapter, the features of the bones forming the skull will be discussed:

Frontal, occipital, temporal, parietal, maxillary, zygomatic, sphenoid, ethmoid, nasal, inferior nasal concha, palatine, lacrimal, mandible, vomer, and hyoid bones. In addition, the auditory ossicles, i.e., malleus, incus, and stapes are also discussed.

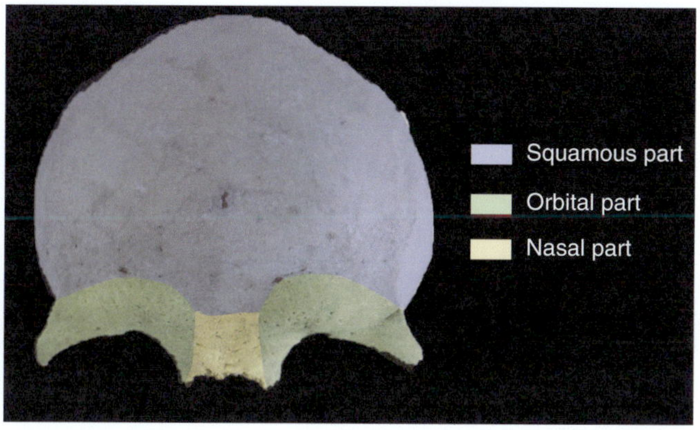

Fig. 2.31 The frontal bone consists of squamous, orbital, and nasal parts

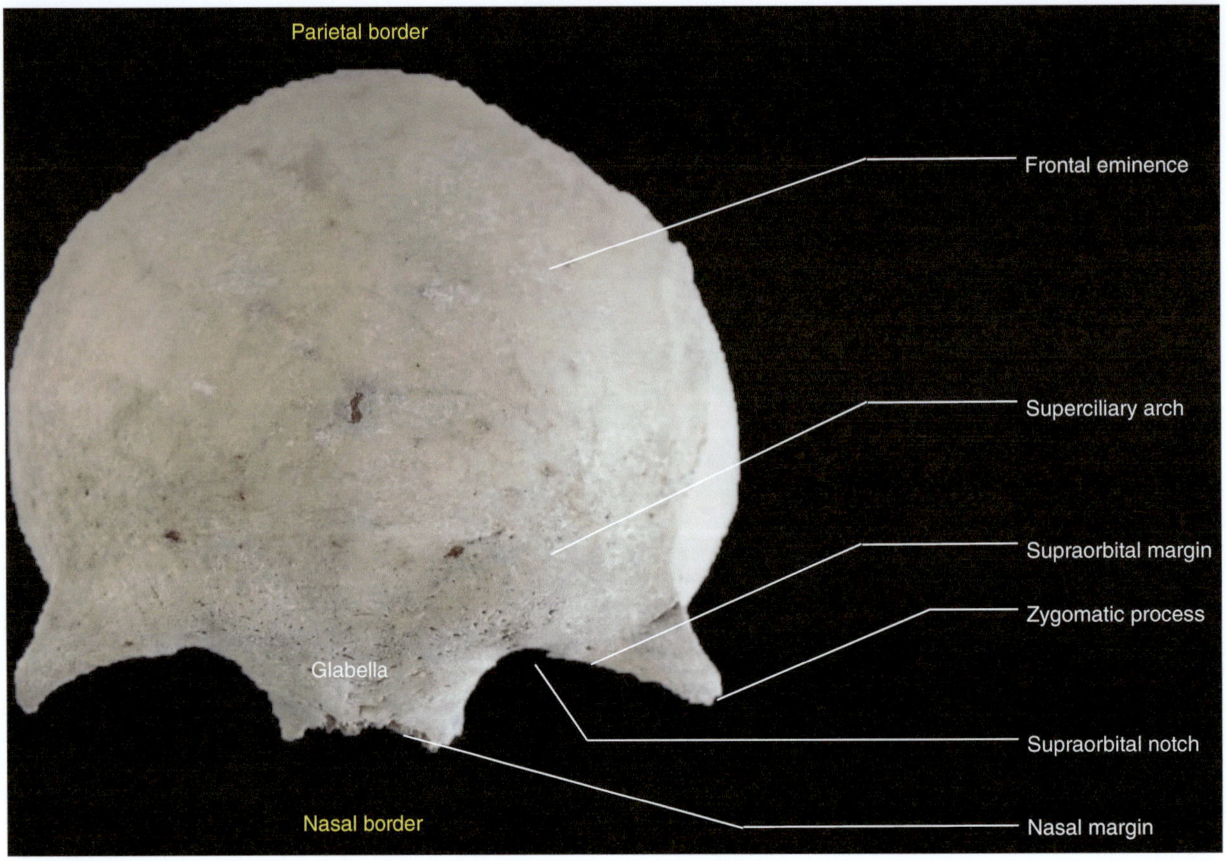

Fig. 2.32 Anterior view of the external surface of the frontal bone

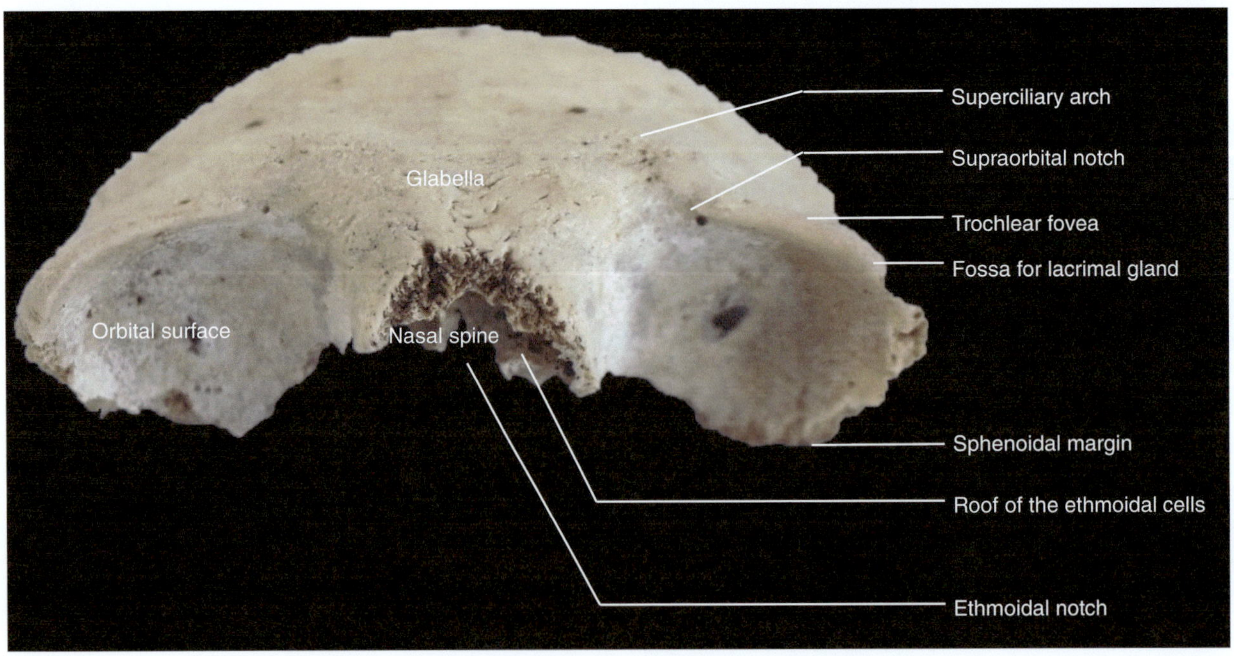

Fig. 2.33 Inferior view of the frontal bone

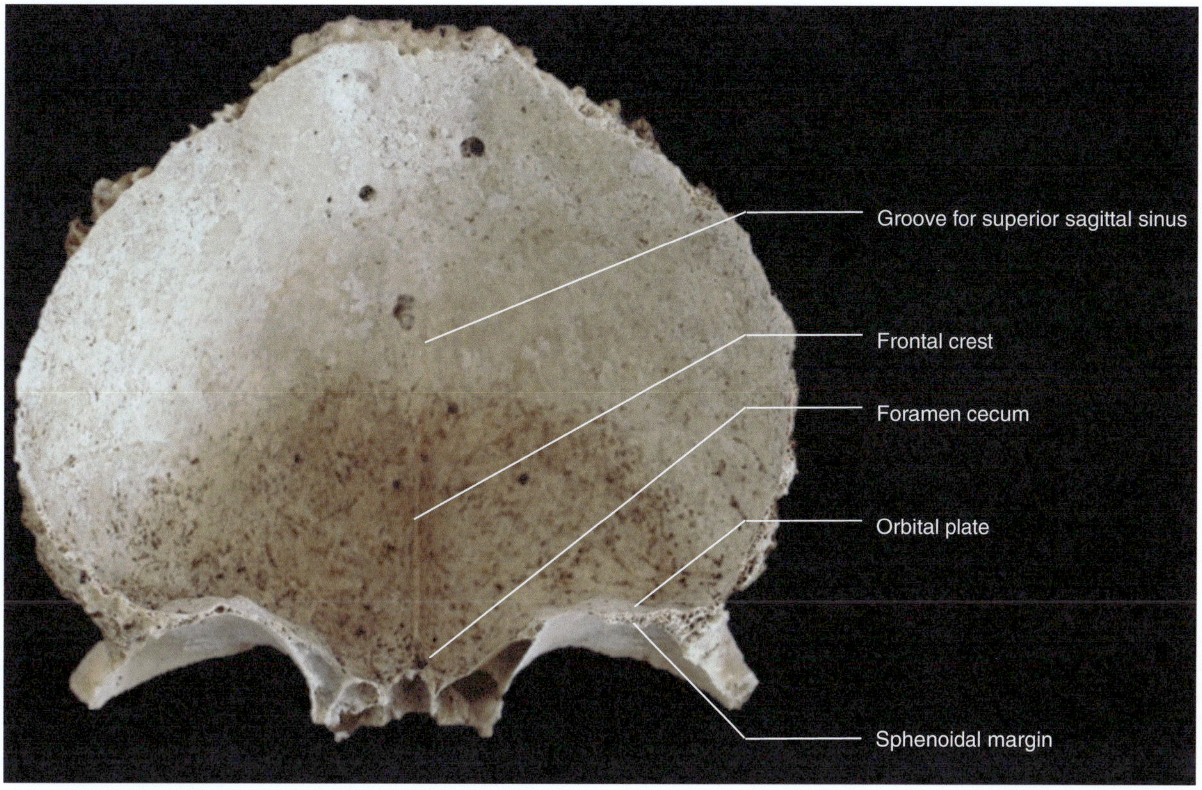

Fig. 2.34 Posterior view (internal surface) of the frontal bone

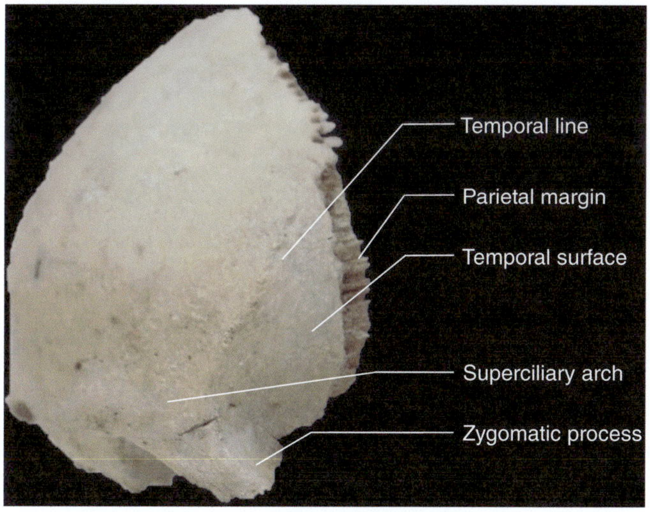

Fig. 2.35 Lateral view of the frontal bone (left side)

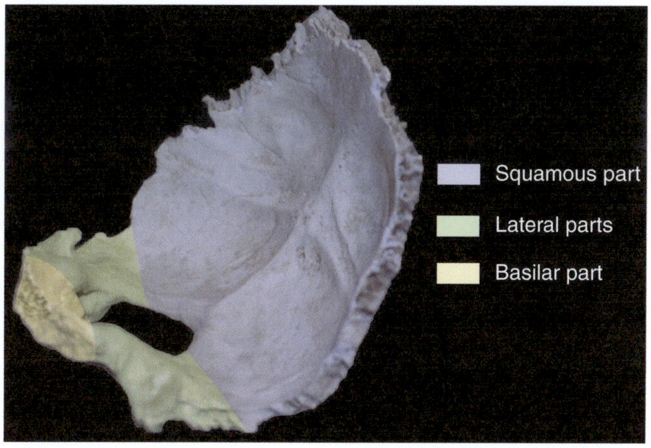

Fig. 2.36 The occipital bone consists of the squamous, lateral, and basilar parts

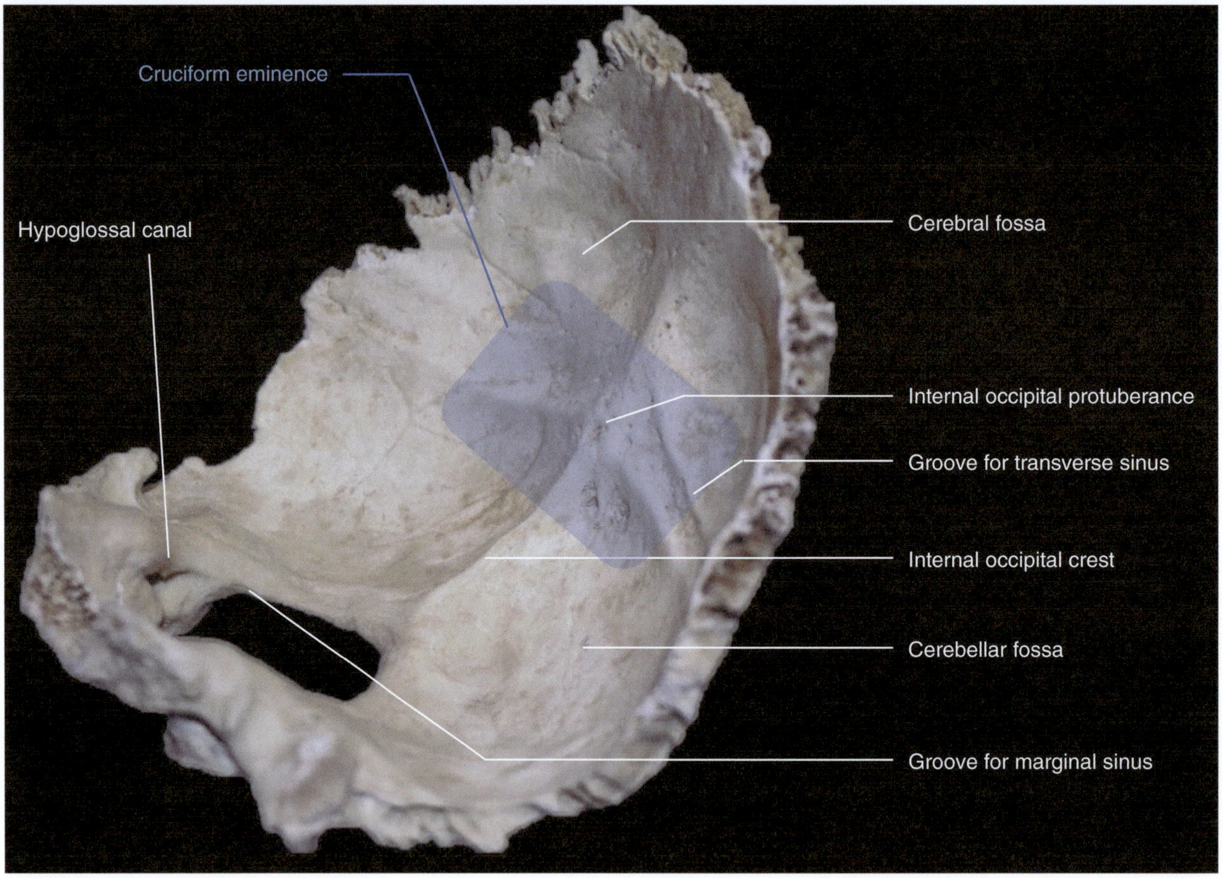

Fig. 2.37 Oblique view of the internal surface of the occipital bone

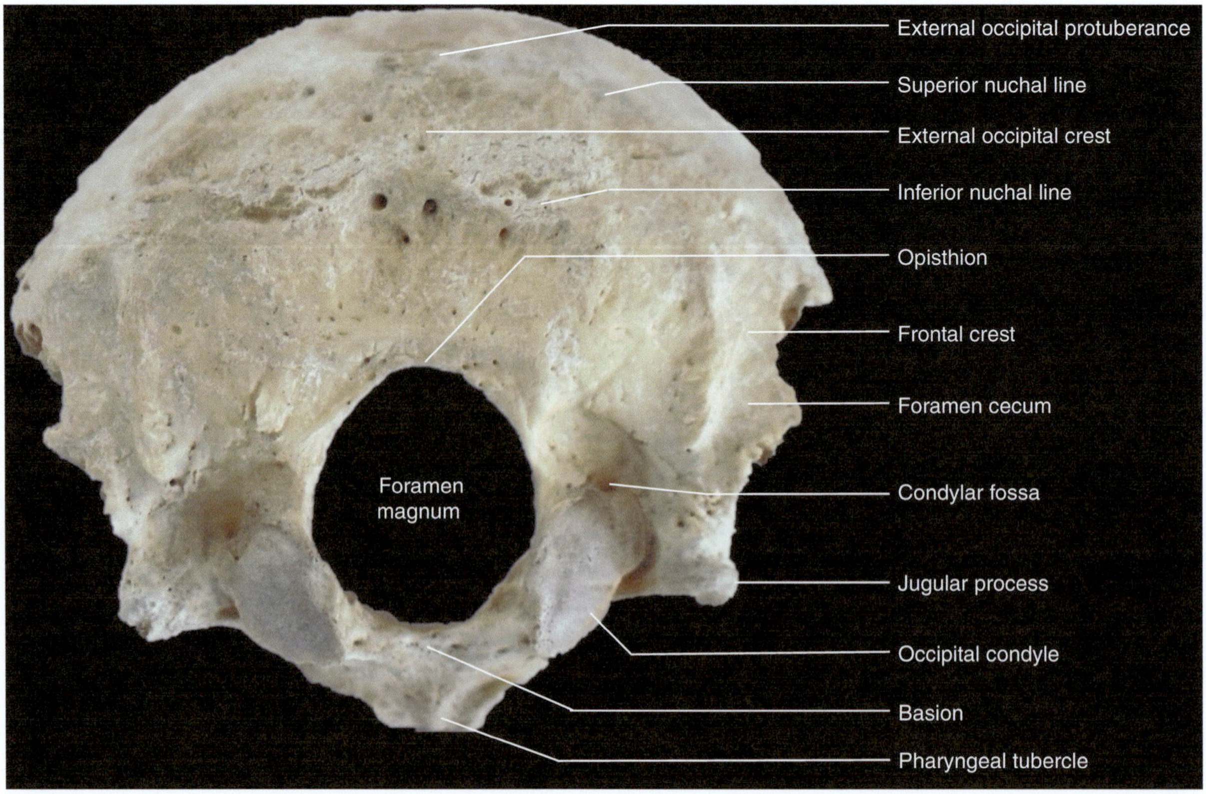

Fig. 2.38 Inferior view of the external surface of the occipital bone

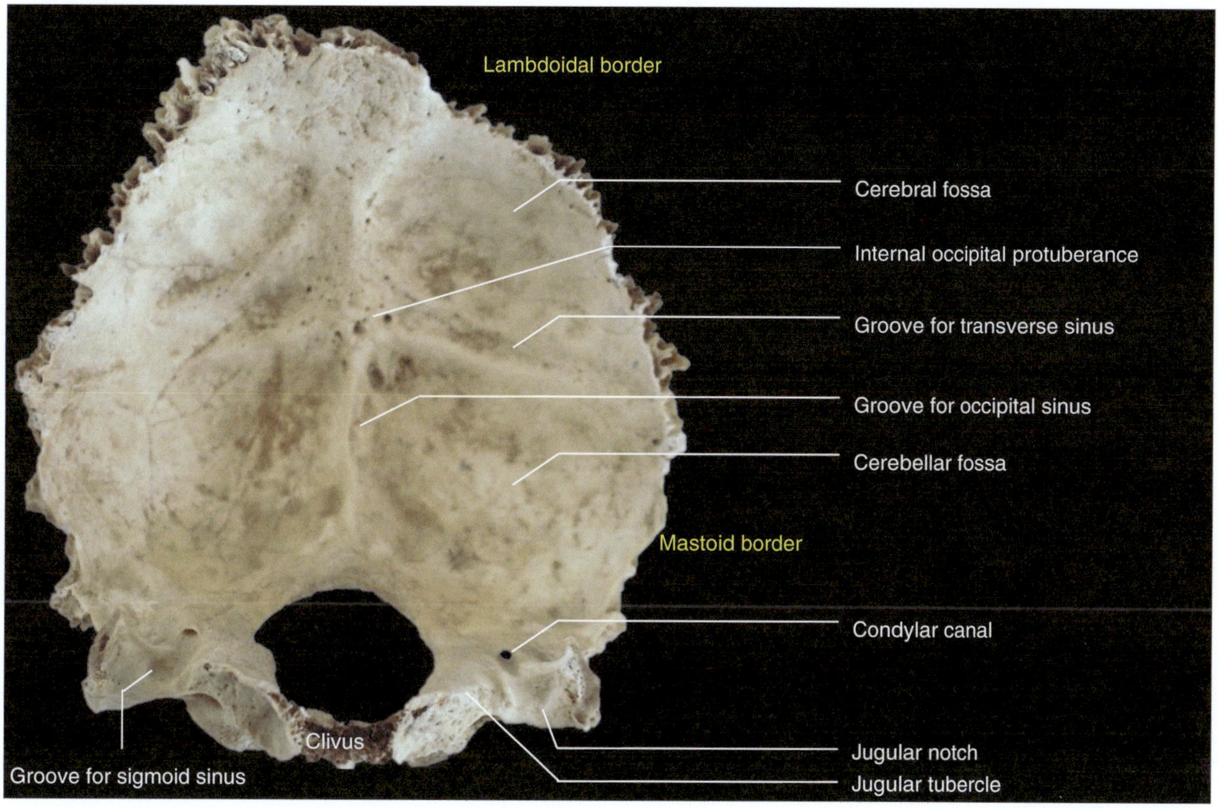

Fig. 2.39 Anterior view of the internal surface of the occipital bone

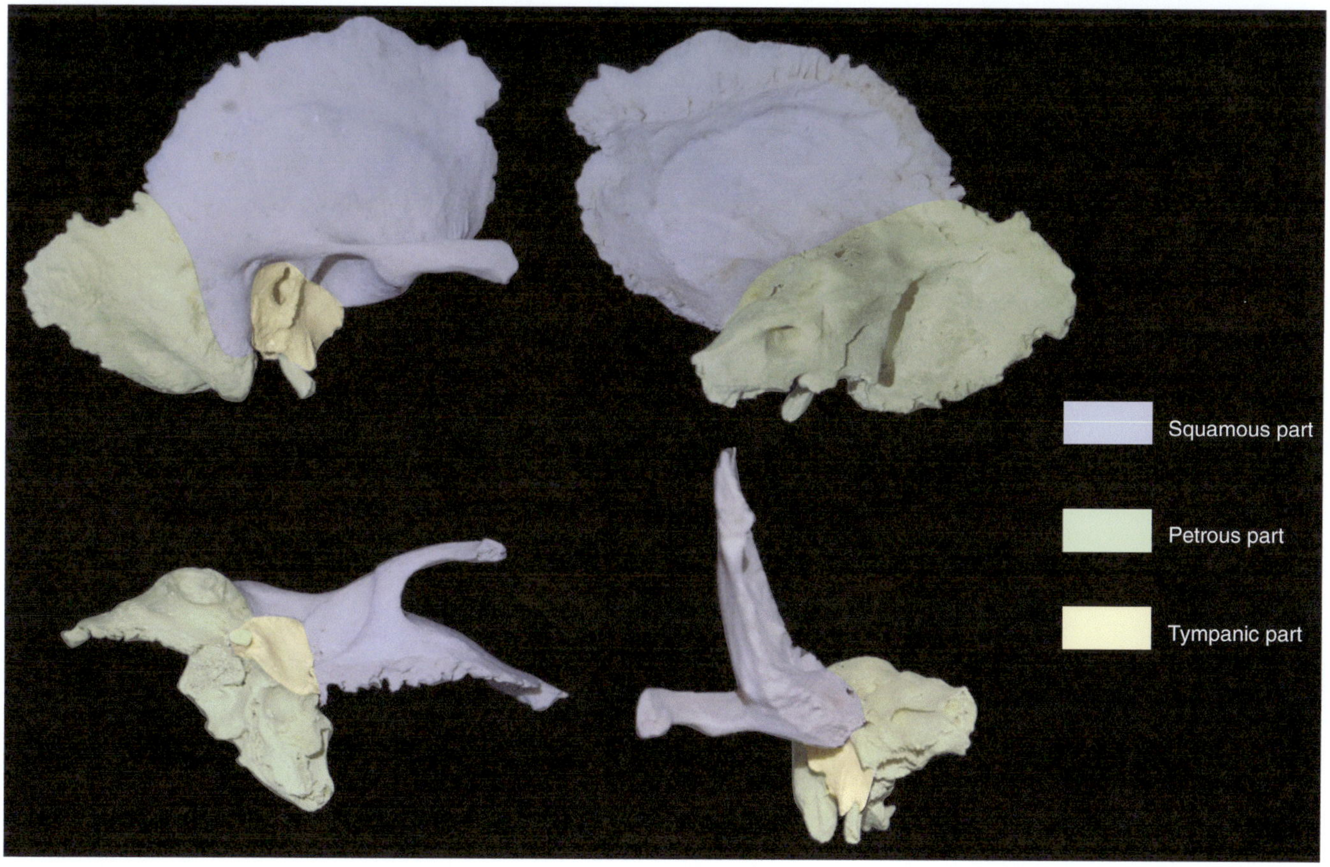

Fig. 2.40 Temporal bone consists of squamous, petrous, and tympanic parts

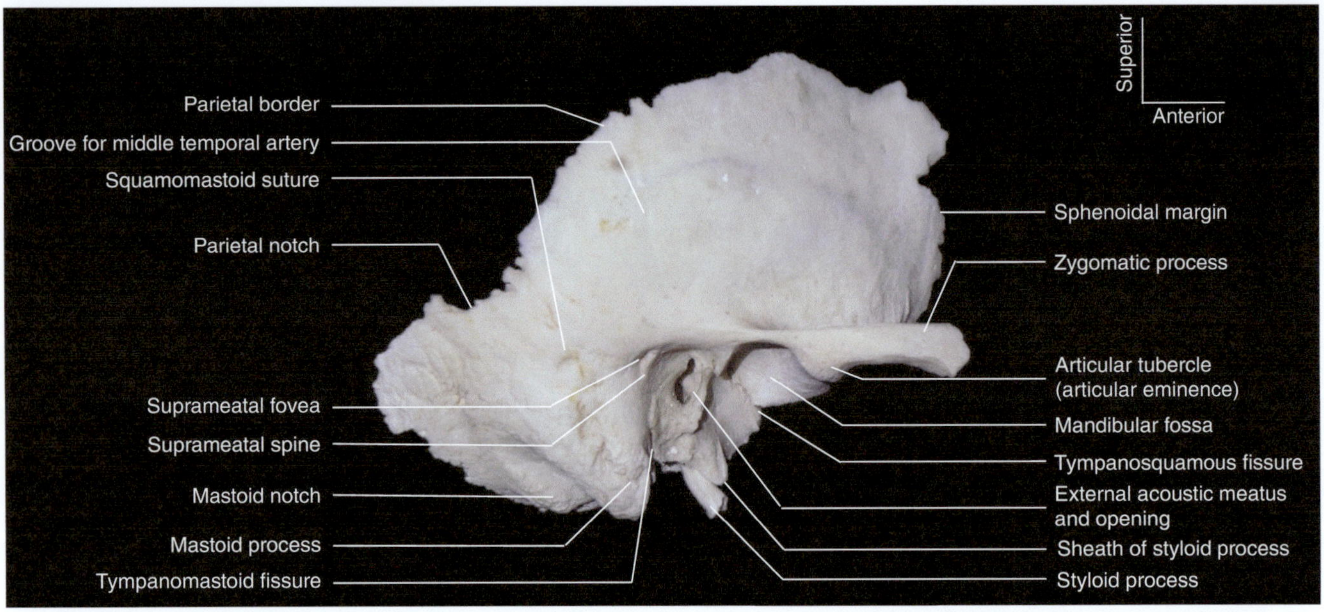

Fig. 2.41 External surface of the right temporal bone. The suprameatal spine is a projection for attachment of the auricular cartilage

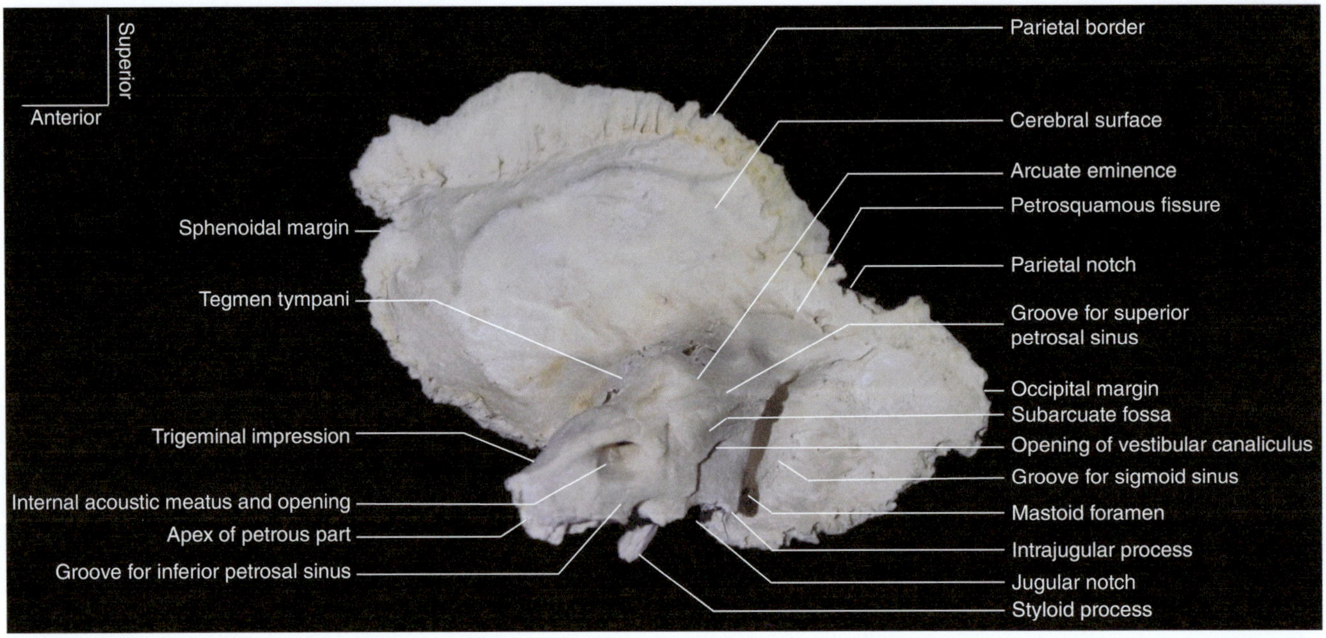

Fig. 2.42 Internal surface of the right temporal bone

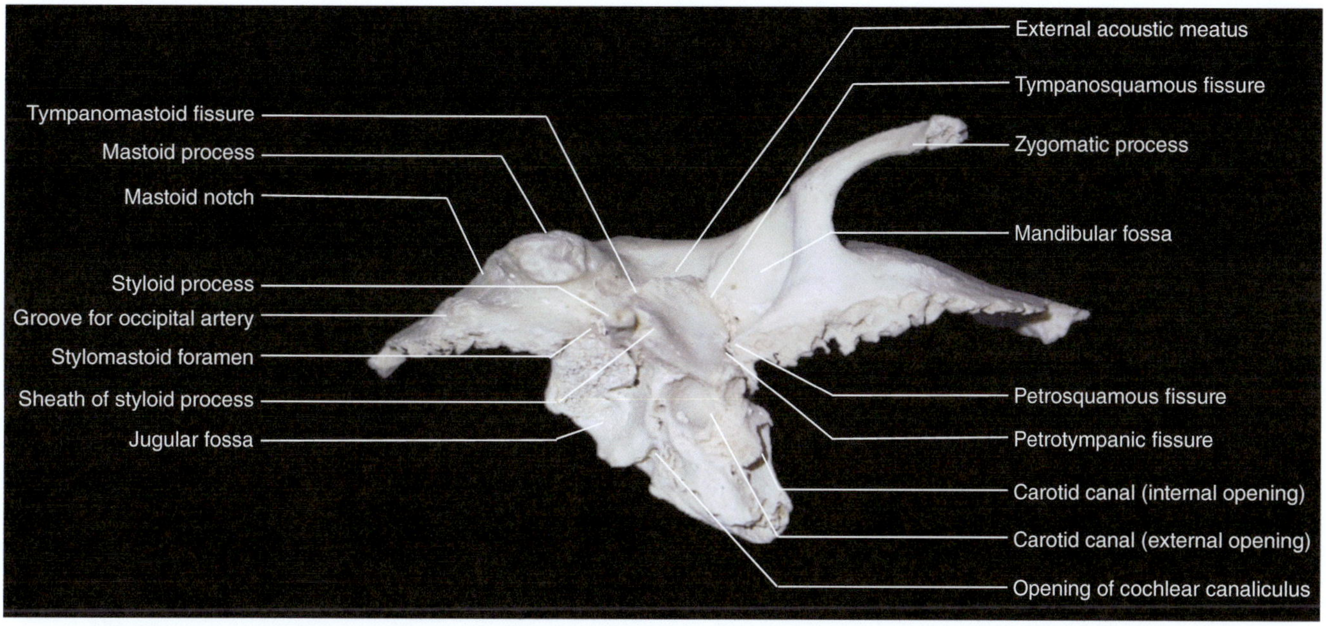

Fig. 2.43 Inferior view of the right temporal bone. Within the mandibular fossa, the tympanosquamous fissure runs laterally, and the tegmental crest divides into a petrosquamous fissure (anterior to the tegmental crest) and petrotympanic fissure (posterior to the tegmental crest) medially

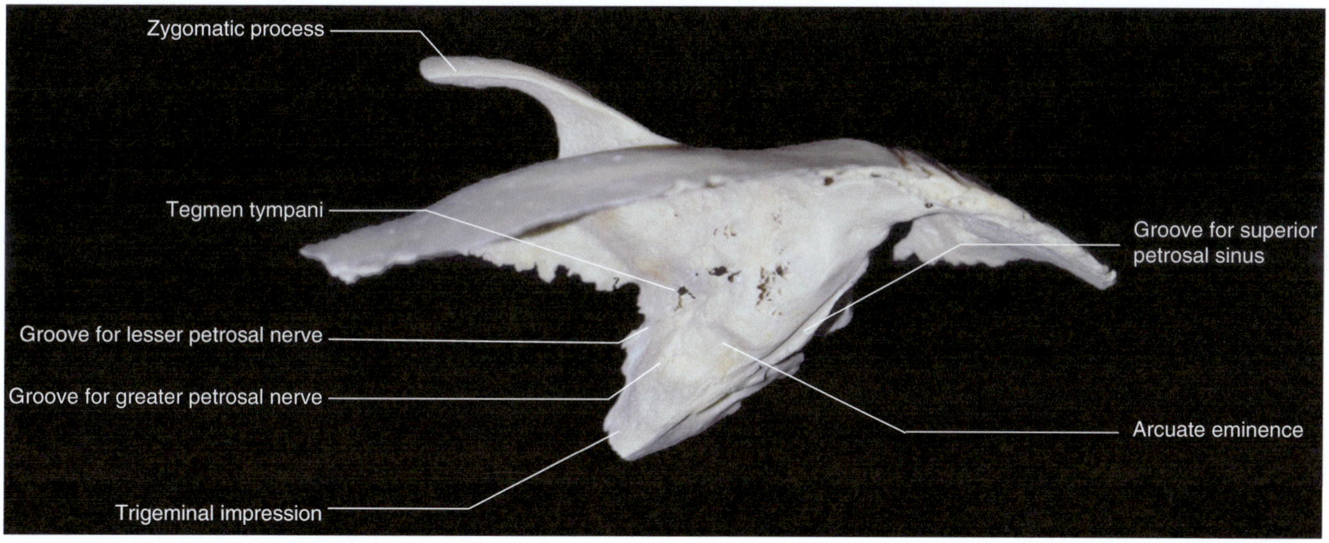

Fig. 2.44 Superior view of the right temporal bone

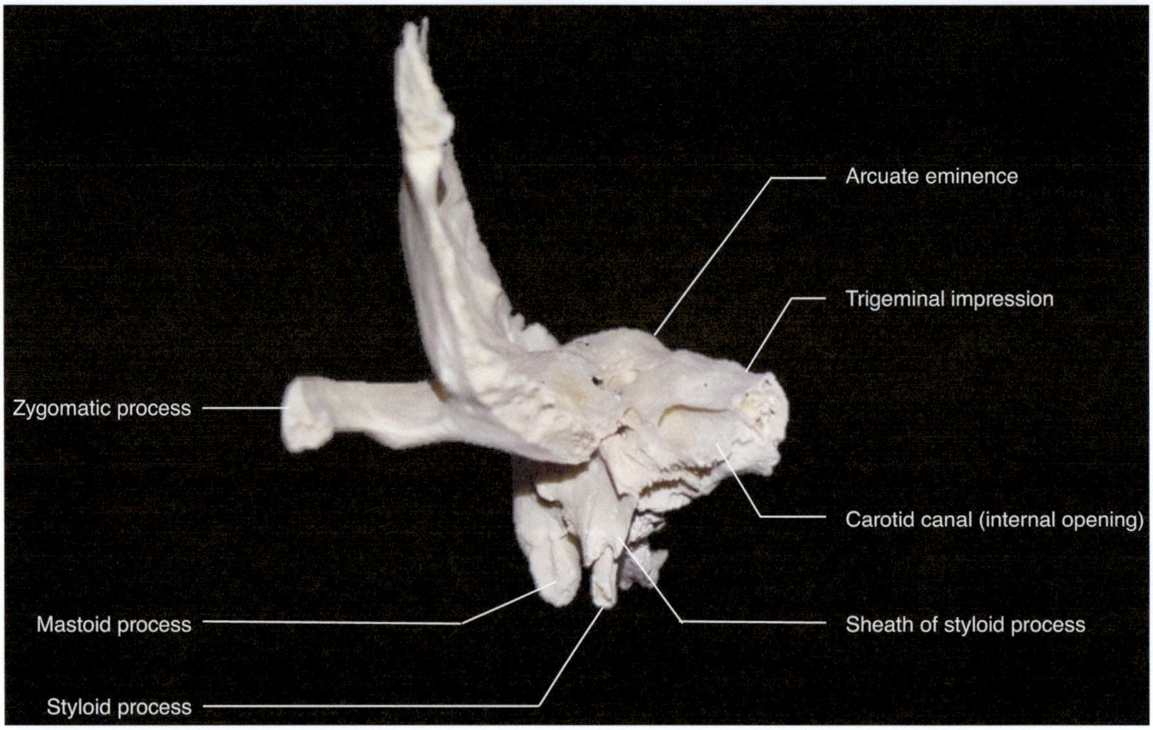

Fig. 2.45 Anterior view of the right temporal bone

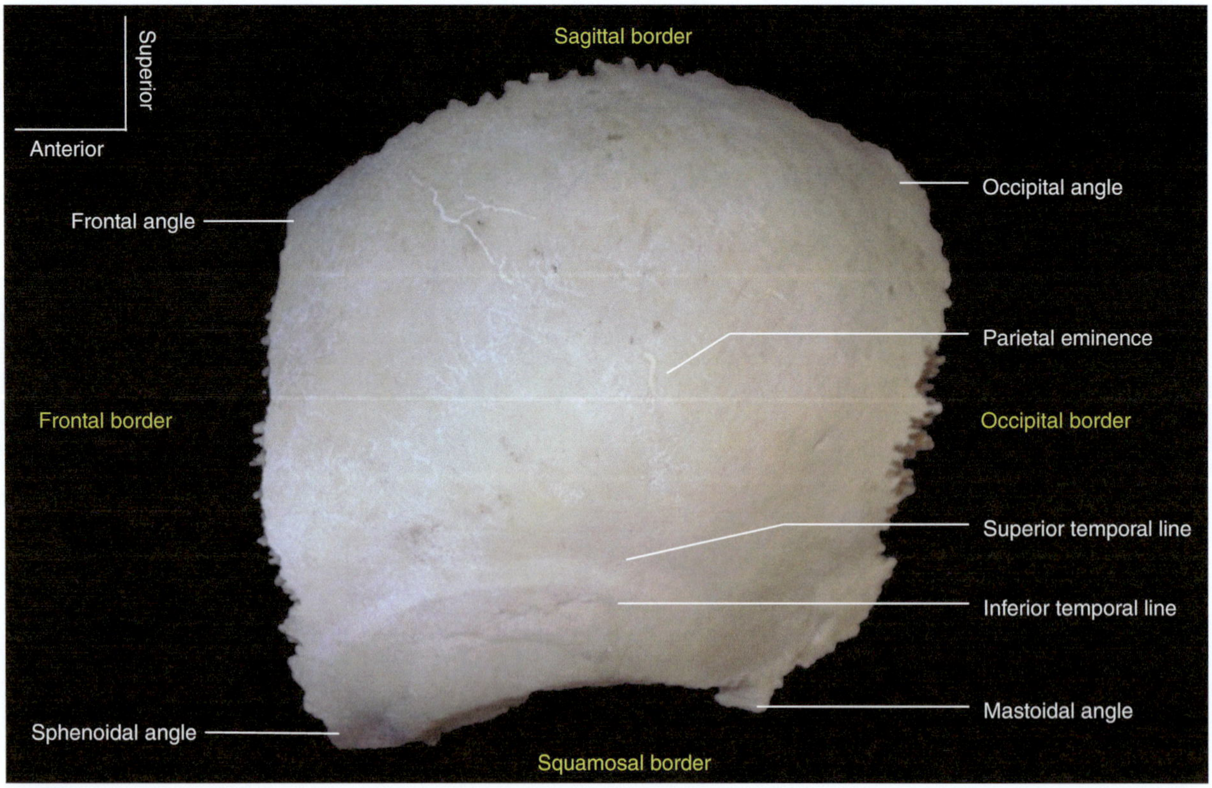

Fig. 2.46 External surface of the left parietal bone

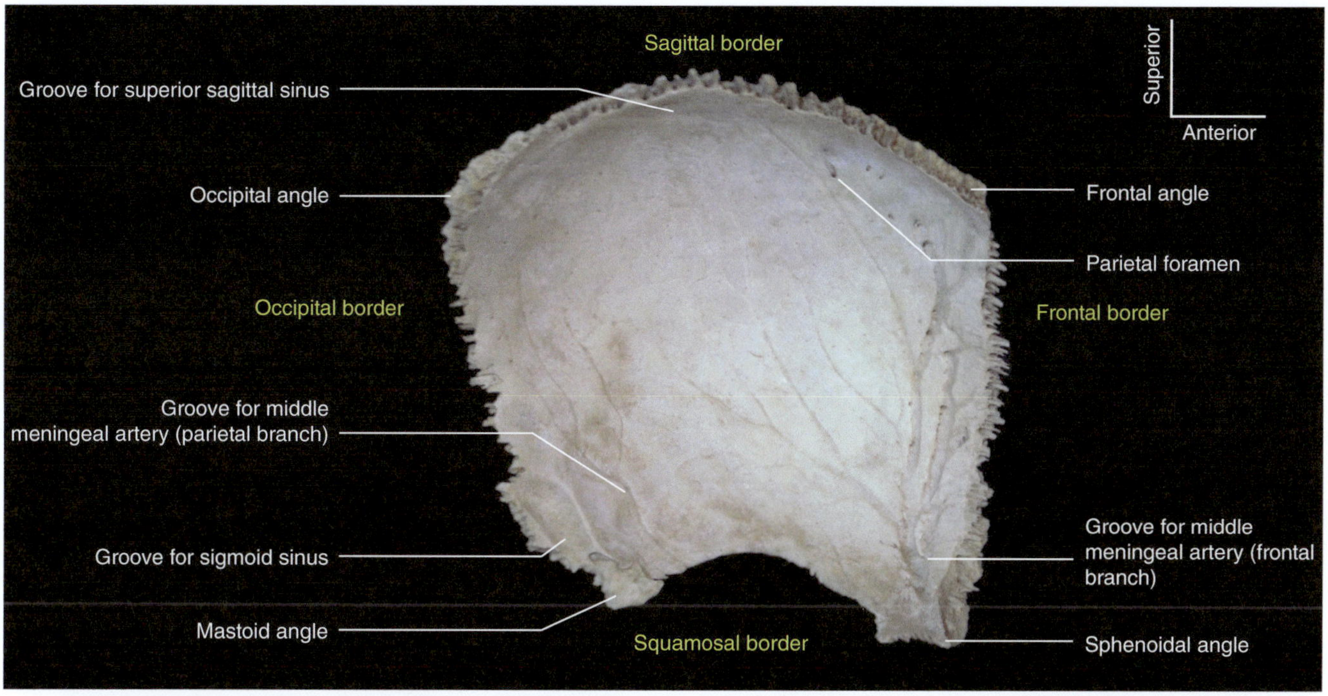

Fig. 2.47 Internal surface of the left parietal bone

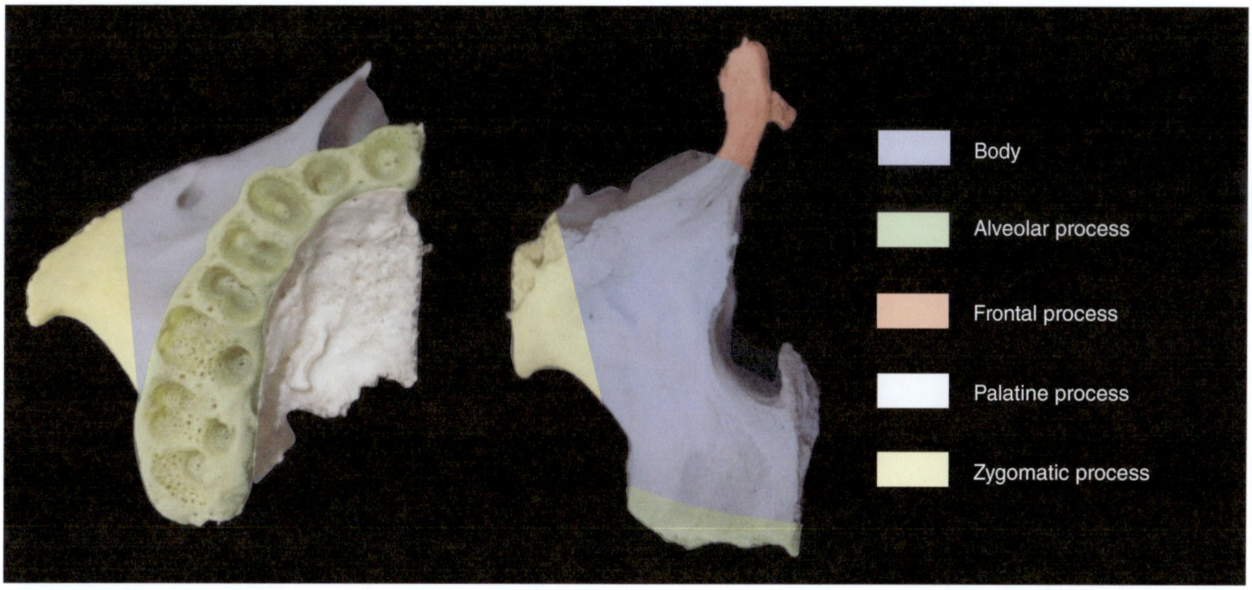

Fig. 2.48 The maxilla consists of a body, alveolar process, frontal process, palatine process, and zygomatic process

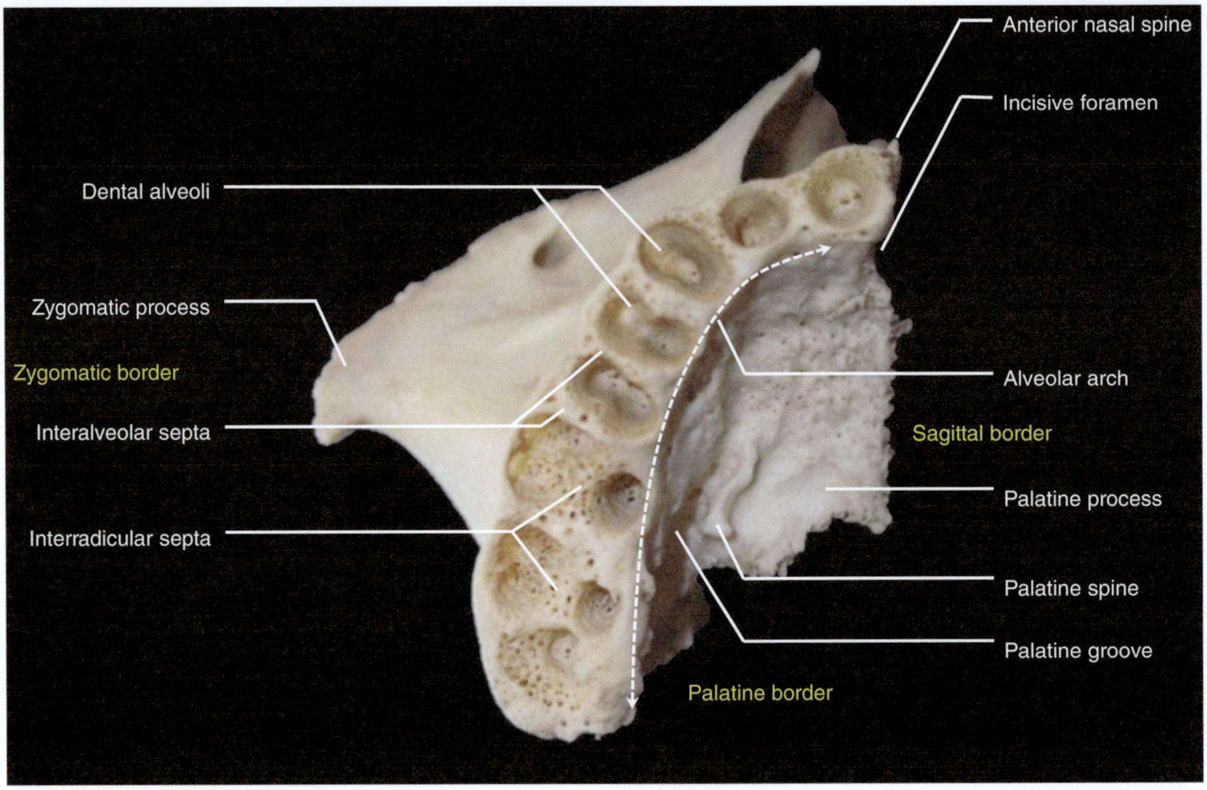

Fig. 2.49 Inferior view of the right maxilla

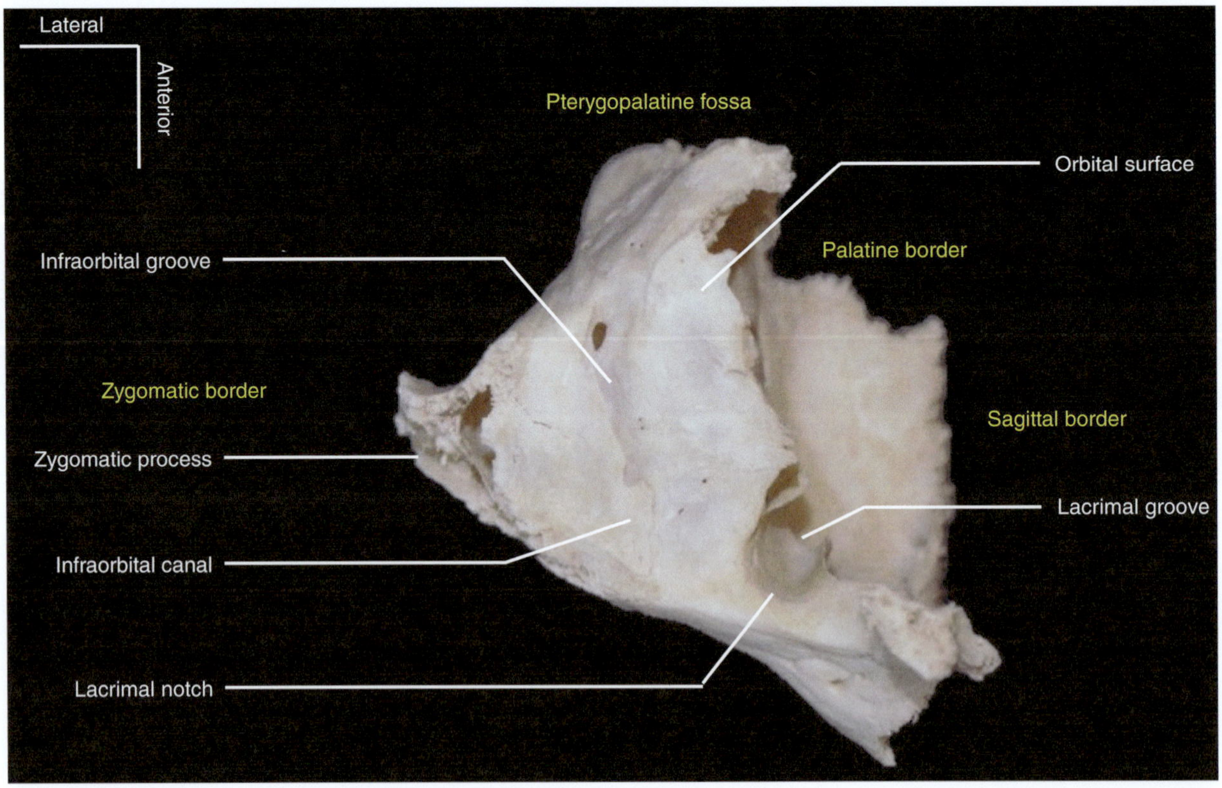

Fig. 2.50 Superior view of the right maxilla

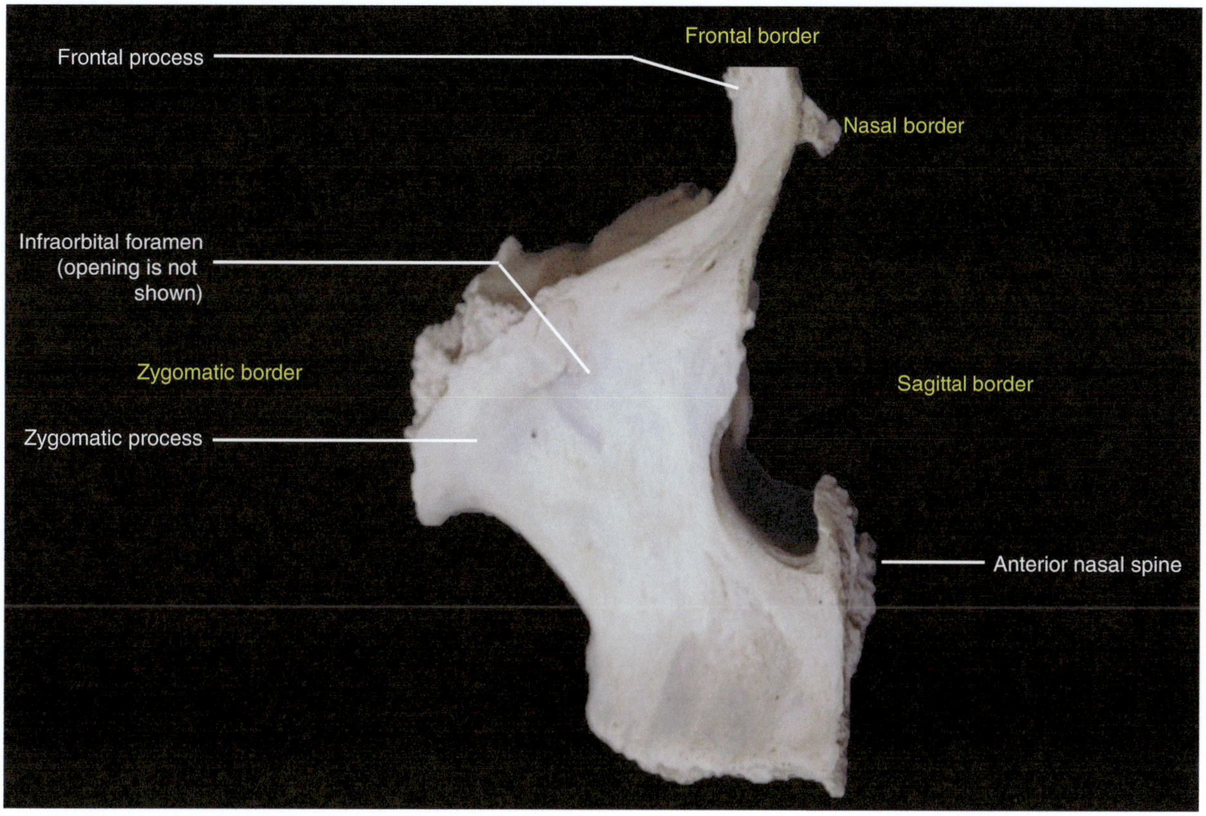

Fig. 2.51 Anterior view of the right maxilla

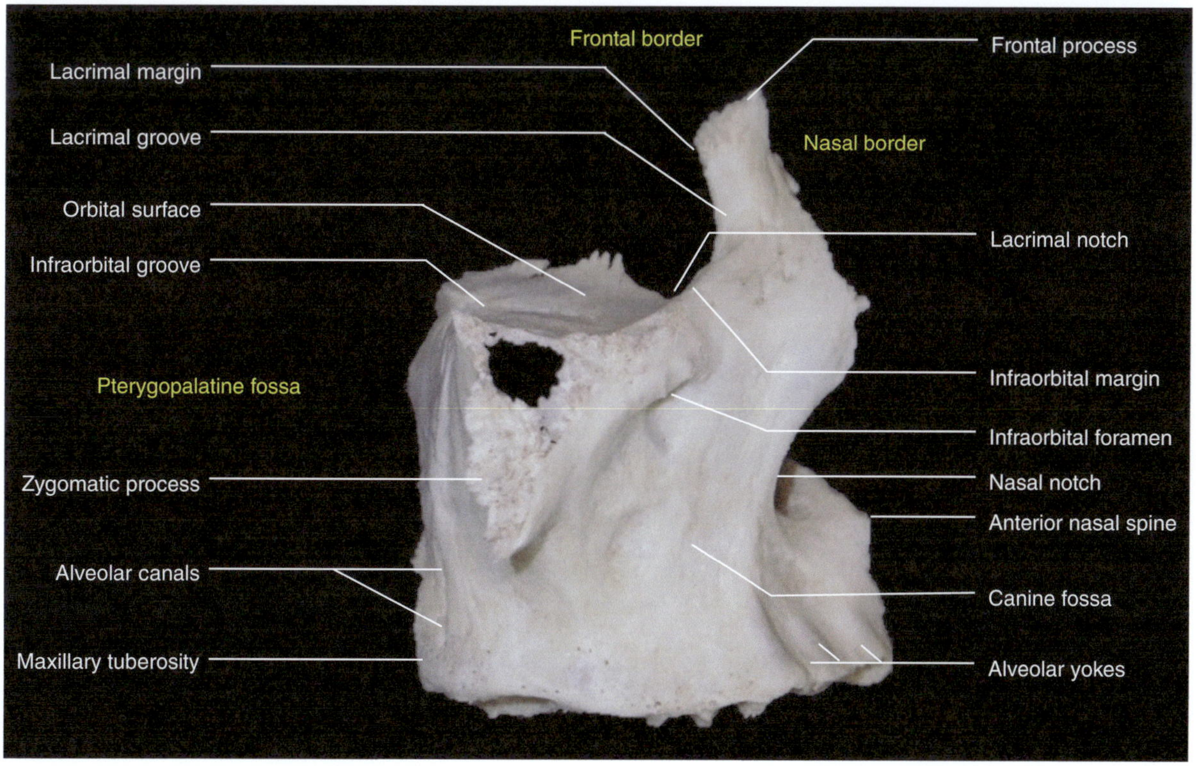

Fig. 2.52 Lateral view of the right maxilla

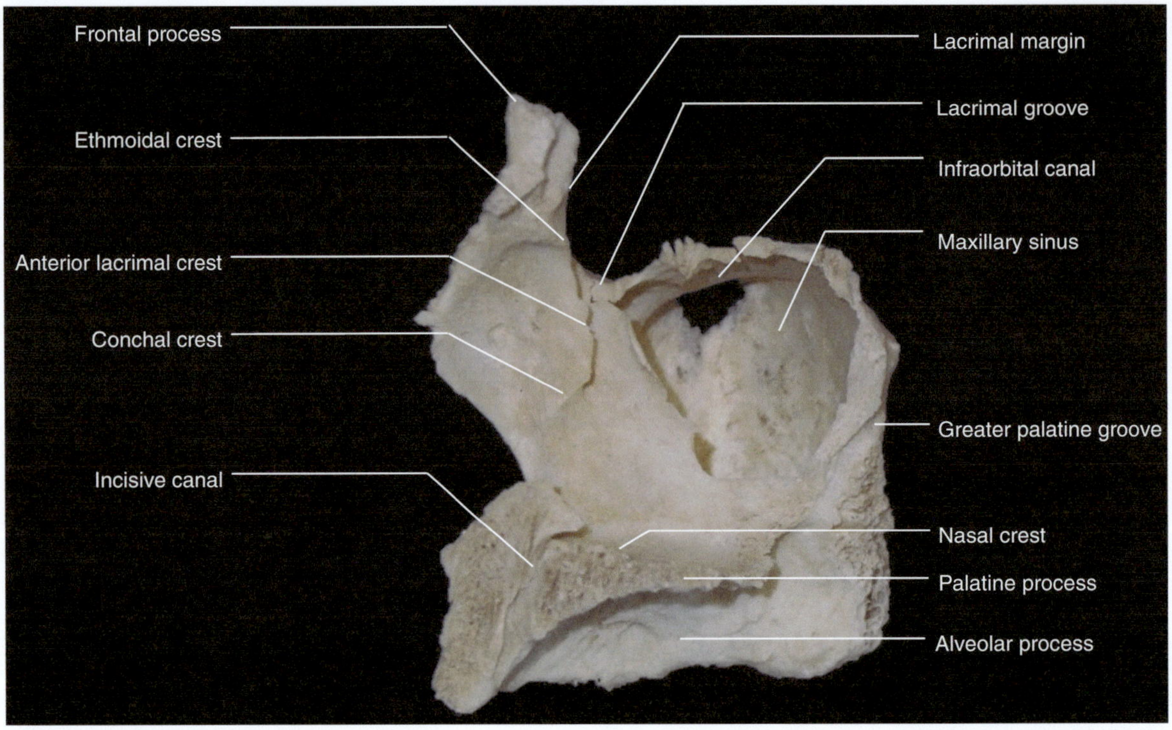

Fig. 2.53 Medial view of the right maxilla

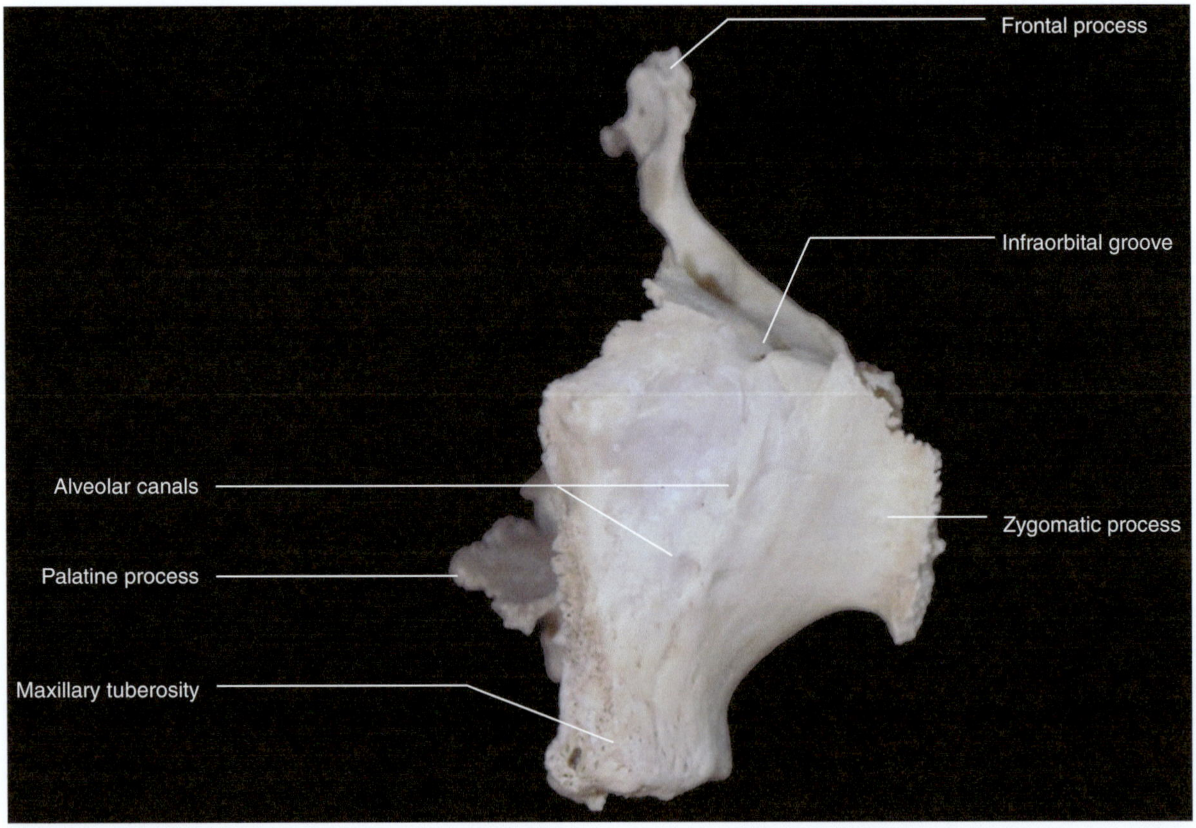

Fig. 2.54 Posterior view of the right maxilla

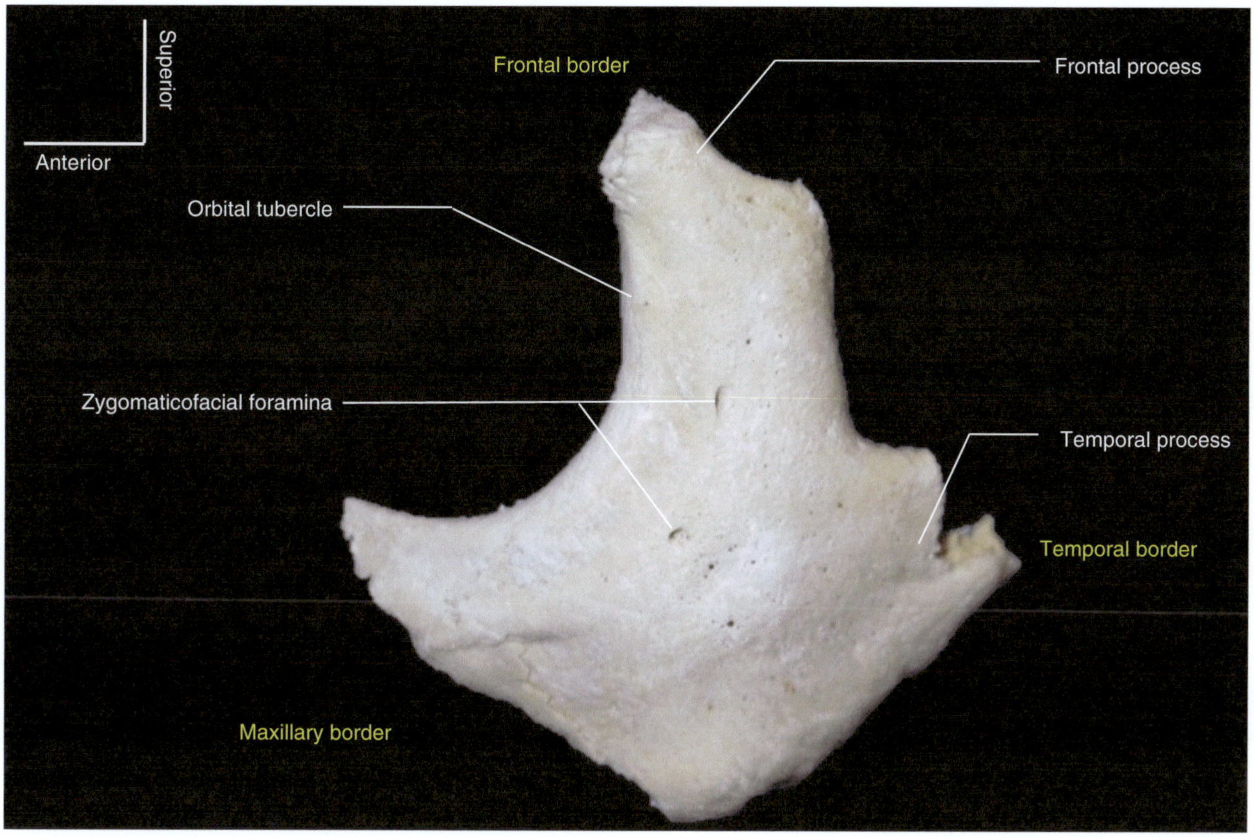

Fig. 2.55 Lateral view of the left zygoma

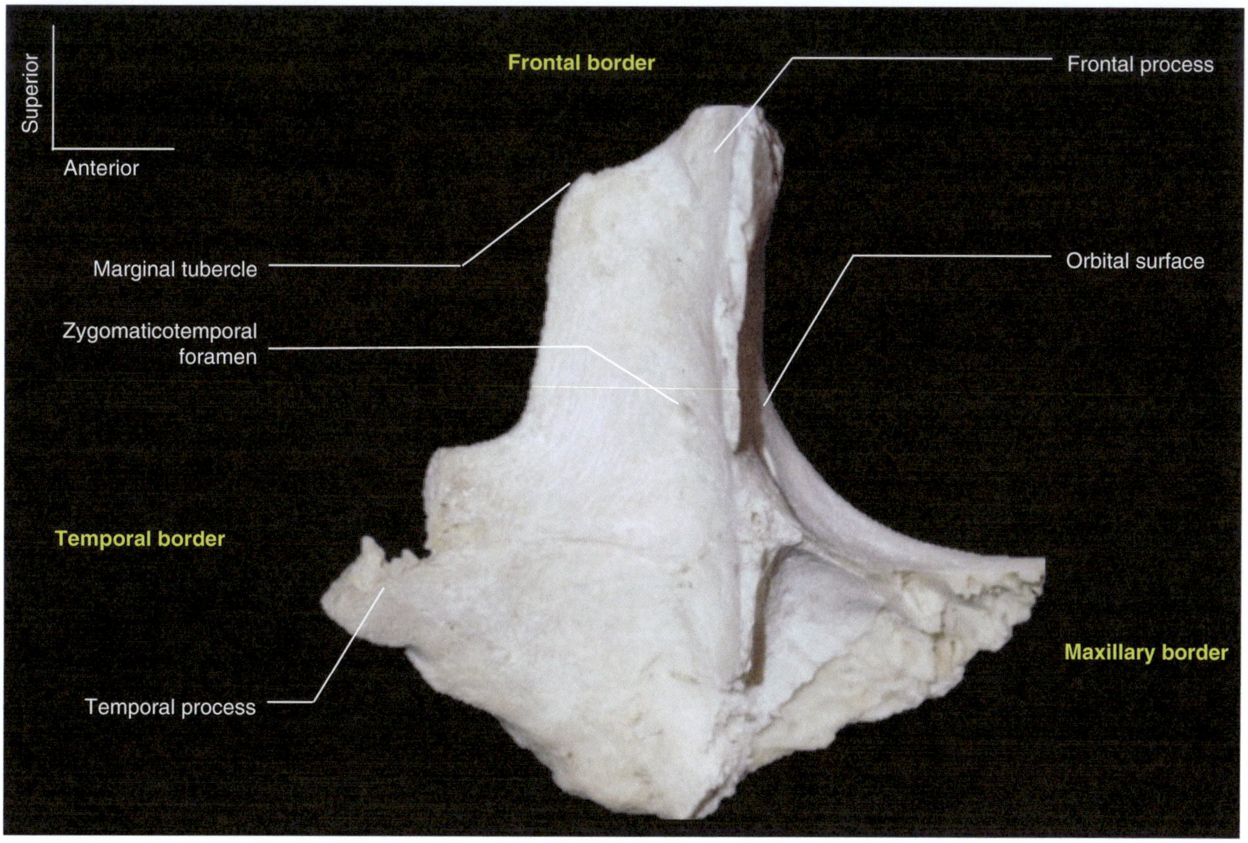

Fig. 2.56 Medial view of the left zygoma

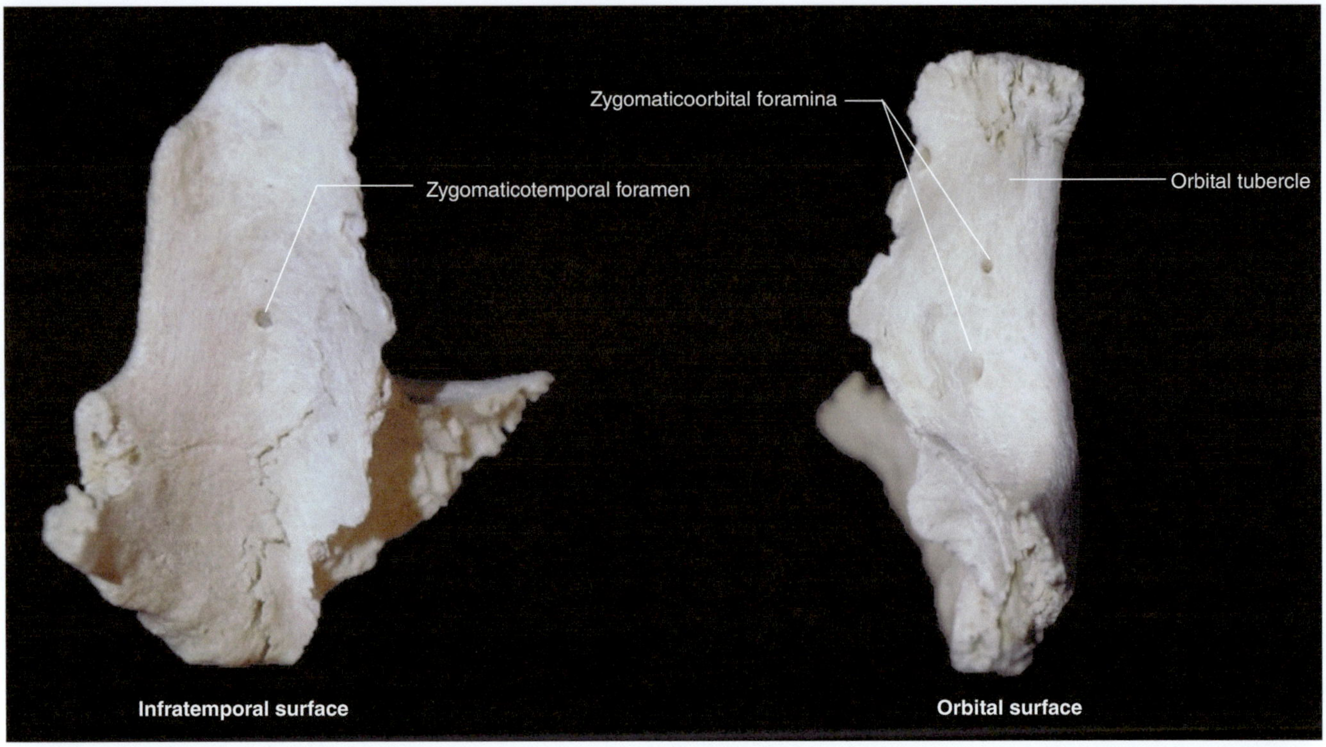

Fig. 2.57 Left zygoma. The orbital tubercle is a small eminence within the orbit and is for the attachment of the lateral palpebral ligament

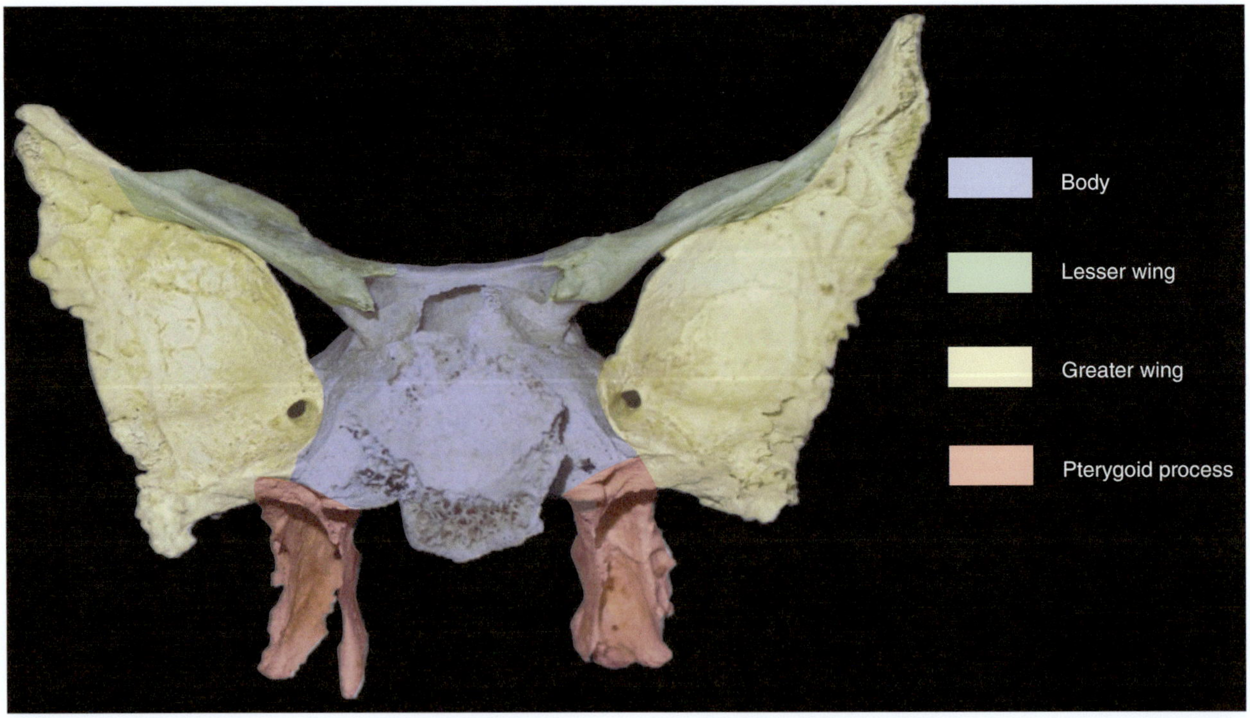

Fig. 2.58 The sphenoid bone consists of a body, lesser wings, greater wings, and pterygoid processes

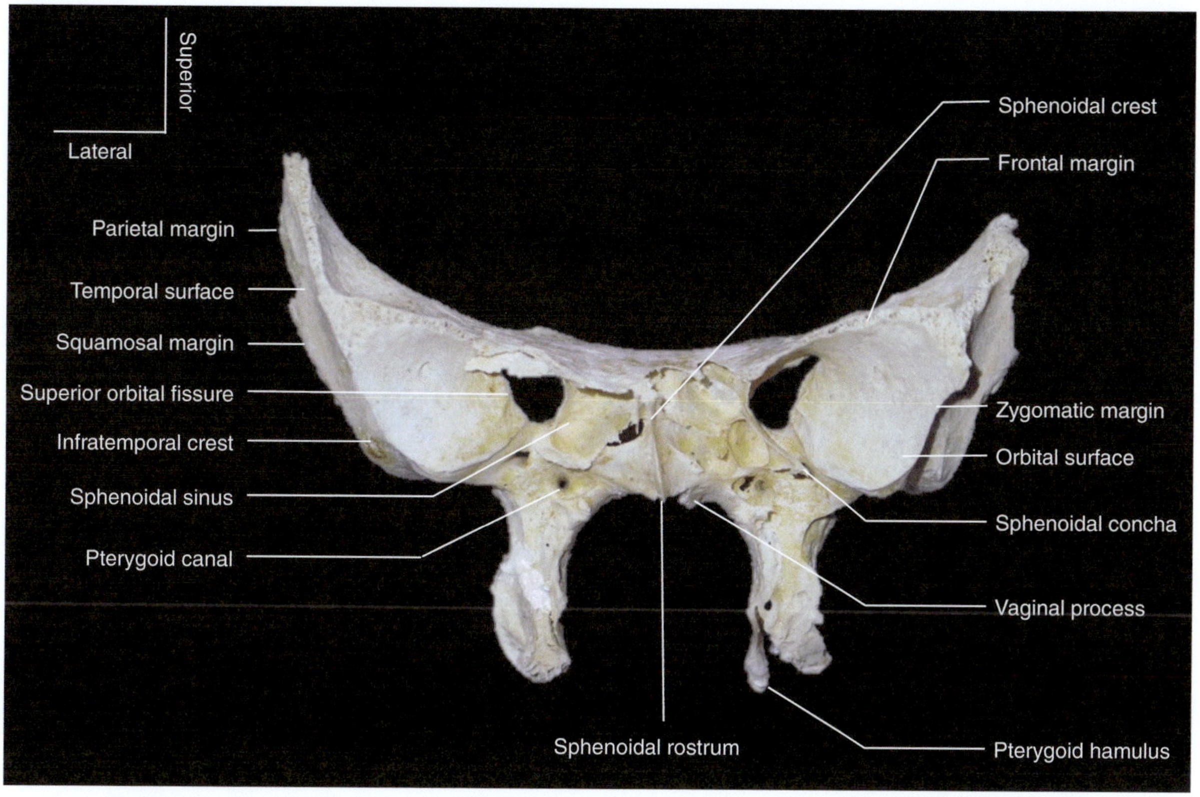

Fig. 2.59 Anterior view of the sphenoid bone

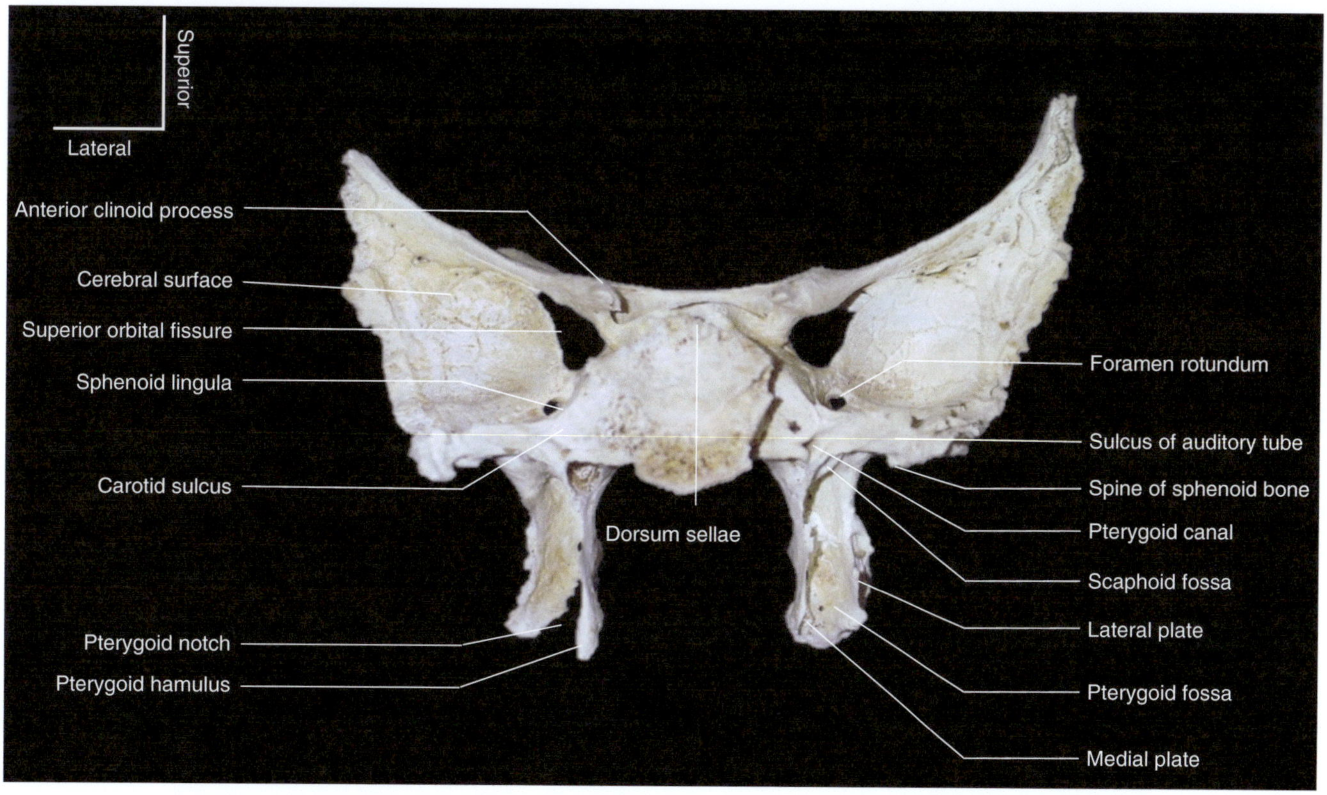

Fig. 2.60 Posterior view of the sphenoid bone

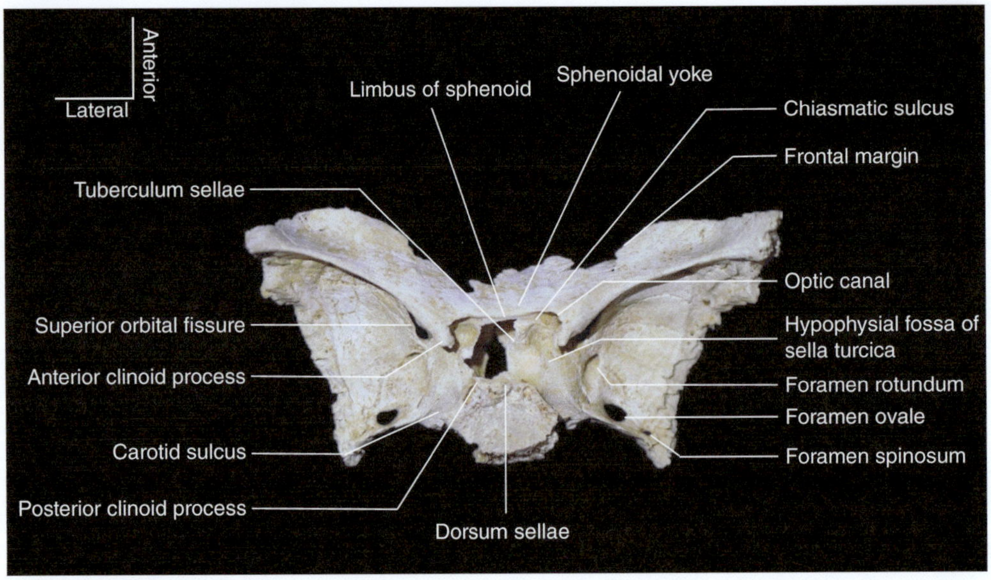

Fig. 2.61 Superior view of the sphenoid bone

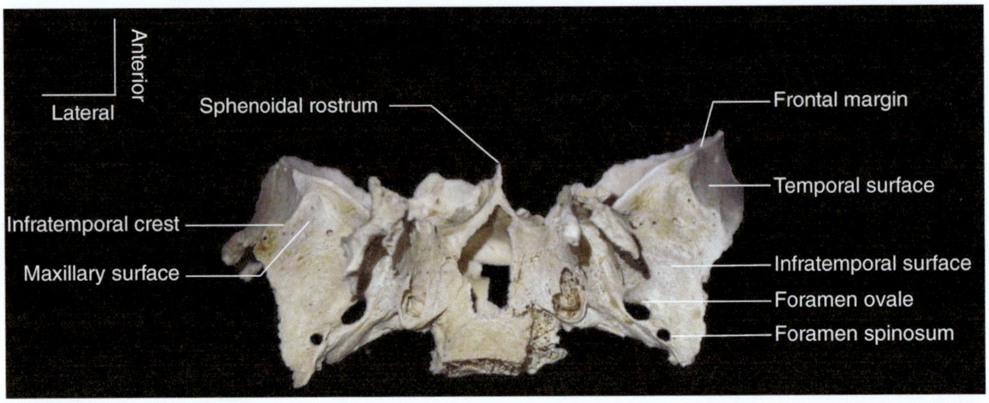

Fig. 2.62 Inferior view of the sphenoid bone

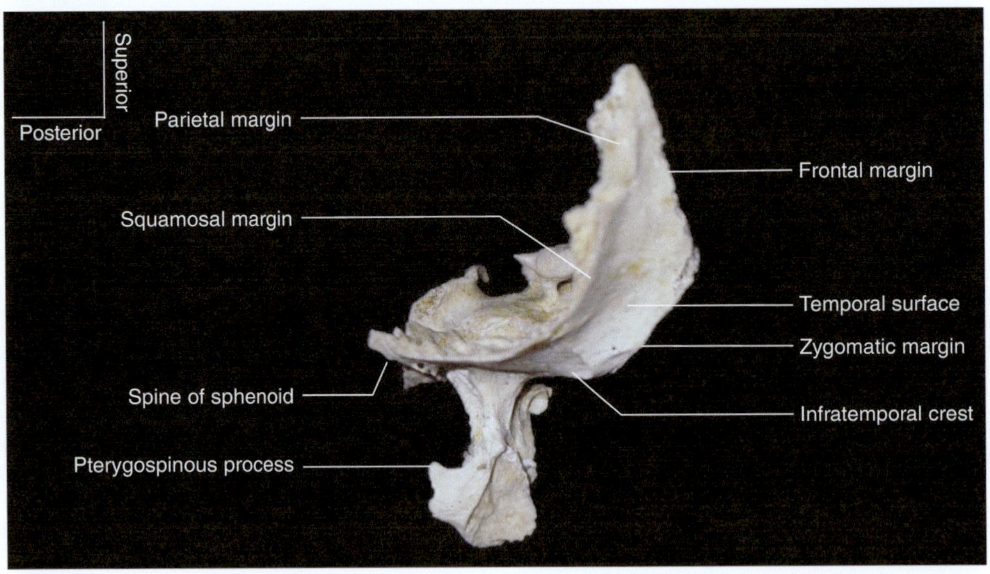

Fig. 2.63 Lateral view of the sphenoid bone (right side)

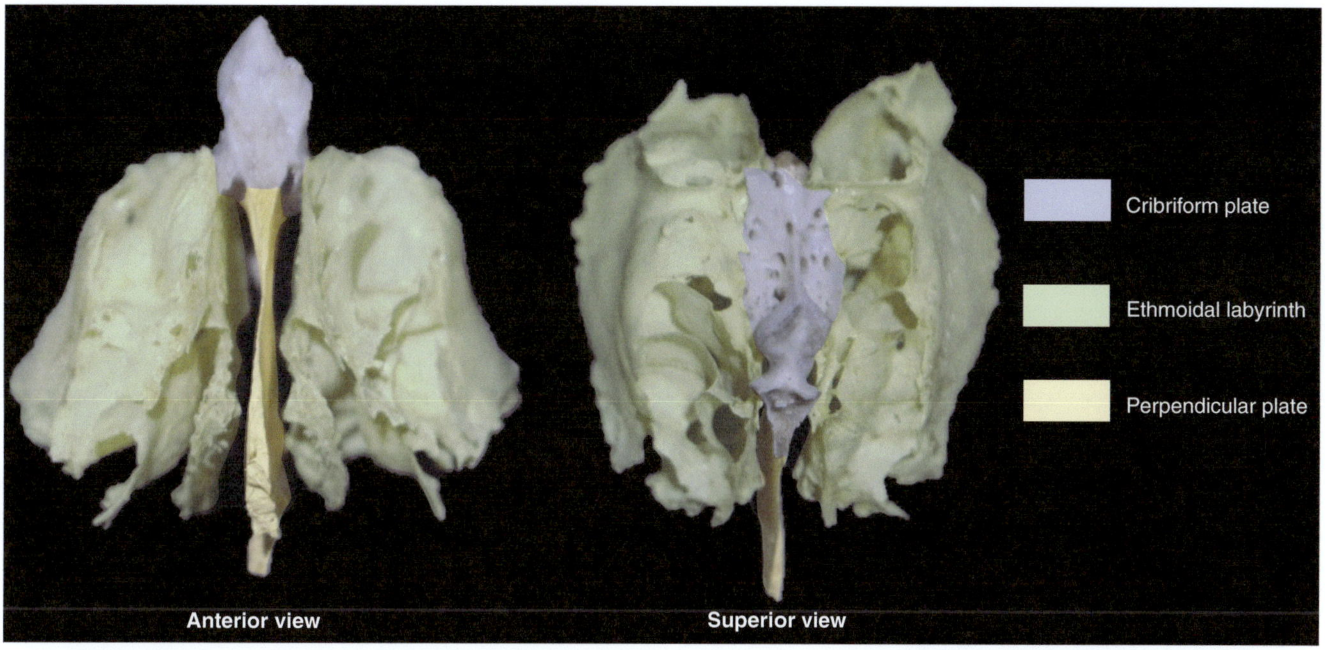

Fig. 2.64 The ethmoid bone consists of the cribriform plate, ethmoidal labyrinth, and perpendicular plate

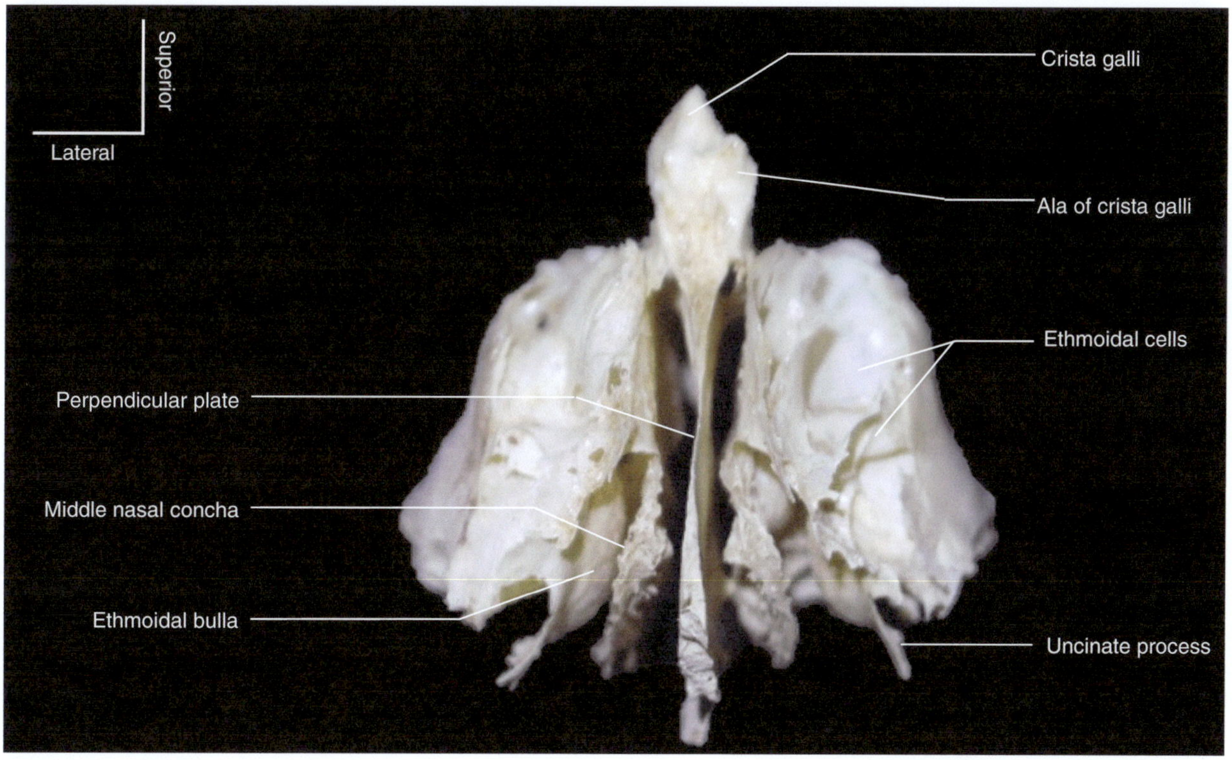

Fig. 2.65 Anterior view of the ethmoid bone

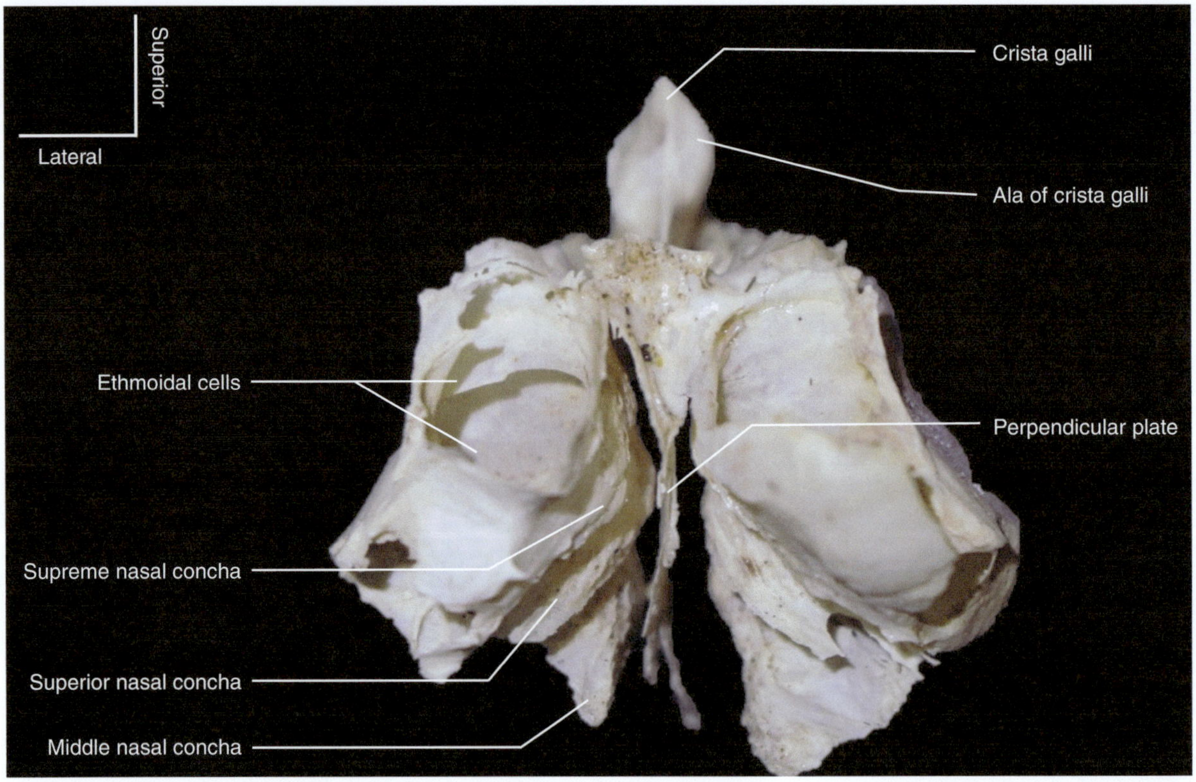

Fig. 2.66 Posterior view of the ethmoid bone

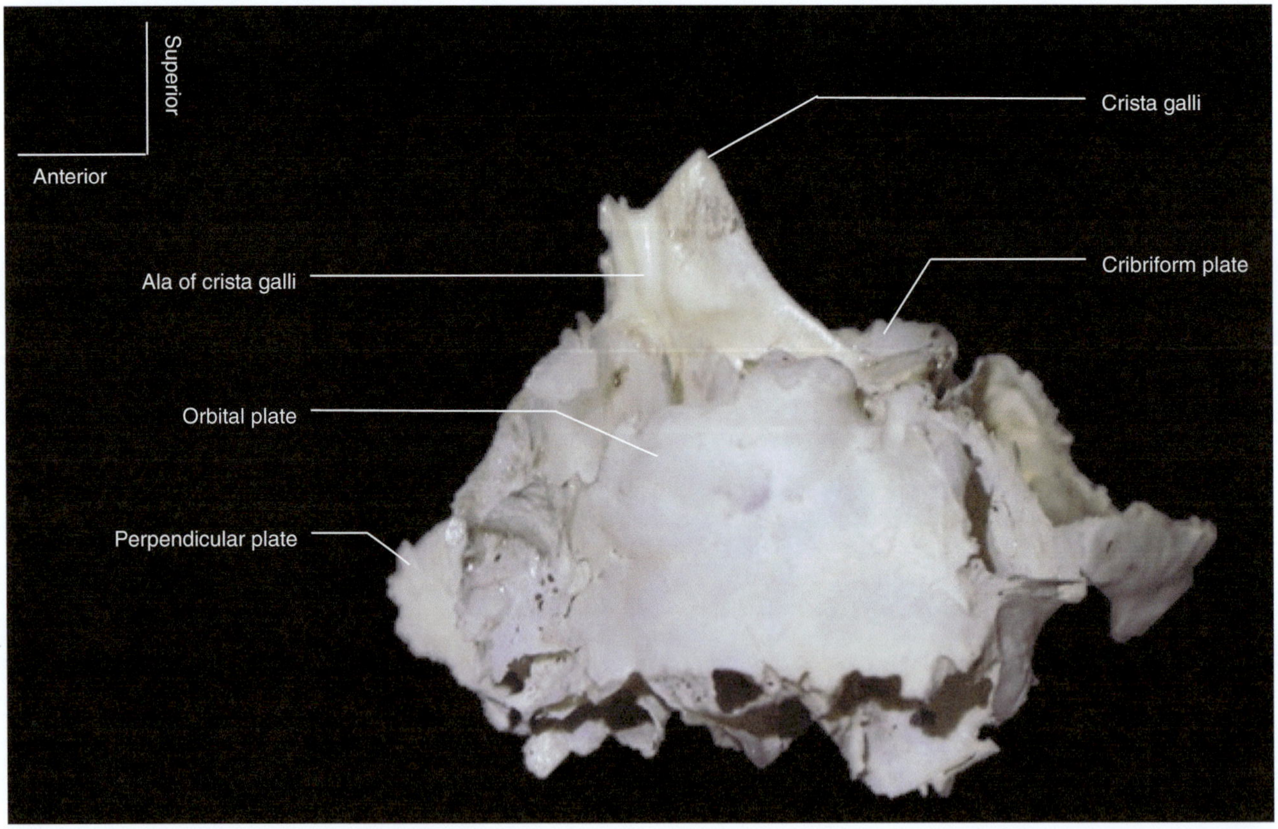

Fig. 2.67 Lateral (left) view of the ethmoid bone

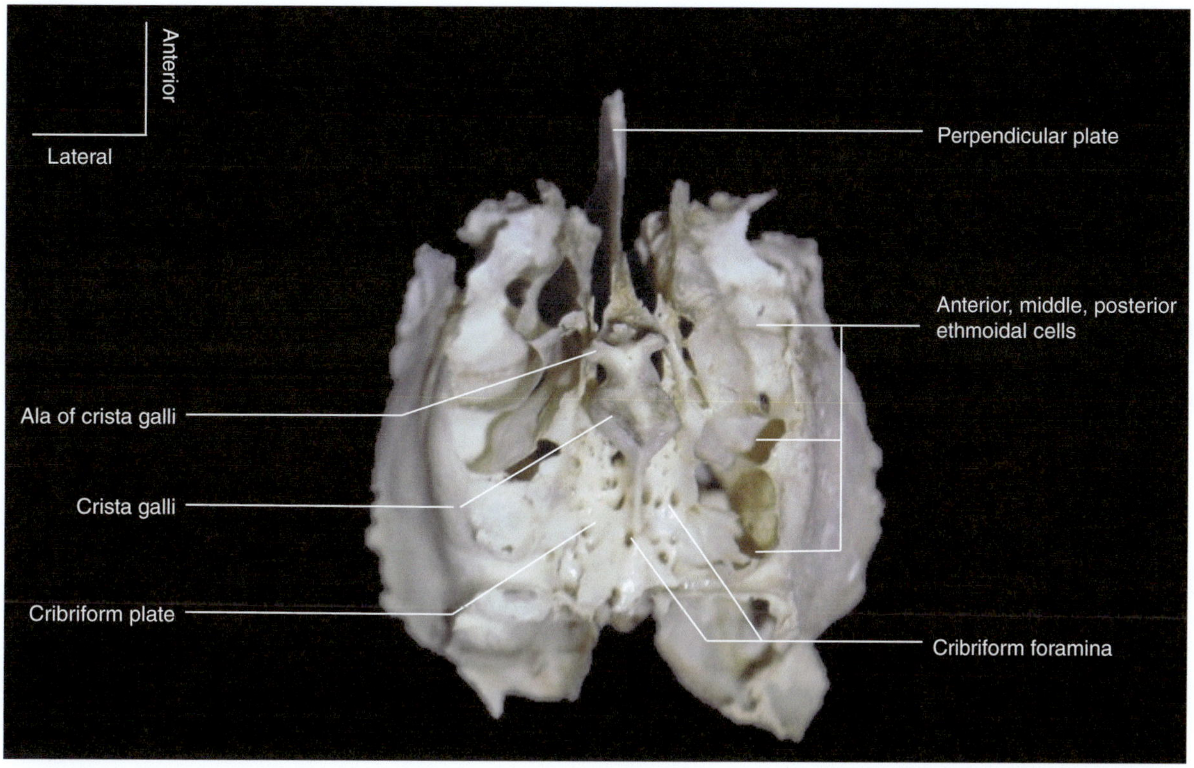

Fig. 2.68 Superior view of the ethmoid bone

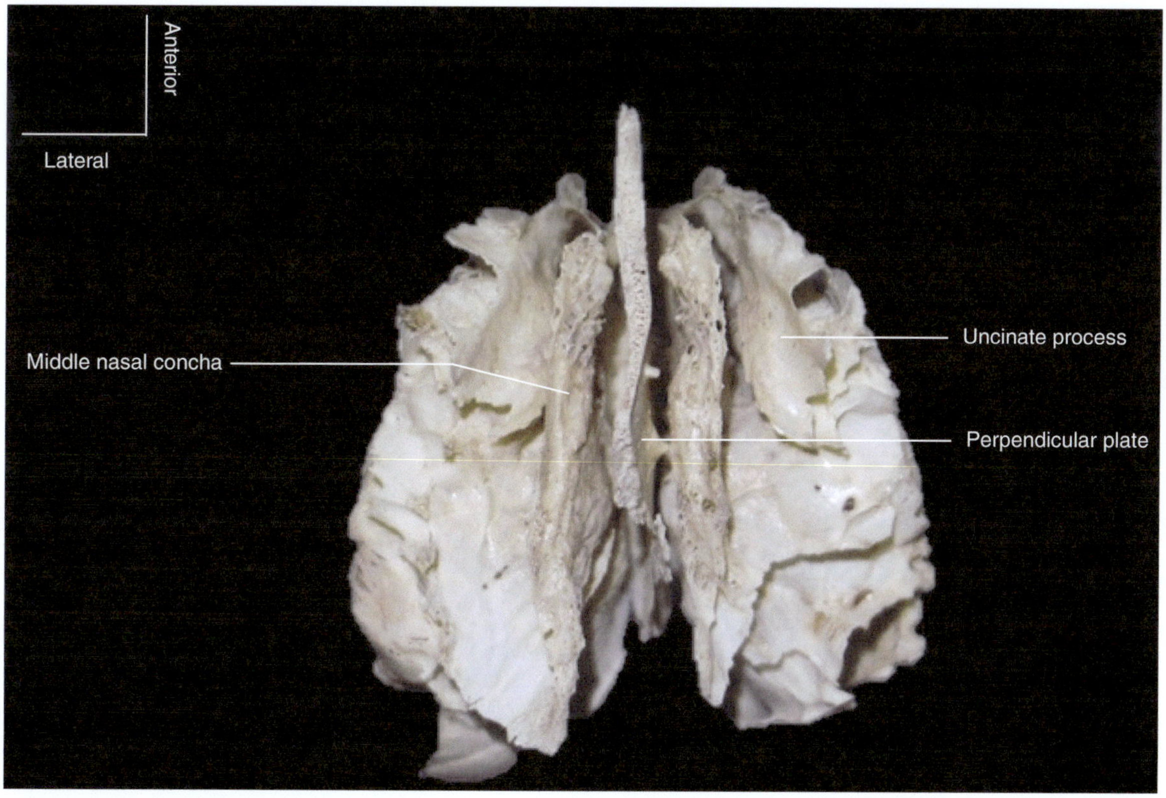

Fig. 2.69 Ethmoid bone inferior view

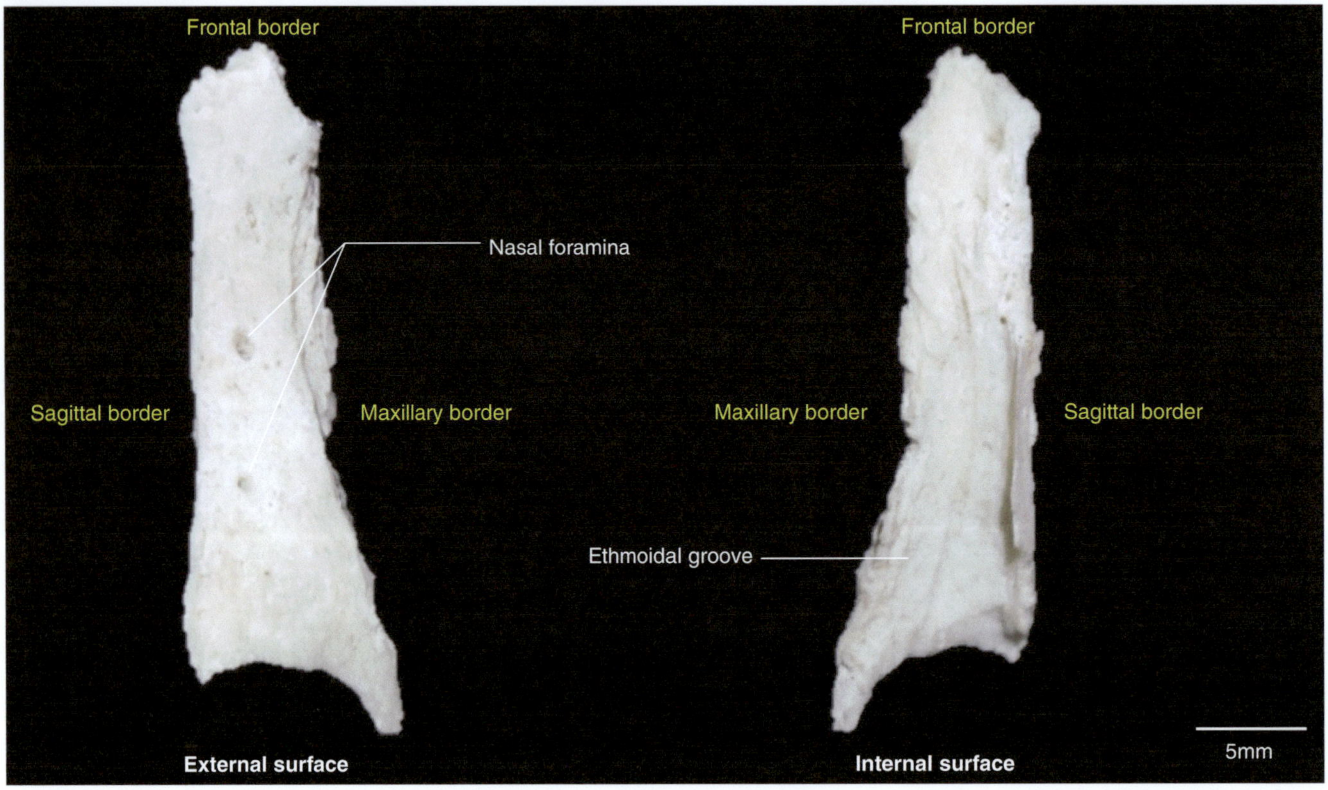

Fig. 2.70 External and internal surfaces of the left nasal bone. The ethmoidal groove accommodates the external nasal branch of the anterior ethmoidal nerve (originally from the nasociliary nerve). The nasal foramina are pathways for small veins

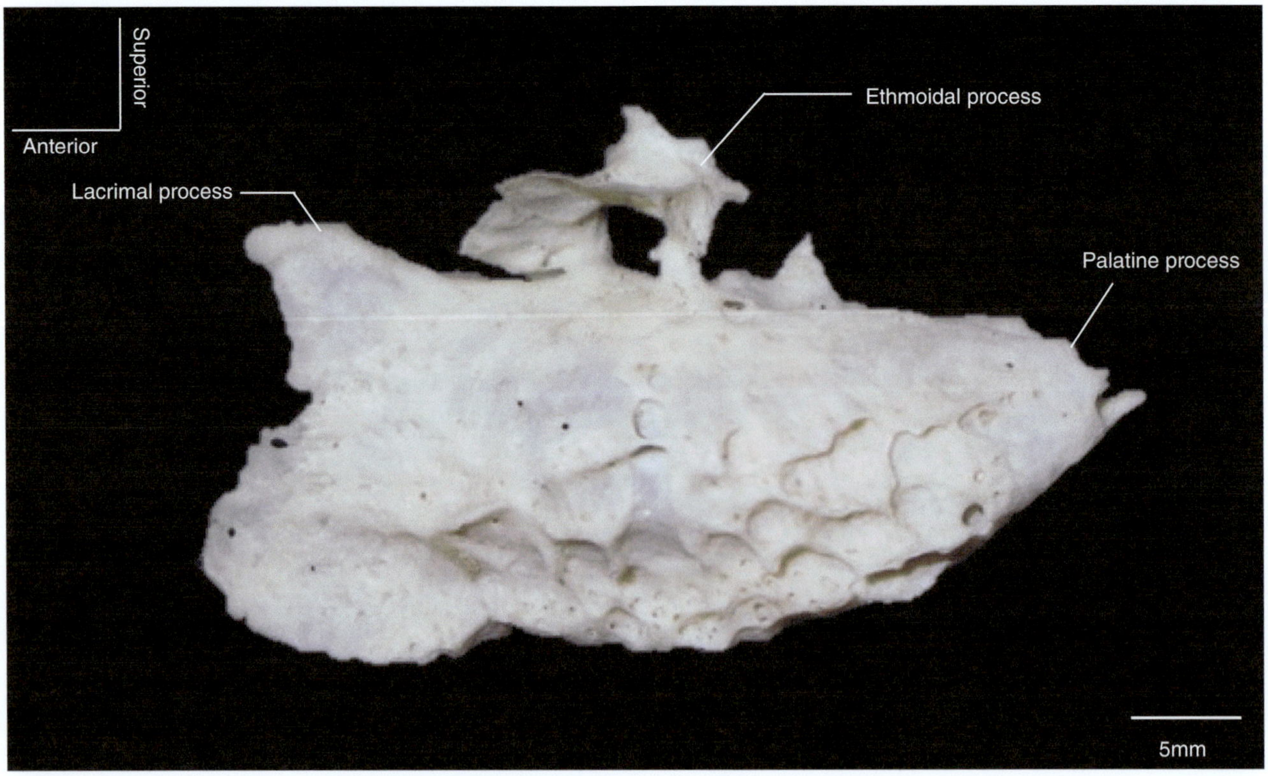

Fig. 2.71 Medial view of the right inferior nasal concha

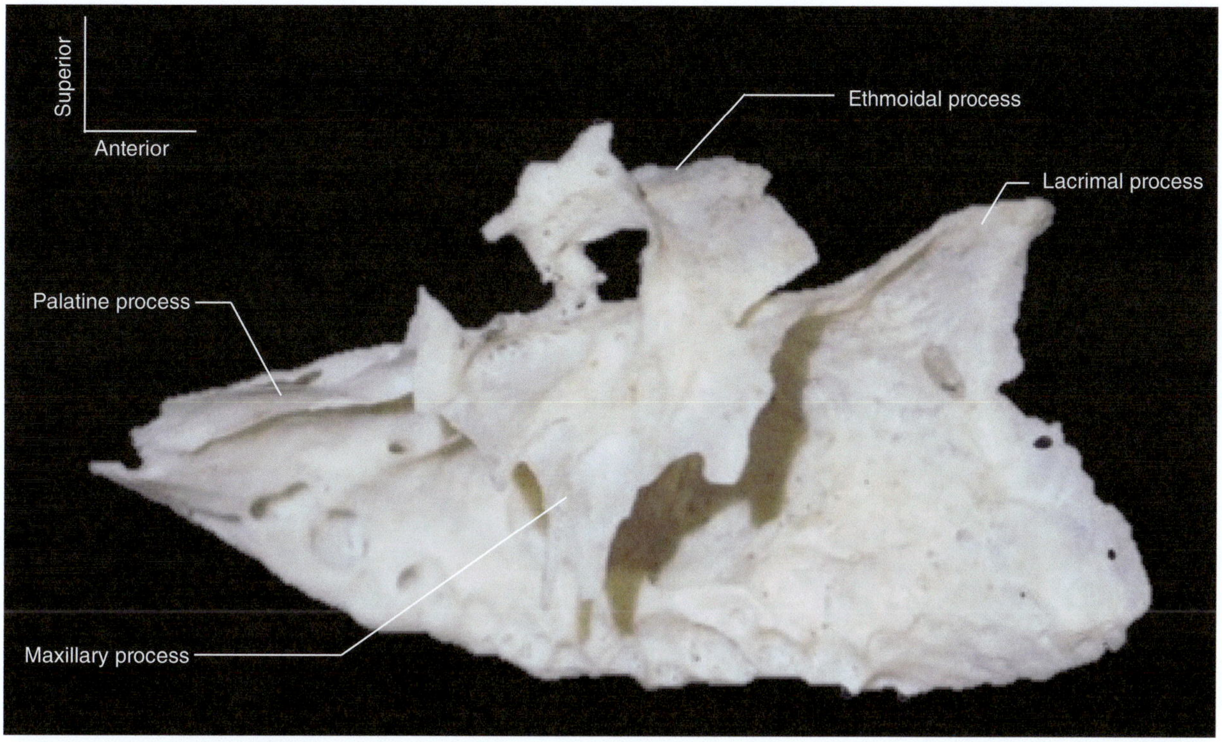

Fig. 2.72 Lateral view of the right inferior nasal concha

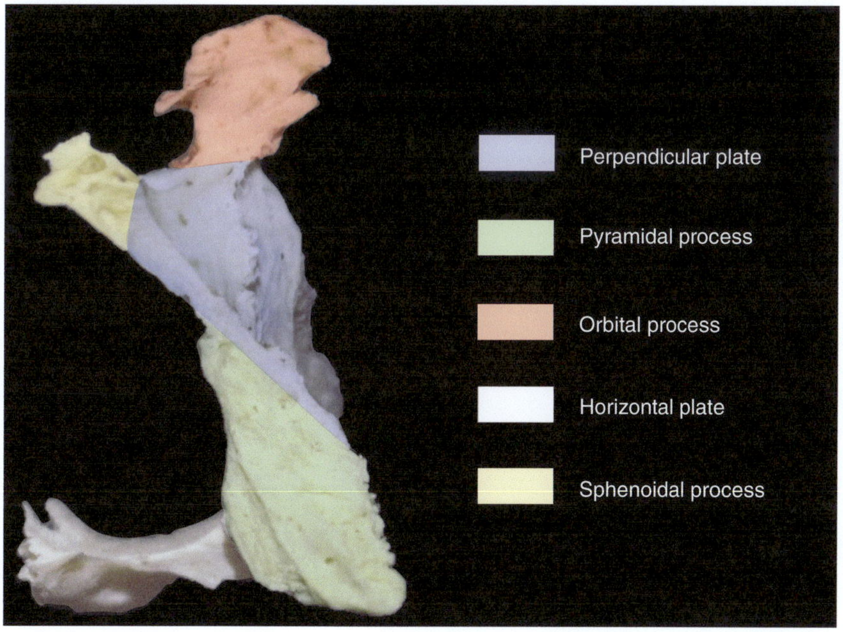

Fig. 2.73 The palatine bone consists of the perpendicular plate, pyramidal process, orbital process, horizontal process, and sphenoidal process

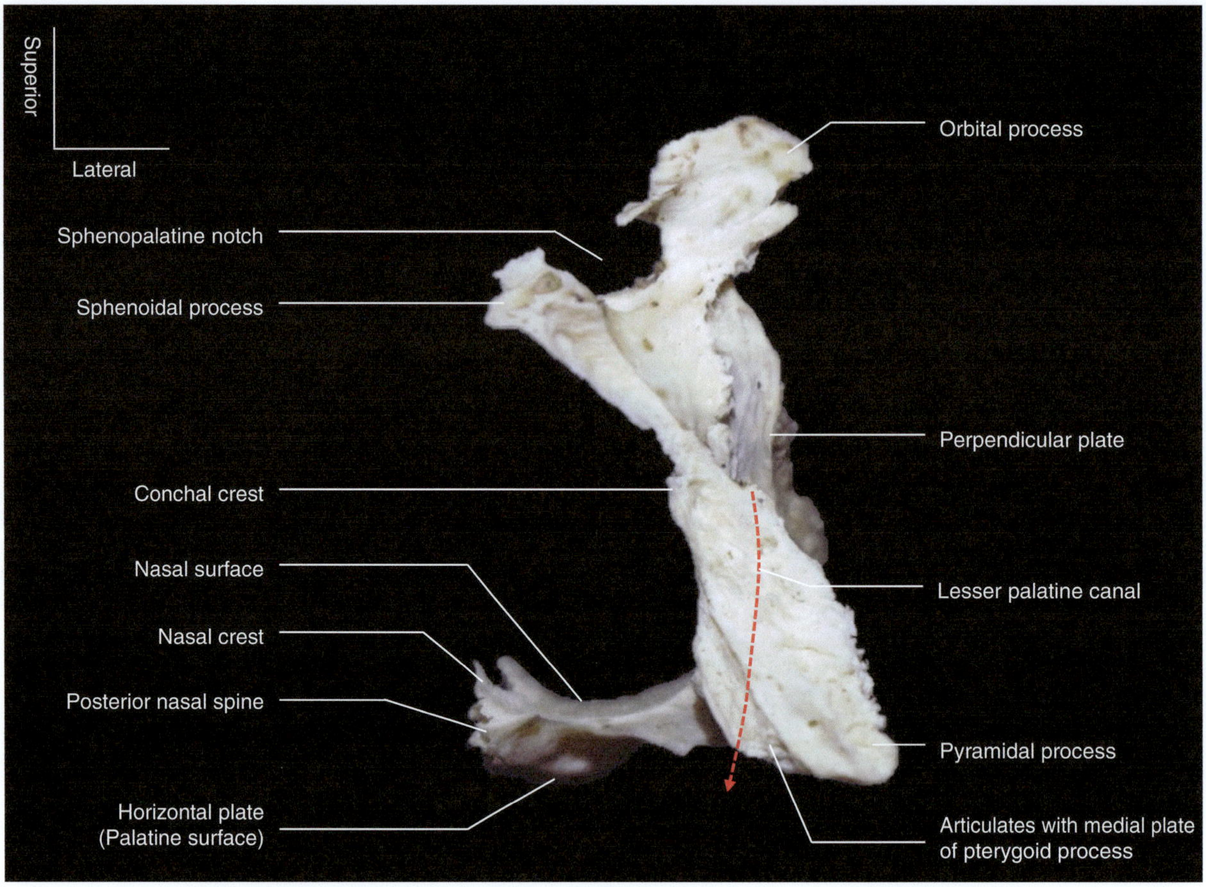

Fig. 2.74 Posterior view of the right palatine bone

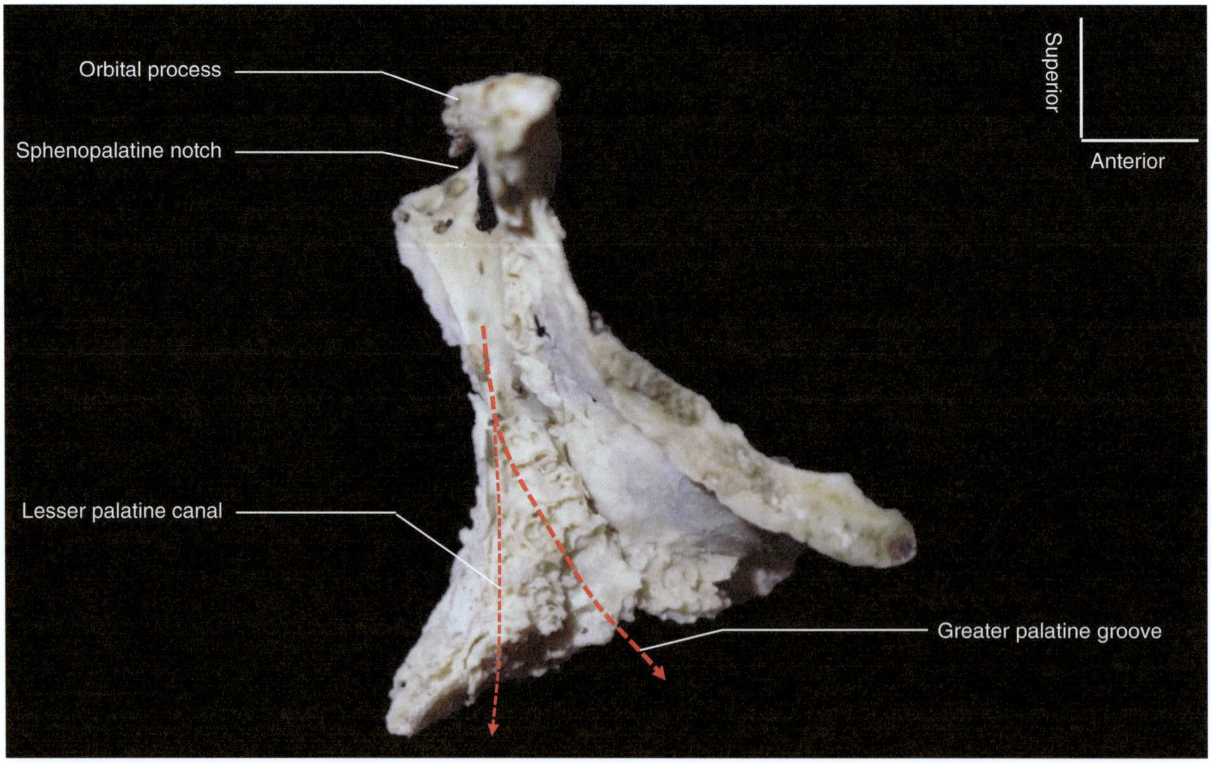

Fig. 2.75 Lateral view of the right palatine bone

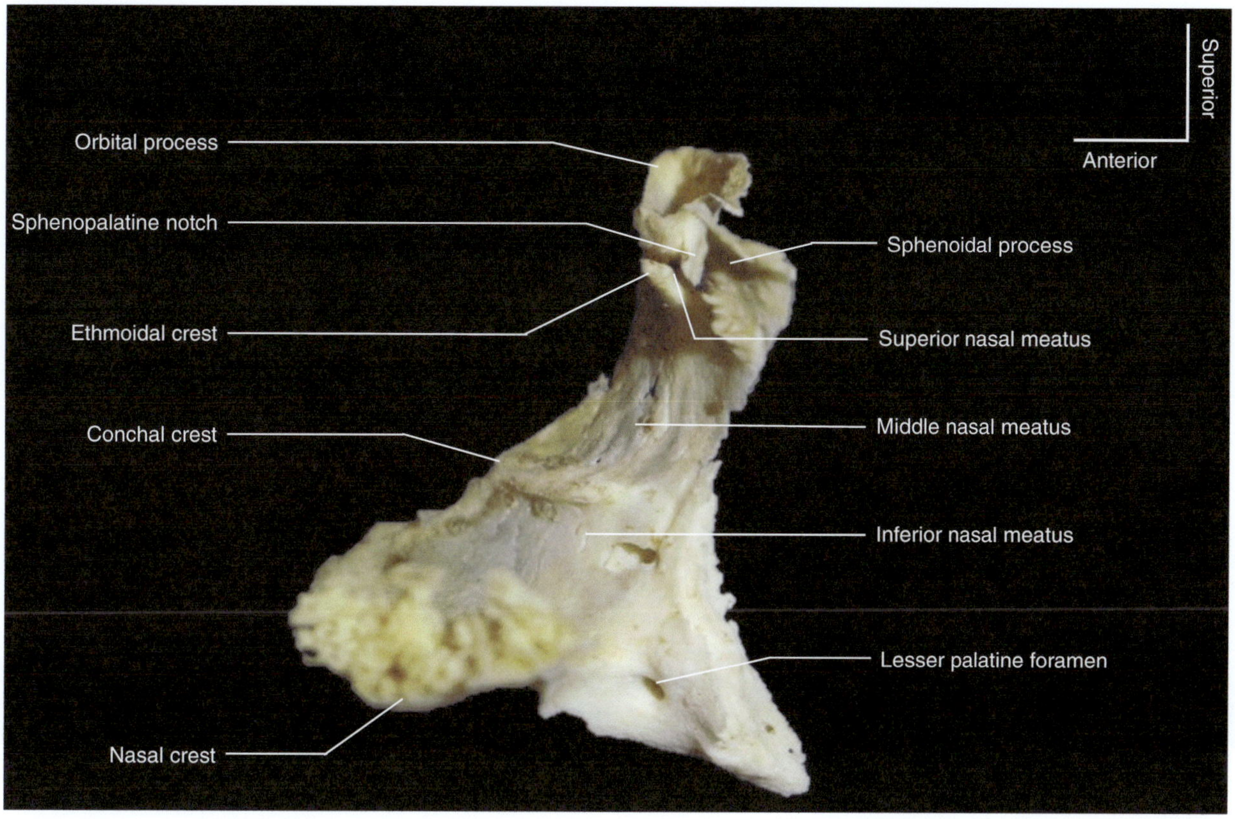

Fig. 2.76 Medial view of the right palatine bone

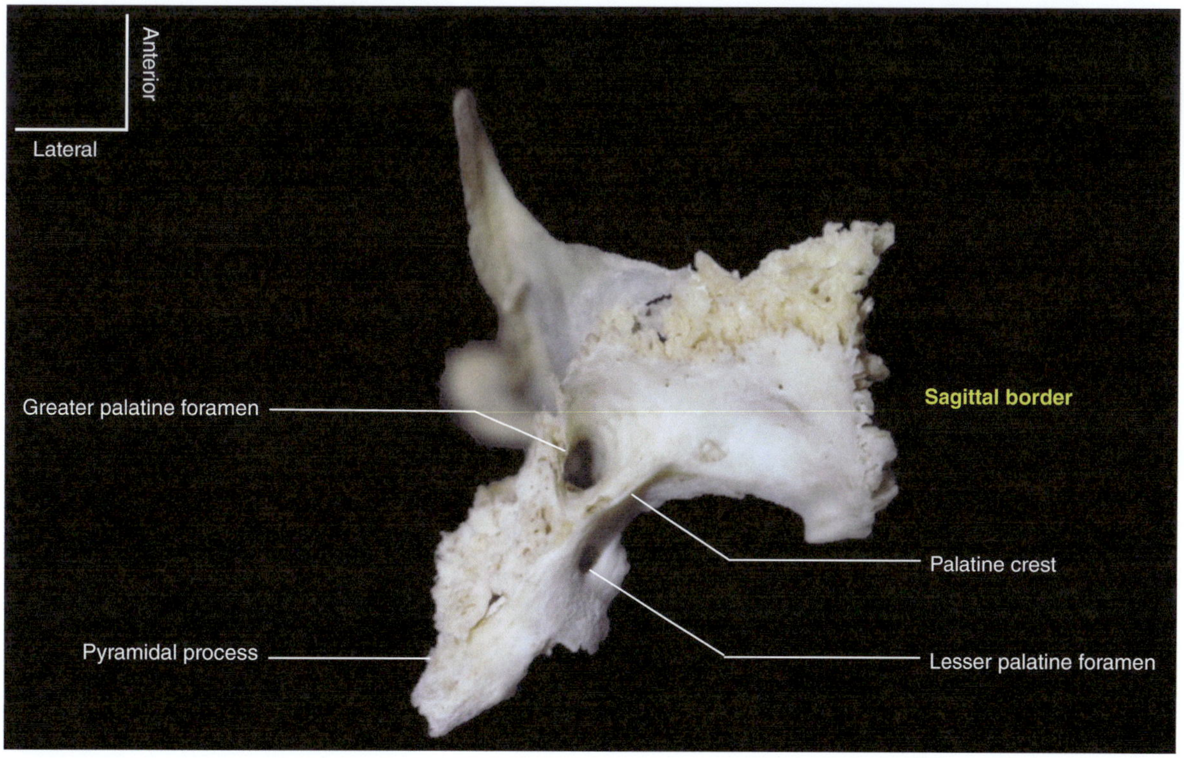

Fig. 2.77 Inferior view of the right palatine bone

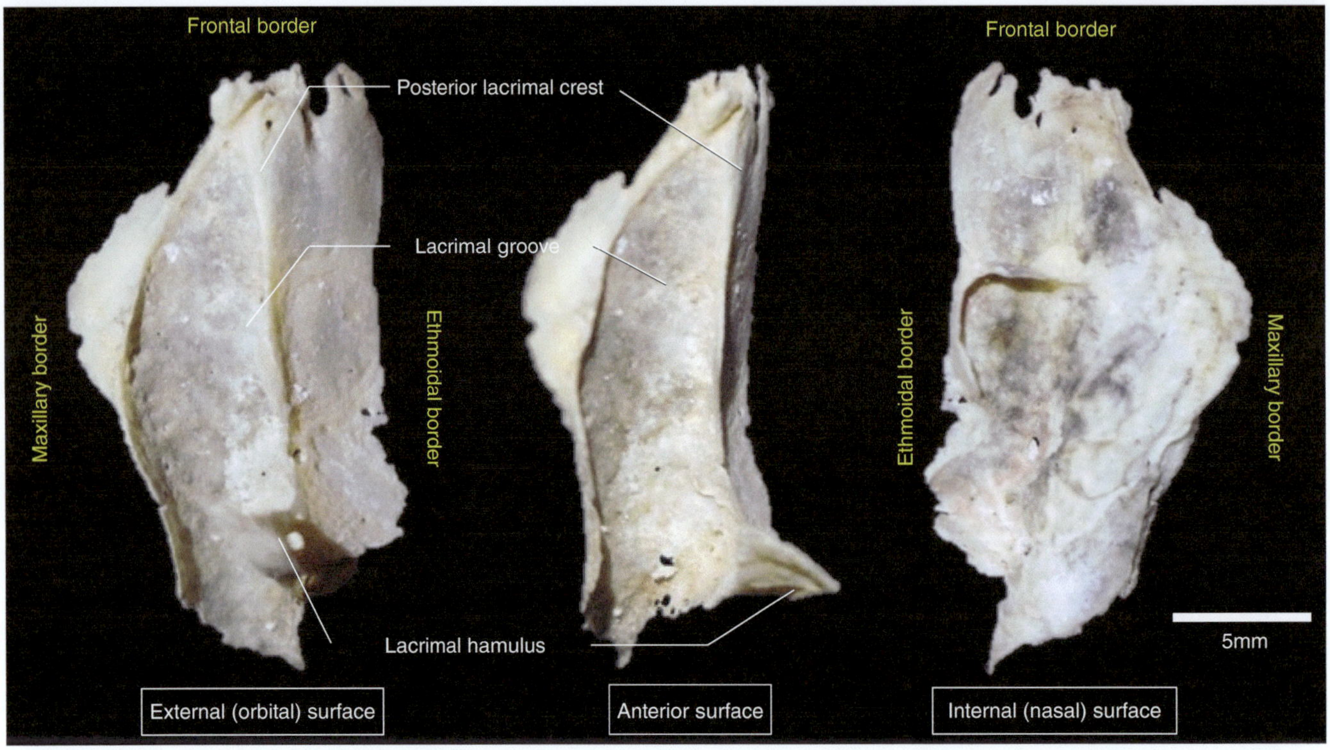

Fig. 2.78 The left lacrimal bone. The lacrimal groove forms the fossa for the lacrimal sac together with the lacrimal groove of the maxillary bone

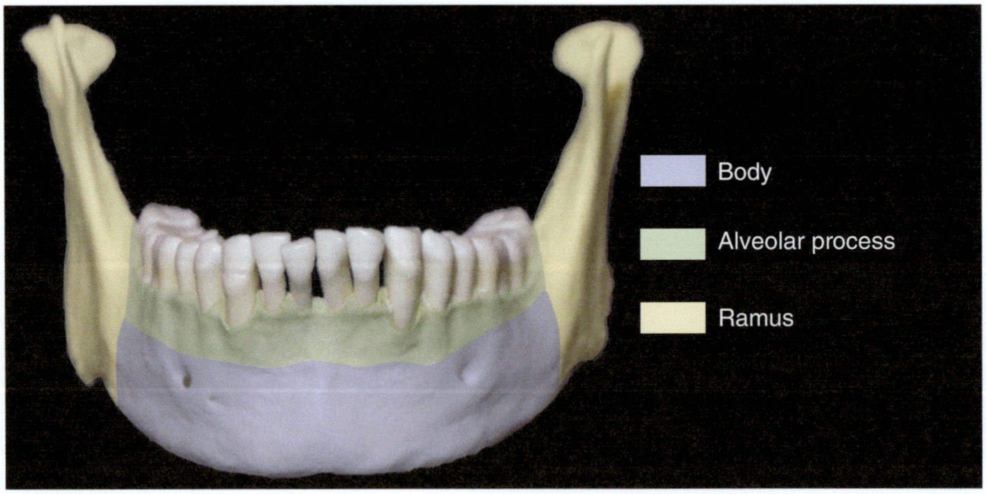

Fig. 2.79 The mandible consists of a body, ramus, and alveolar part (alveolar process of the mandible)

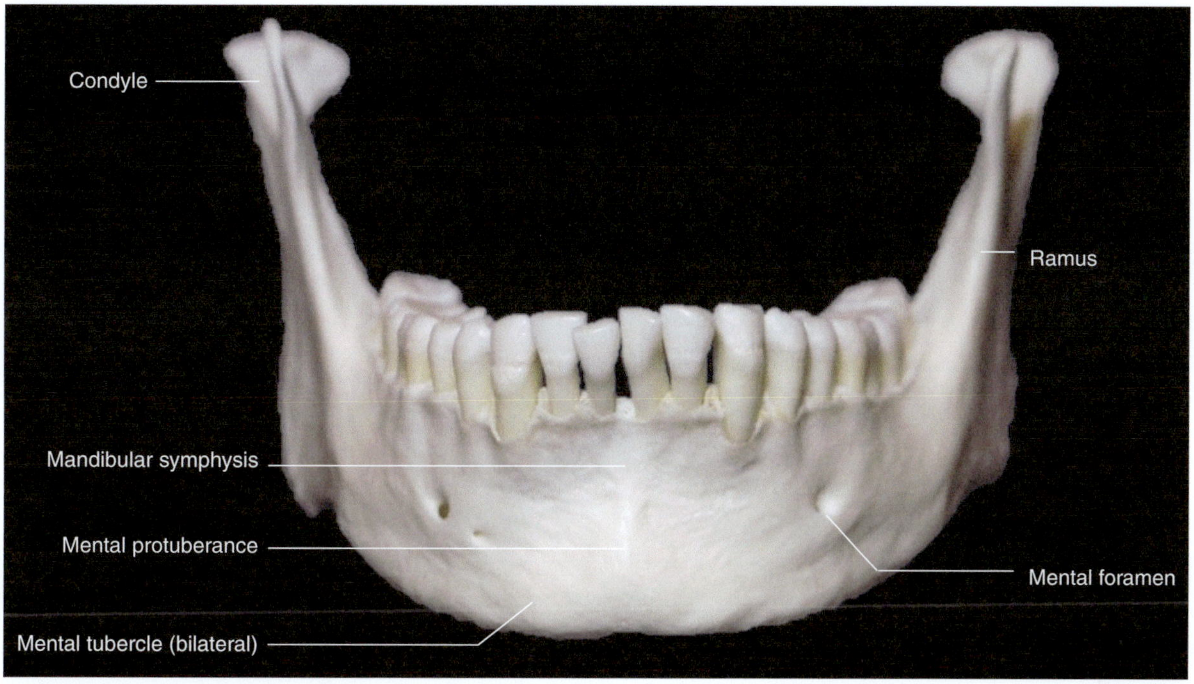

Fig. 2.80 Anterior view of the mandible

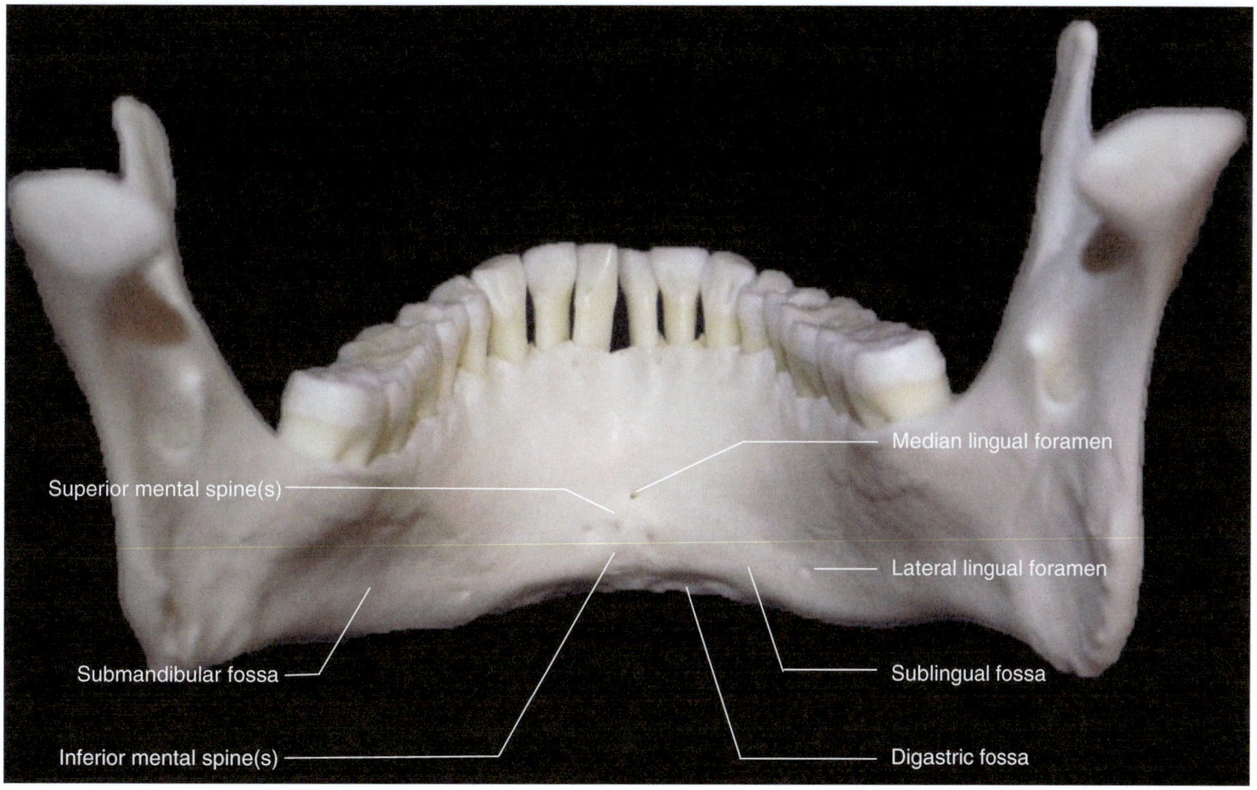

Fig. 2.81 Posterior view of the mandible

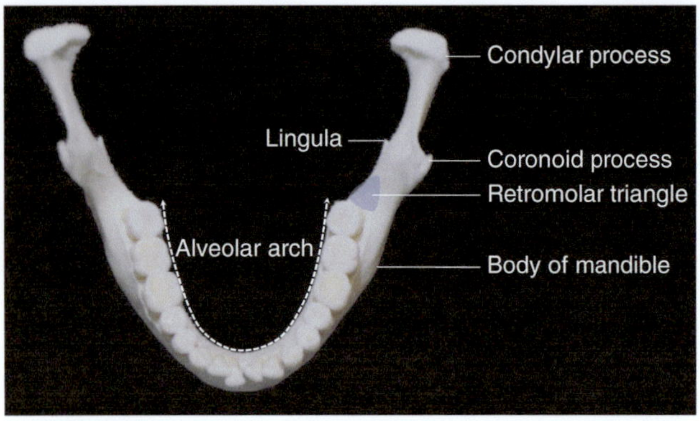

Fig. 2.82 Superior view of the mandible

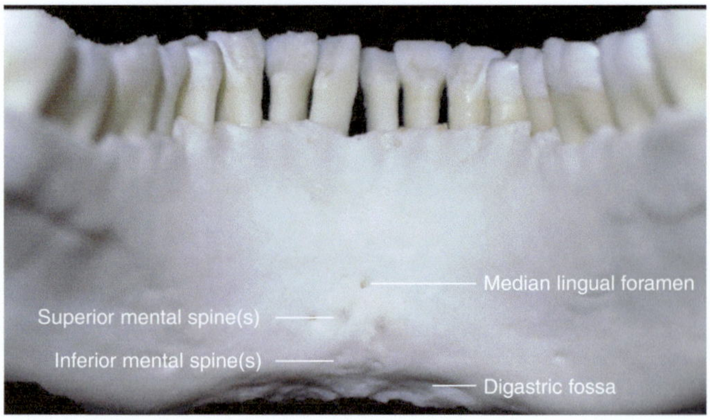

Fig. 2.83 Magnified posterior view of the mandible

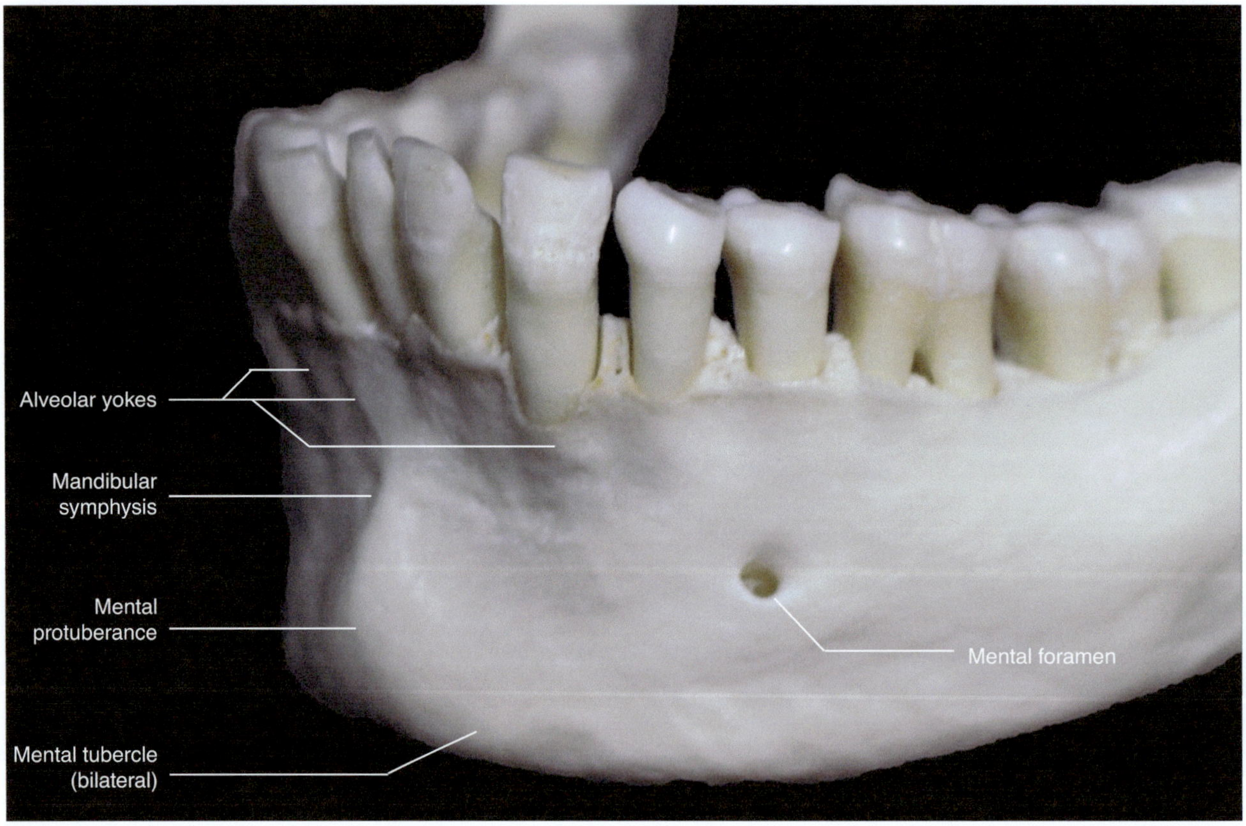

Fig. 2.84 Magnified anterolateral view of the mandible. The teeth are embedded in the dental alveoli which result in the the formation of the alveolar yokes on the buccal/labial sides

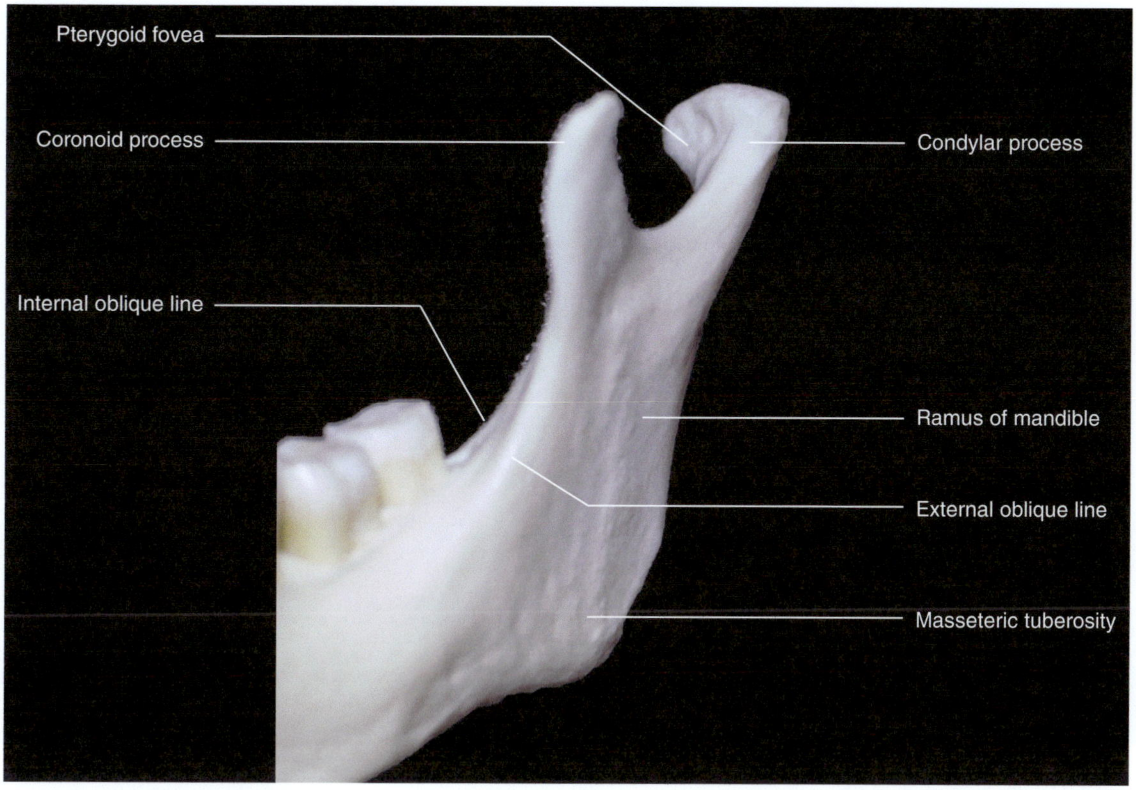

Fig. 2.85 Anterolateral view of the mandibular ramus

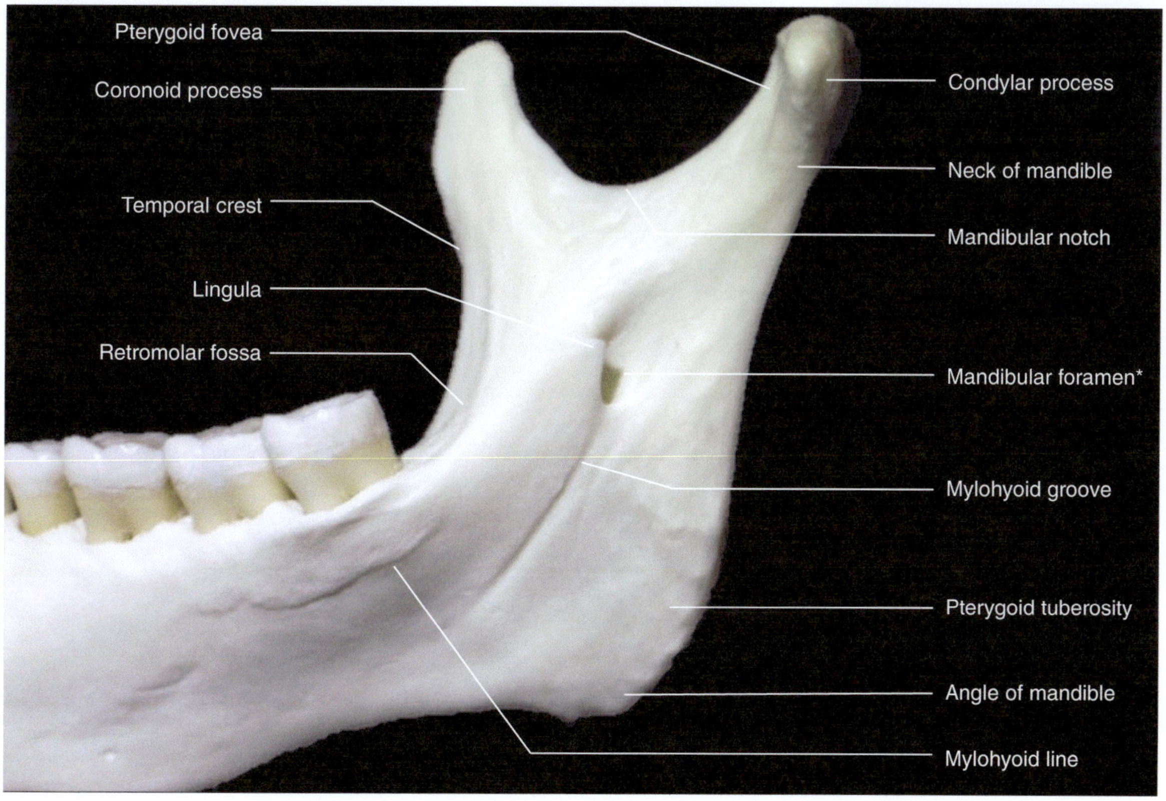

Fig. 2.86 Medial view of the mandible. *The 2nd edition of Terminologia Anatomica uses inferior alveolar foramen for the mandibular foramen (the mandibular foramen is listed as a synonym). FIPAT. (2019) TerminologiaAnatomica 2nd ed. FIPAT.library.dal.ca. Federative International Programme for Anatomical Terminology

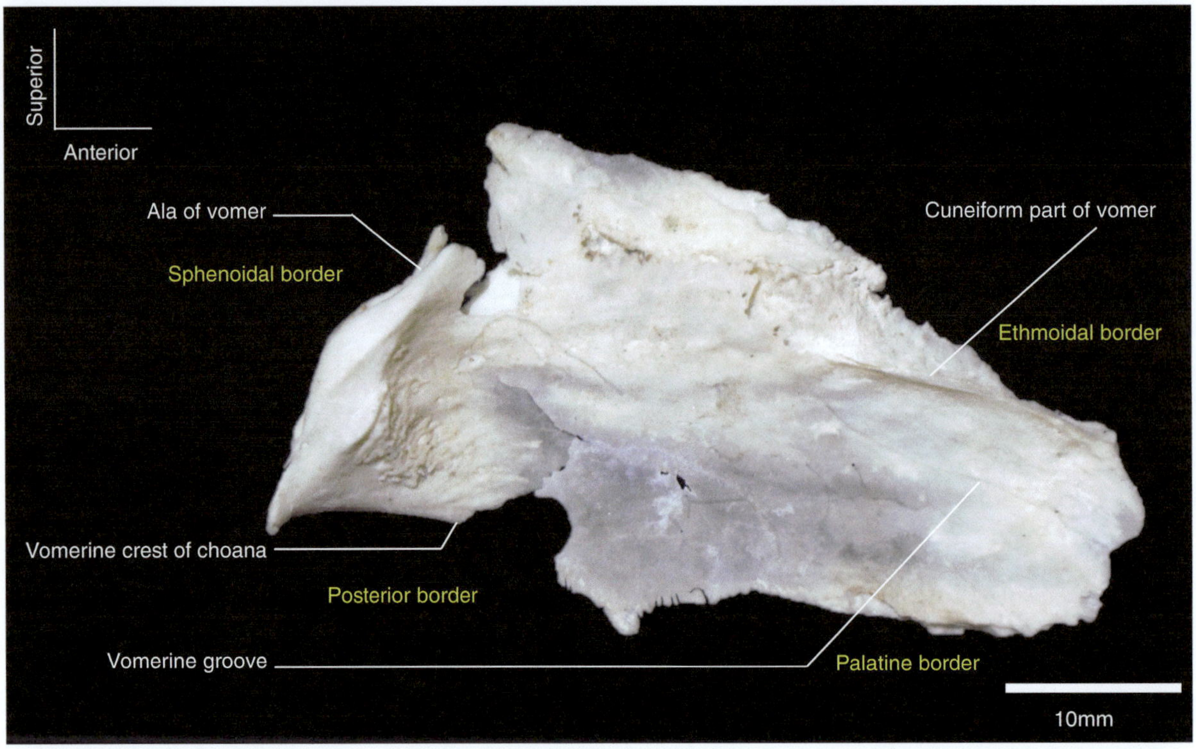

Fig. 2.87 Lateral (right) view of the vomer. The nasopalatine nerve and sphenopalatine vessels run on the vomerine groove

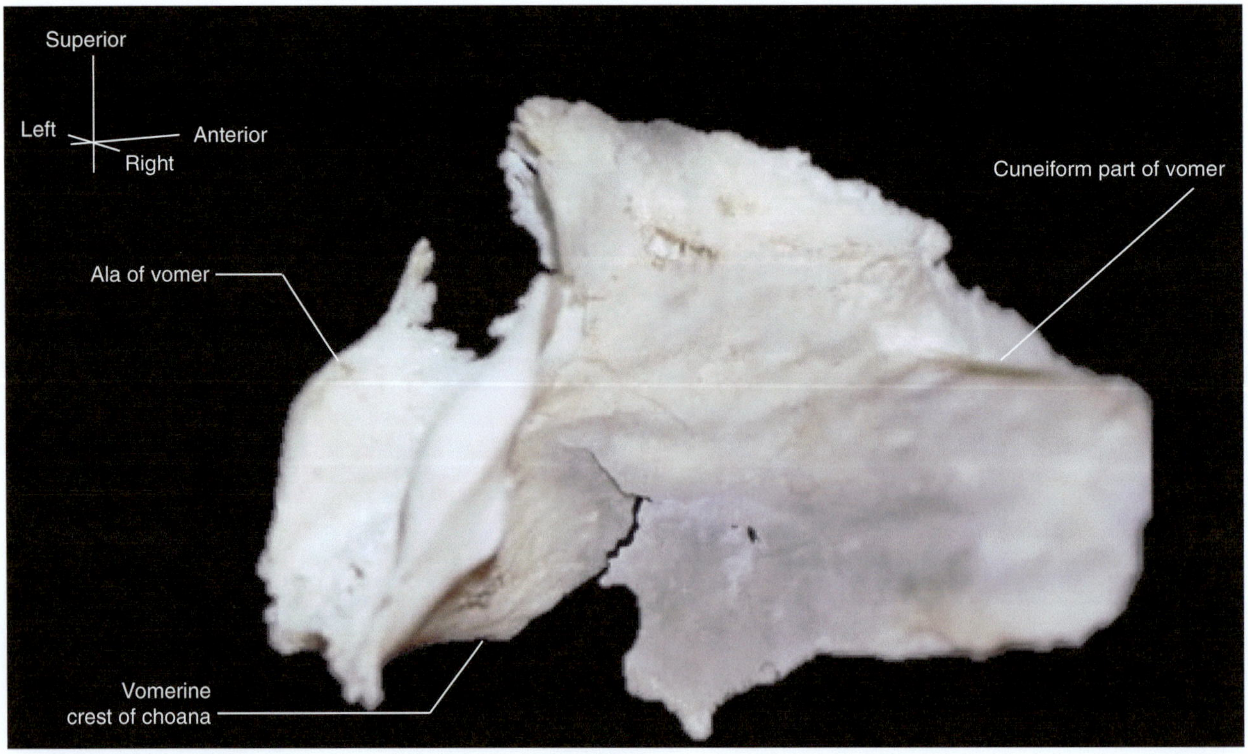

Fig. 2.88 Posterolateral (right) view of the vomer

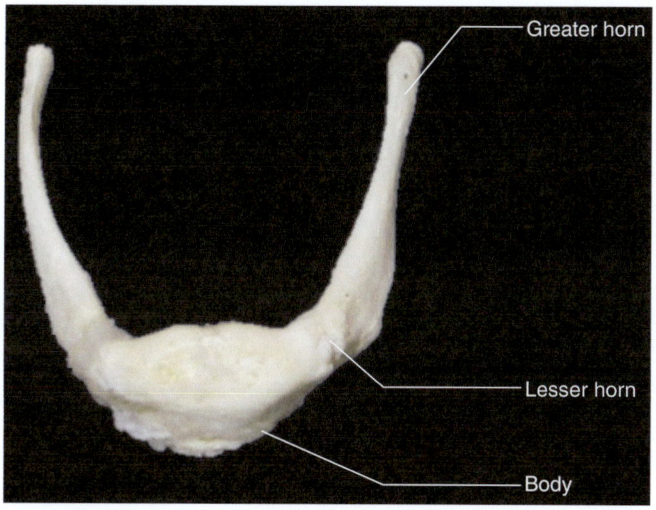

Fig. 2.89 Anterior view of the hyoid bone

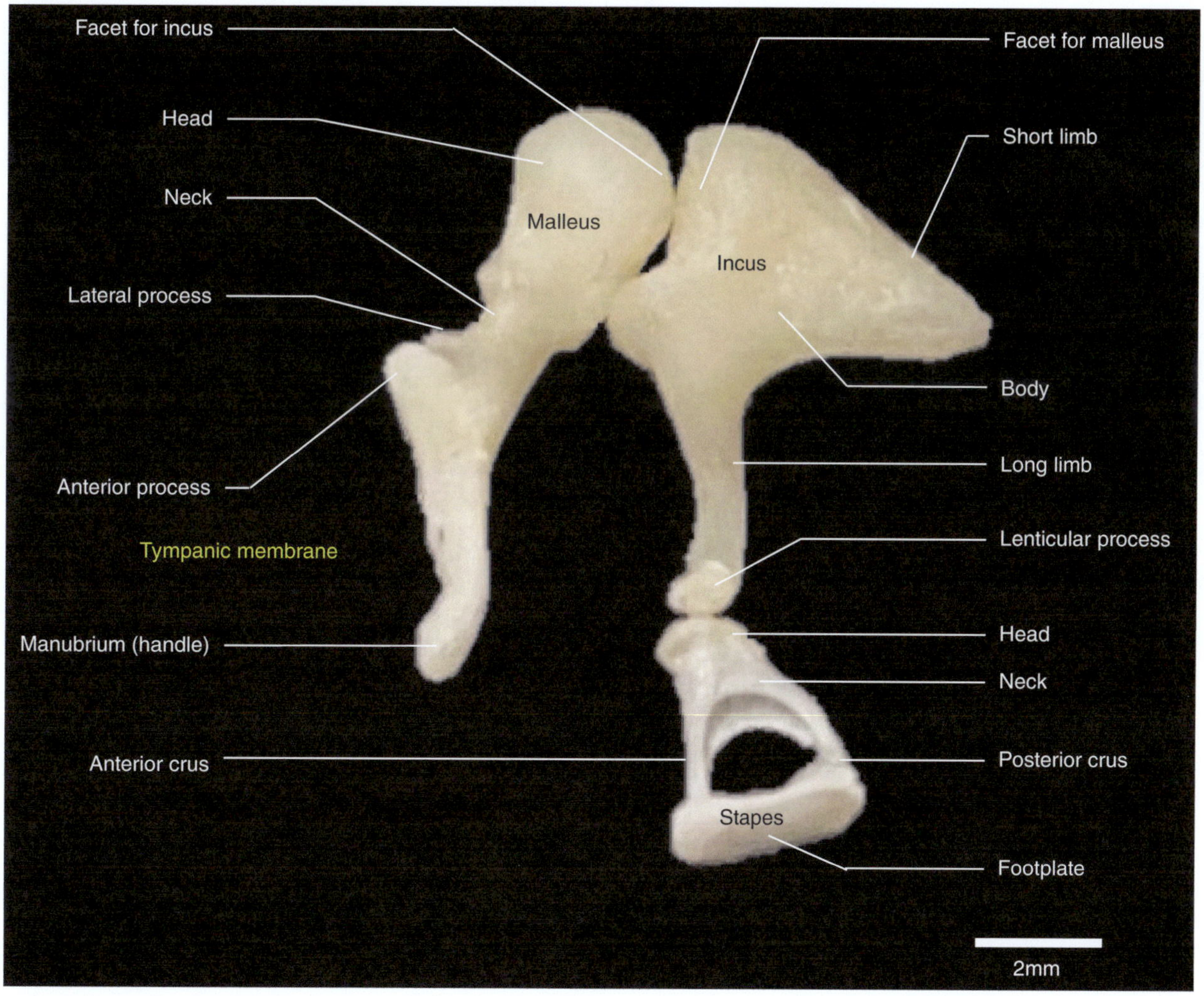

Fig. 2.90 Right auditory ossicles

2.4 Cervical Vertebrae

Summary

There are seven cervical vertebrae. C1, C2, and C7 vertebrae show unique features so they are also known by the names atlas, axis, and vertebra prominens, respectively. The occipital bone, C1 and C2 form the craniocervical junction. Knowledge of normal bony features of each cervical vertebra helps in understanding the regional anatomy and its variations. In this section, the osteology of the cervical vertebrae will be discussed.

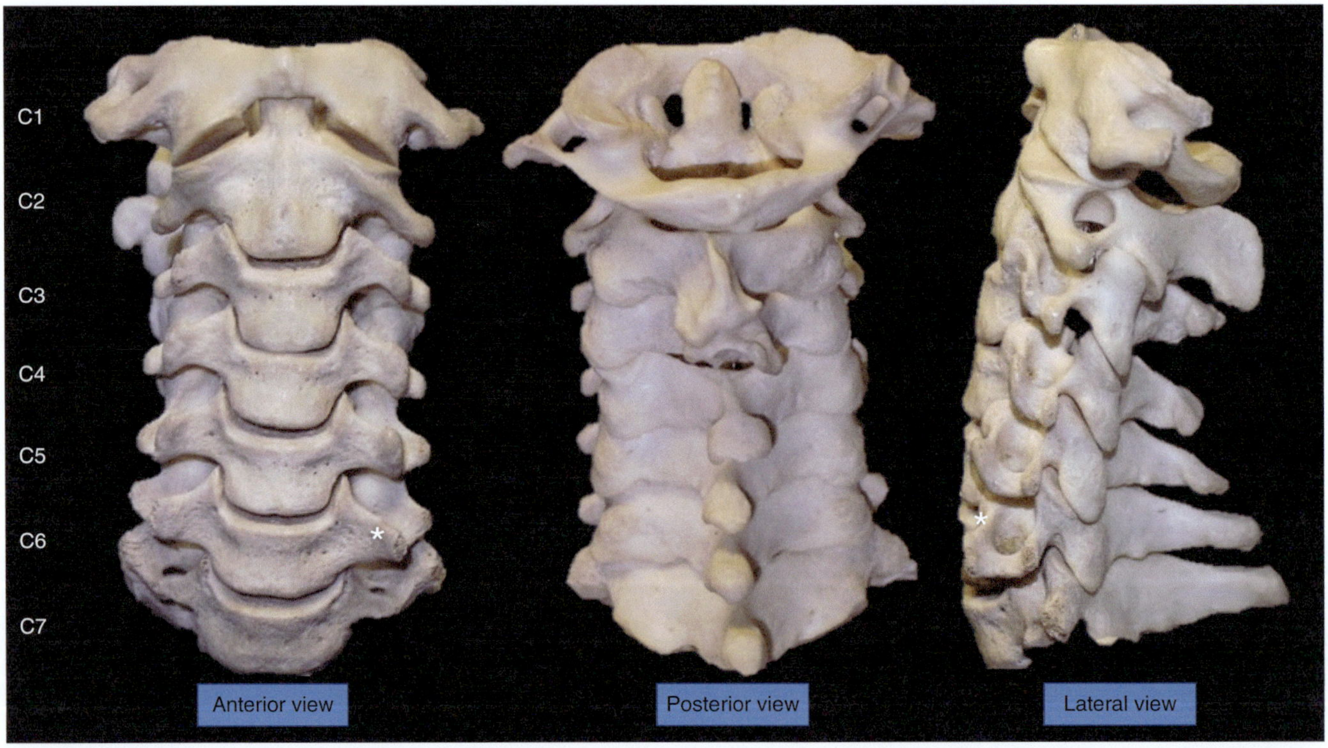

Fig. 2.91 The cervical vertebrae. The superior articular surfaces of C1 articulate with the occipital condyles and the inferior articular facet of C7 joins with the superior articular facet of T1. The philtrum of the upper lip can serve as a landmark for the position of the dens (Fisahn et al. 2018). The carotid tubercle (of Chassaignac) (*) i.e., the anterior tubercle of C6 is used as an anatomical landmark for regional anesthesia such as a brachial plexus blockade

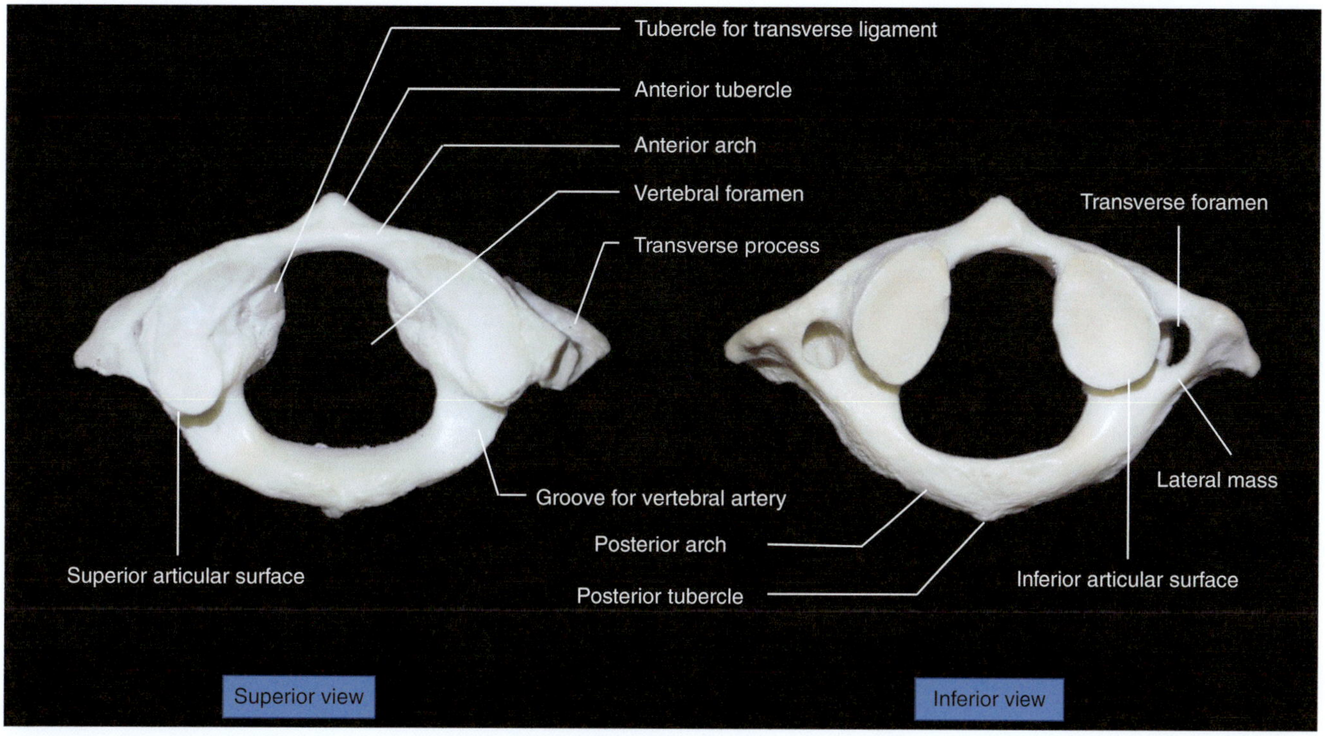

Fig. 2.92 Superior and inferior views of the first cervical vertebra (atlas)

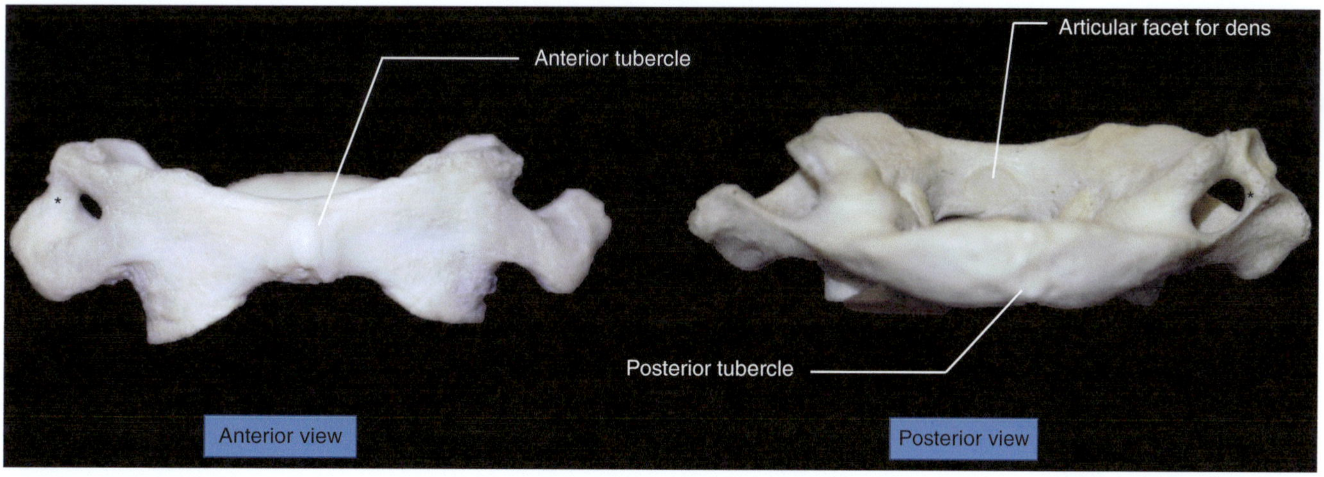

Fig. 2.93 Anterior and posterior views of the first cervical vertebra (atlas). A lateral ponticle of the transverse process* (anatomical variation) is observed on the right side

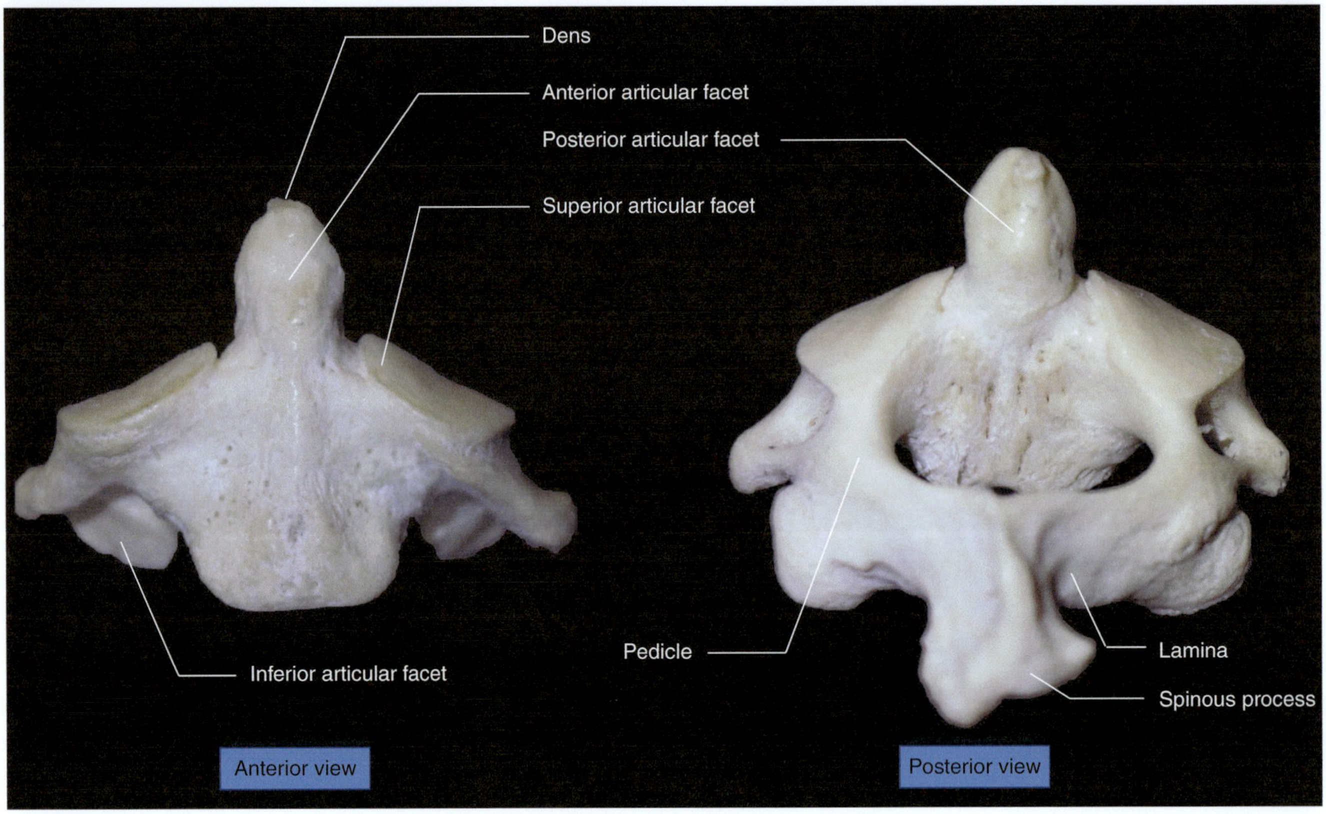

Fig. 2.94 Anterior and posterior views of the second cervical vertebra (axis)

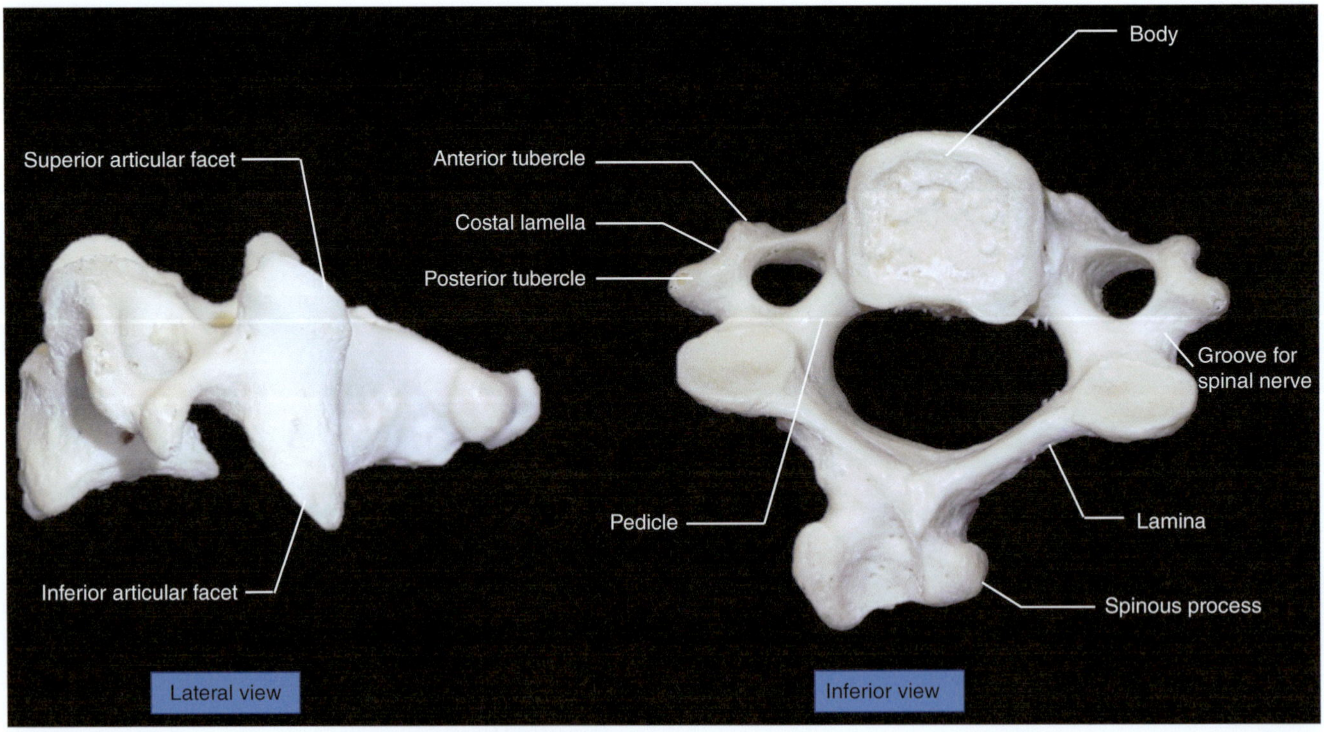

Fig. 2.95 Lateral and inferior views of the third and fifth cervical vertebrae

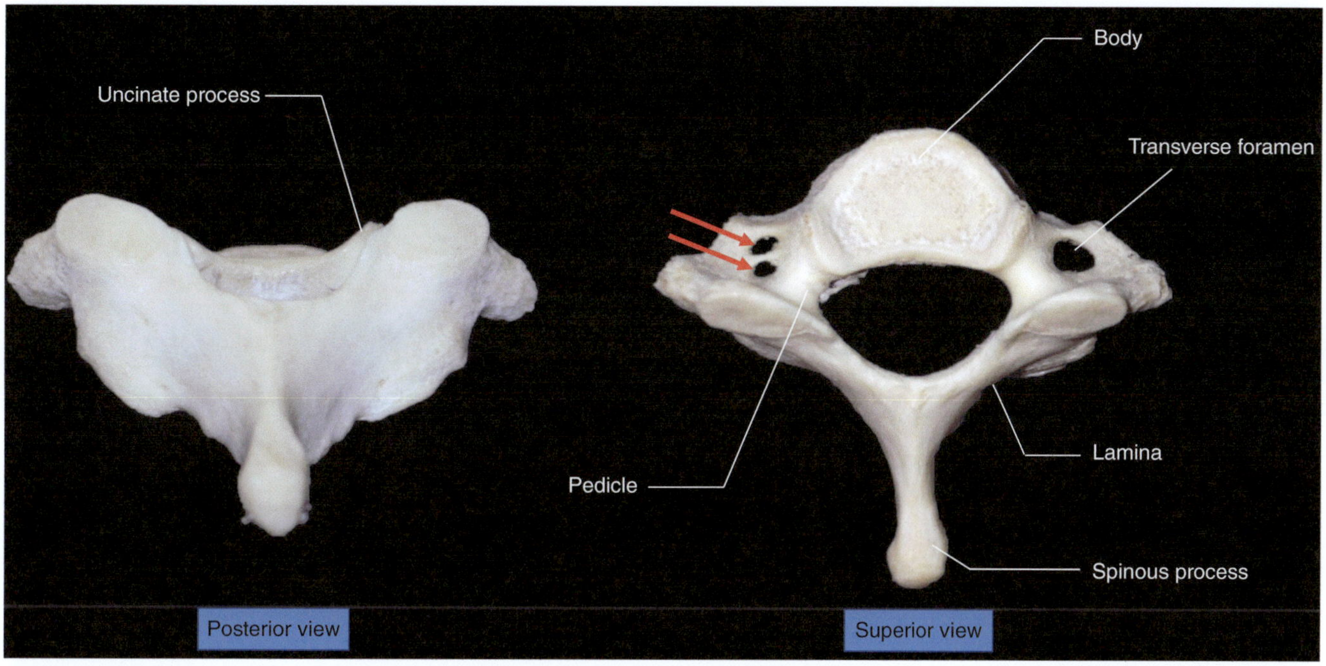

Fig. 2.96 Posterior and superior views of the seventh cervical vertebra, also known as the vertebra prominens, with similar features as the C3–C6 vertebrae but with a more prominent spinous process. The specimen shown has a septated right transverse foramen (arrows). The vertebral arteries usually enter the transverse foramina of C6 and ascend to C1. The transverse foramina of C7 usually transmit vertebral veins and not the vertebral arteries

Reference

Fisahn C, Montalbano MJ, Iwanaga J, Moisi M, Loukas M, Chapman JR, Oskouian RJ, Tubbs RS. A new superficial landmark for the odontoid process: a cadaveric study. Anat Sci Int. 2018;93(2):203–6. https://doi.org/10.1007/s12565-017-0390-1.

3 Anatomy of the Oral Cavity

3.1 Surface Anatomy of the Oral Cavity

Summary
In this section, the surface structures of the oral cavity, which are necessary to understand the mimetic muscles and floor of the mouth, will be reviewed.

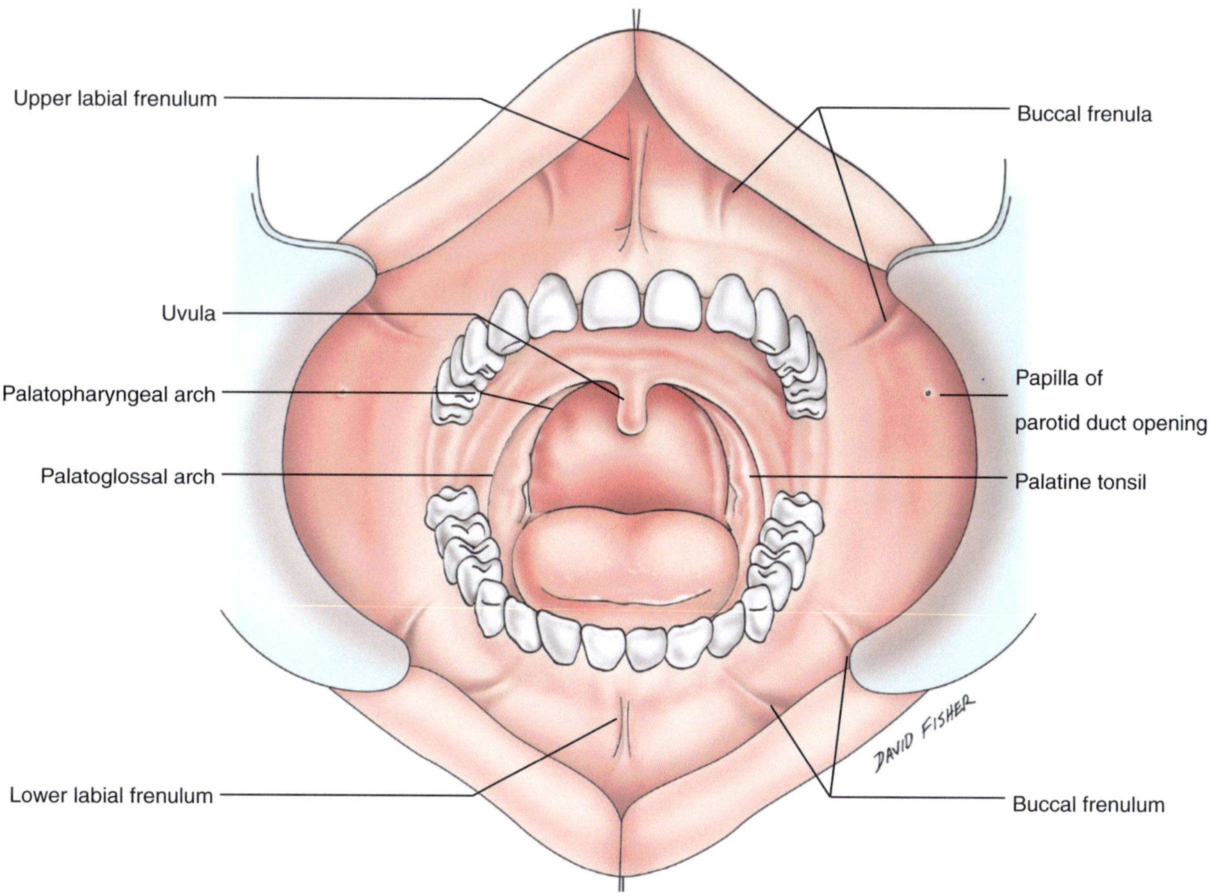

Fig. 3.1 Surface anatomy of the oral cavity. © Fisher/Tubbs 2020. All Rights Reserved

J. Iwanaga, R. S. Tubbs, *Atlas of Oral and Maxillofacial Anatomy*, https://doi.org/10.1007/978-3-030-78327-3_3

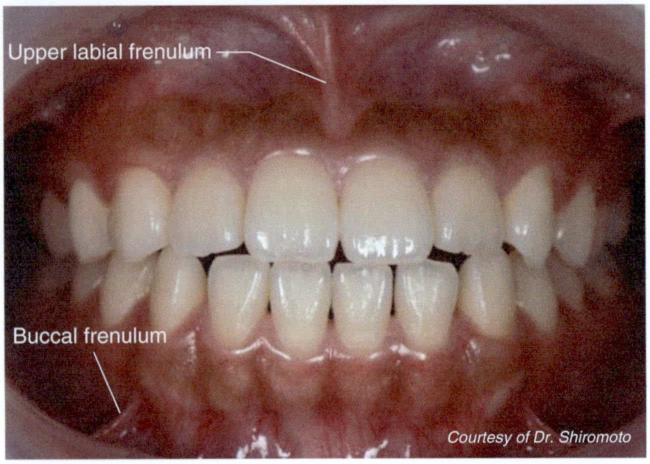

Fig. 3.2 Frontal view

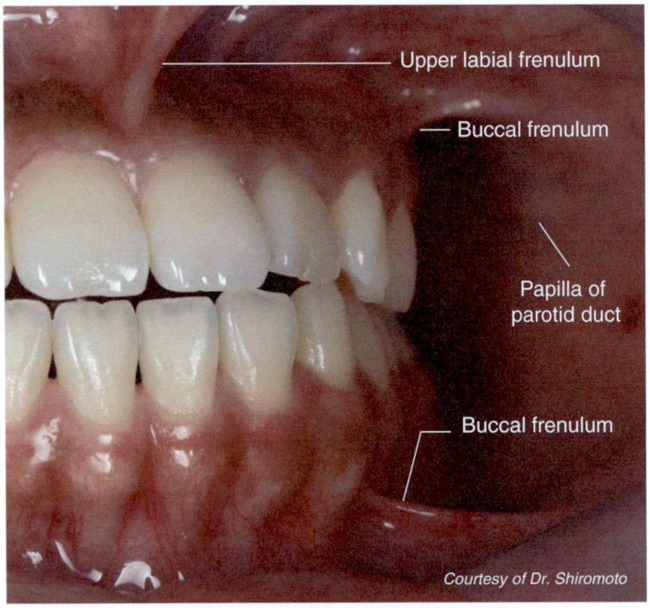

Fig. 3.3 Surface anatomy of the oral vestibule

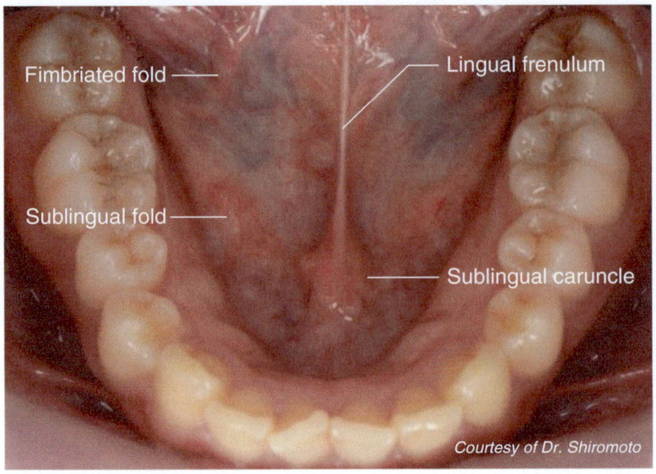

Fig. 3.4 Surface anatomy of floor of the mouth

3.2 Related Mimetic Muscles

Summary
Maxillofacial surgery necessitates a comprehensive anatomical knowledge of the mimetic muscles and thus these have been well depicted in anatomy and surgical textbooks. However, extraoral views of the mimetic muscles are not applicable for dentistry or oral surgery as these specialties need an intraoral perspective. For a better understanding, intraoral dissection of the mimetic muscles is necessary. In this chapter, the mimetic muscles are shown via intraoral dissection that is the same view as dentists and oral surgeons see in their daily practice. Of all mimetic muscles, the incisivus labii inferioris and superioris muscles have not been well described in the literature.

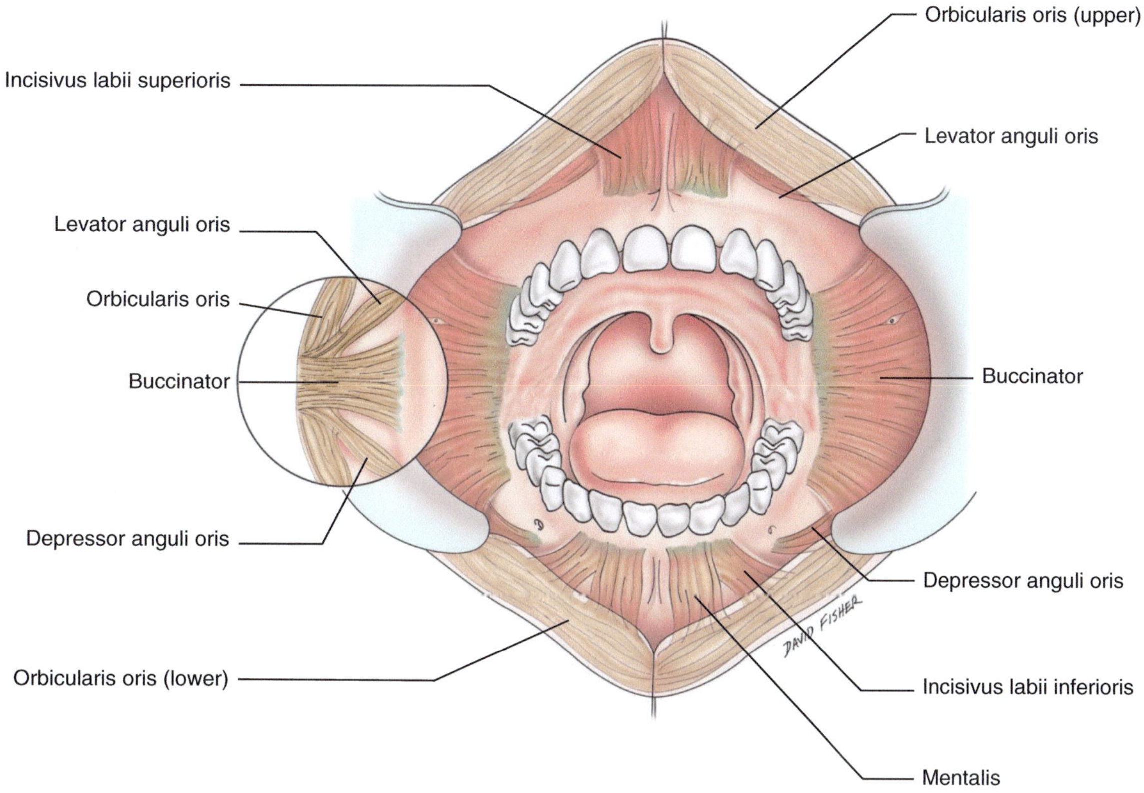

Fig. 3.5 Schema of the mimetic muscles from an oral cavity view. The incisivus labii superioris and inferioris muscles are shown. These muscles contribute to the oral vestibule of the oral cavity.

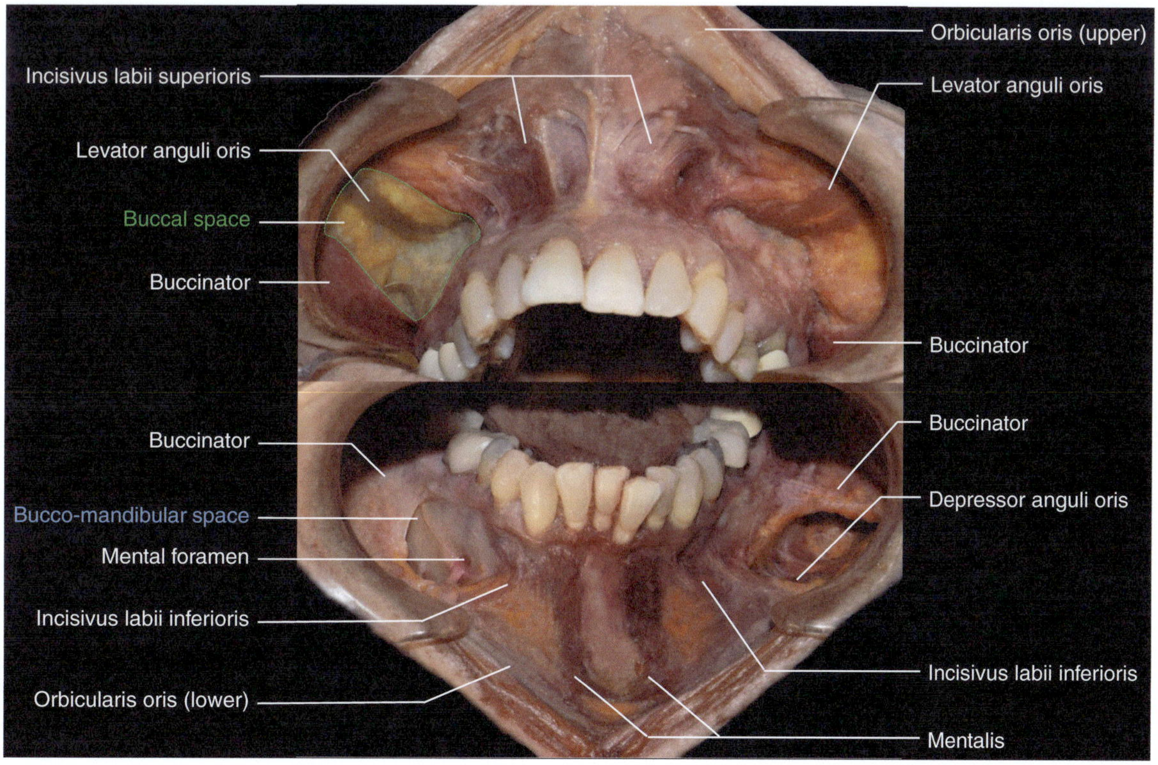

Fig. 3.6 Intraoral dissection of the mimetic muscles. Superiorly, there is an entrance into the buccal space between the buccinator and incisivus labii superioris. Inferiorly, there is entrance into the bucco-mandibular space between the buccinator and incisivus labii inferioris muscles

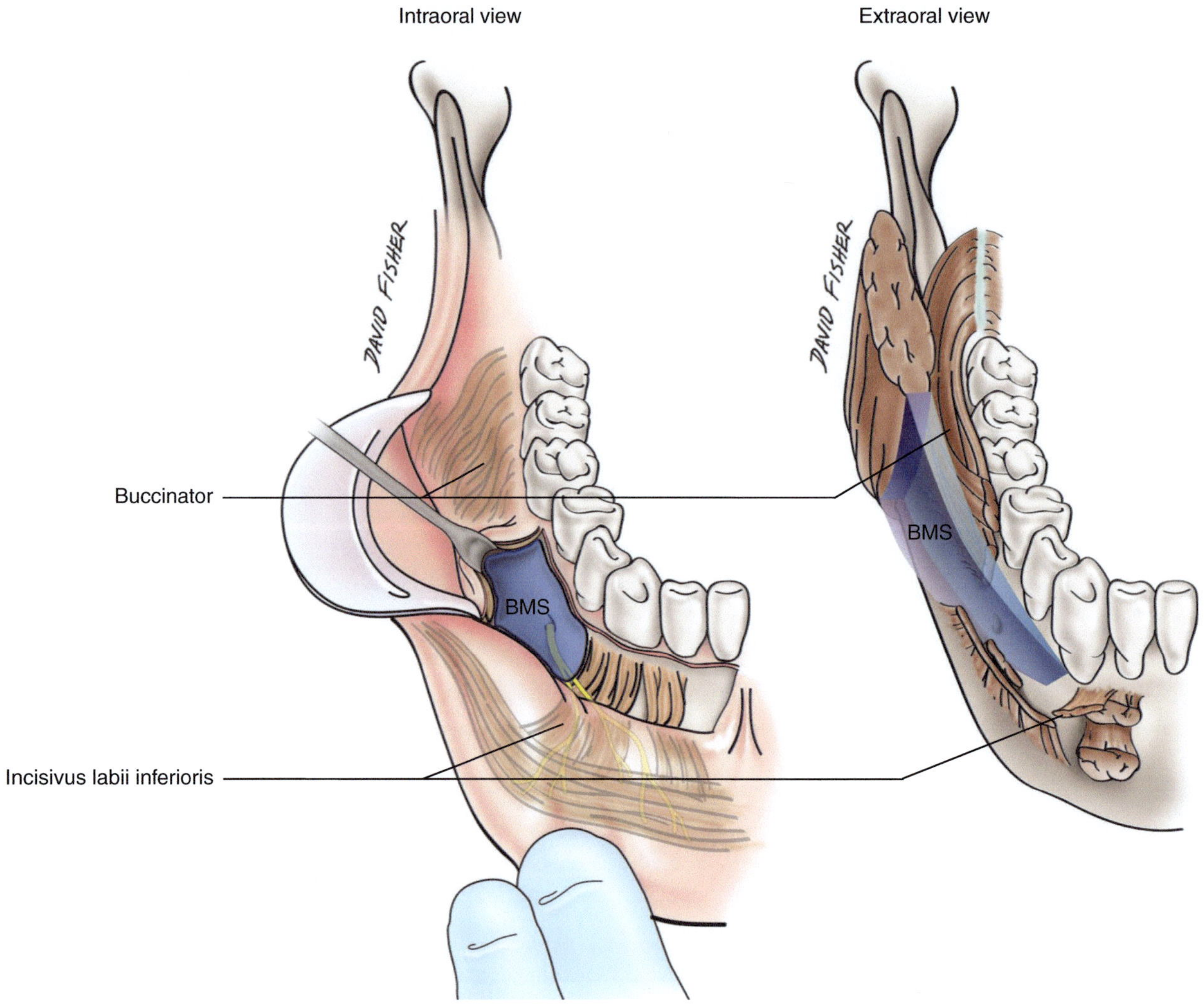

Fig. 3.7 Intraoral and extraoral view of the buccomandibular space (BMS). Intraorally, BMS's entrance into is shown between the buccinator and incisivus labii inferioris muscles. Extraorally the BMS lies lateral to the buccinator and does not have continuation with the buccal space superiorly (Iwanaga et al. 2017).

3.3 Maxilla and Maxillary Sinus

Summary
The maxillary sinus is one of the four paranasal sinuses that is related to both dentistry and rhinology as it is adjacent to the nasal and oral cavities. The maxillary sinus is pyramid-shaped and is the largest of the paranasal sinuses. The floor of the maxillary sinus is formed by the palatine and alveolar processes of the maxilla and lies inferolateral to the nasal cavity, which is normally positioned from the mesial part of the upper first premolar to the distal part of the upper third molar with the lowest at the first and second molar teeth. In implant dentistry, the maxillary sinus is related to augmentation procedures (sinus lift) of the sinus floor and thus a thorough understanding of surrounding structures, e.g., posterior superior alveolar artery, is vital for avoiding complications.

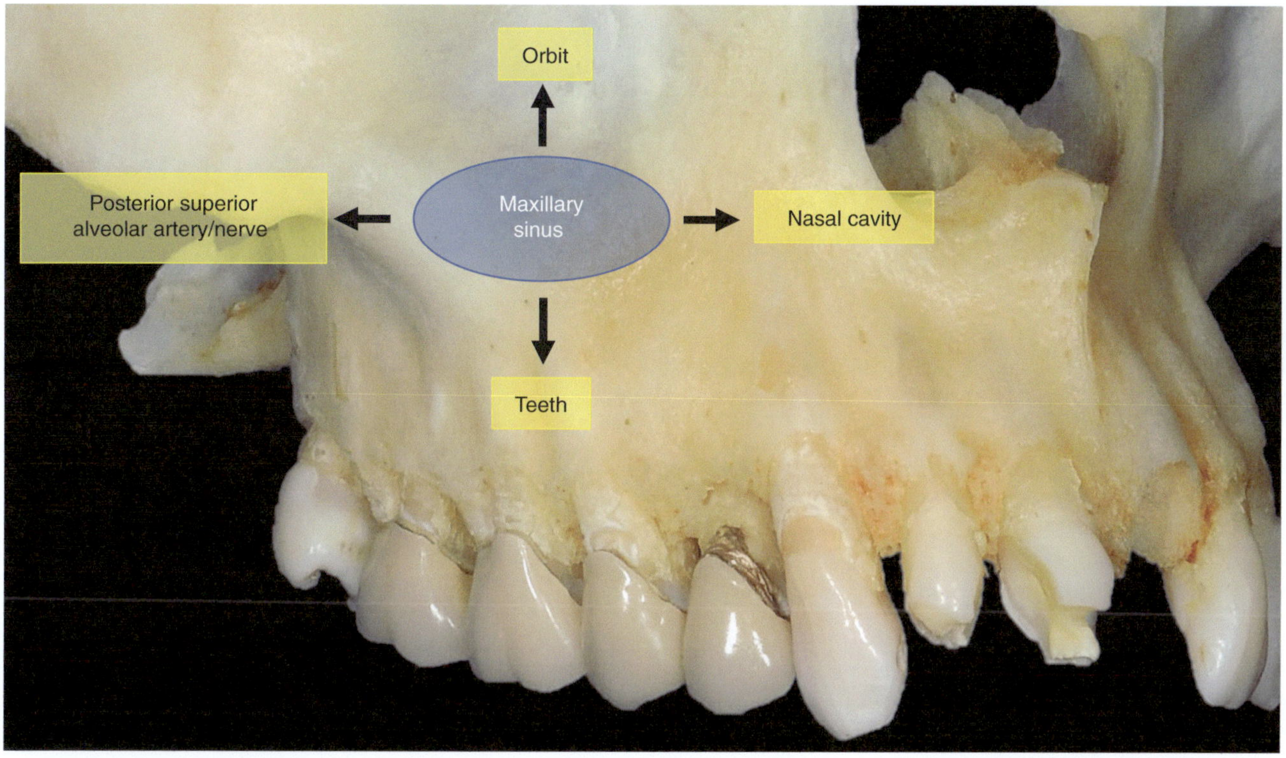

Fig. 3.8 The maxillary sinus is one of the four paranasal sinuses and is surrounded by various structures such as the nasal cavity medially, the posterior superior alveolar nerve/vessels posterolaterally, the apices of the molar teeth inferiorly, and the orbit superiorly

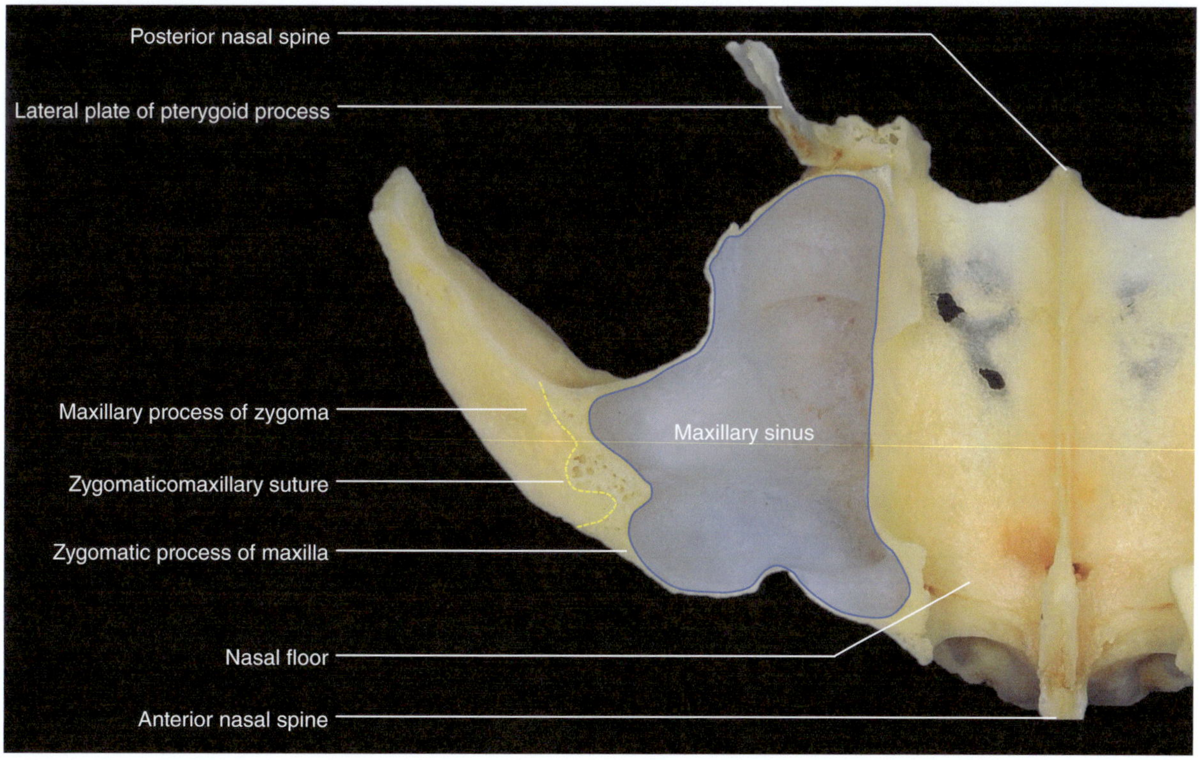

Fig. 3.9 Superior view of the floor of the maxillary sinus. The maxillary sinus is located within the maxilla with the zygoma laterally. The maxillary process of the zygoma articulates with the zygomatic process of the maxilla. The mean volume of the maxillary sinus in adults is 12.5 ml (range 5.0 to 22 ml), and the mean length, width and height are 27.96 mm, 19.57 mm, and 25.33 mm, respectively (Gosau et al. 2009; Lovasova et al. 2018)

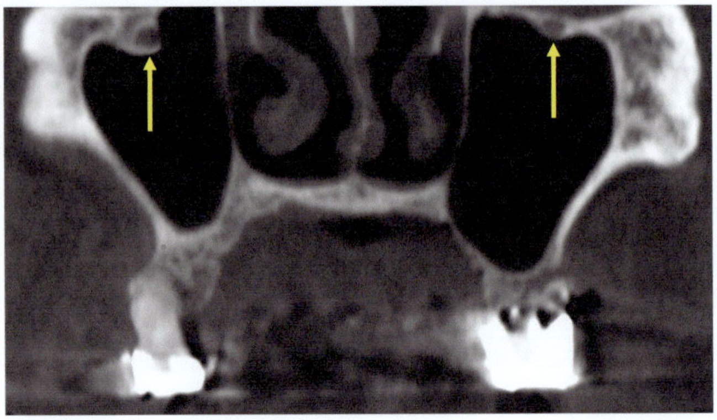

Fig. 3.10 Coronal CT image of the maxillary sinuses. The infraorbital canals (arrows) run right above the superior wall of the maxillary sinus. Within the canal, the infraorbital nerve and vessels travel to emerge from the infraorbital foramina. In this image, the nasal septum is slightly deviated to the left side

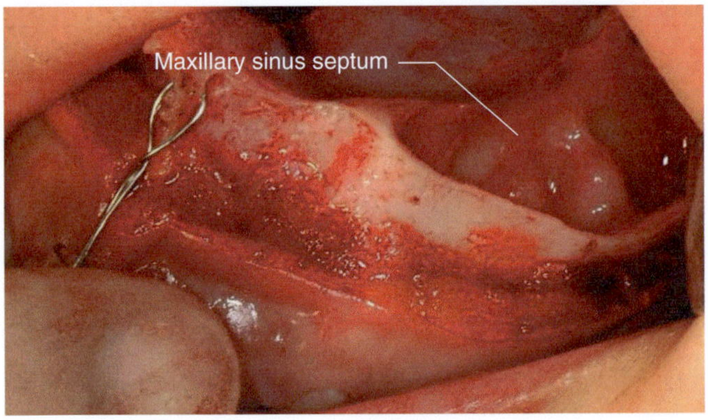

Fig. 3.12 Maxillary sinus septum following down-fracture of the maxilla during Le Fort I osteotomy (Courtesy of Dr. Ibaragi)

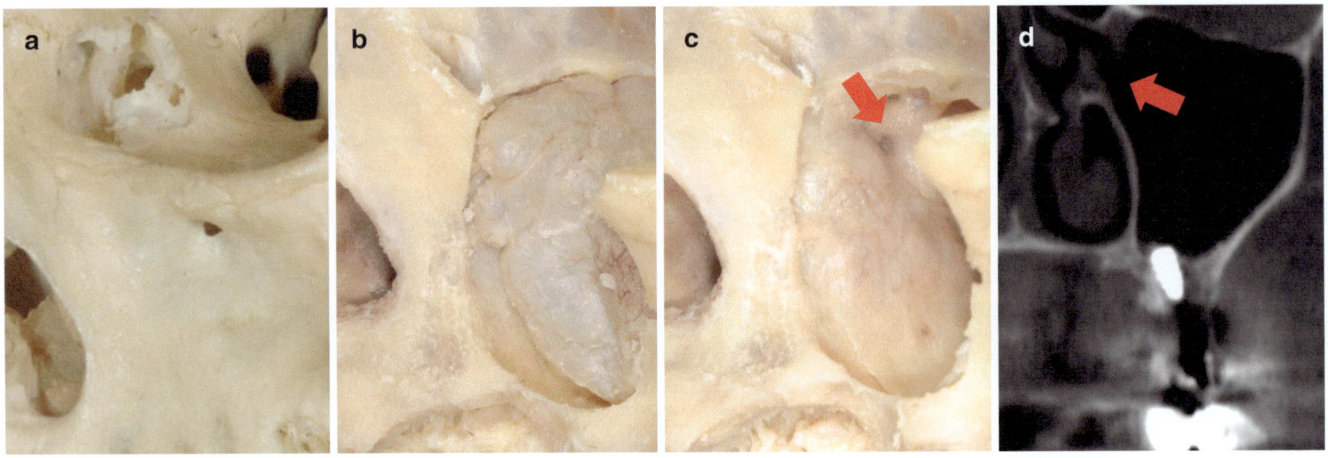

Fig. 3.11 Left maxillary sinus with anterior cadaveric views (**a**–**c**) and coronal CBCT image (**d**). (**a**) The maxillary sinus wall is still intact but the ostium is not visible; (**b**) The superior and anterior walls of the maxillary sinus have been removed and the sinus membrane is shown but the ostium is not visible (**b**); The sinus membrane is removed and the ostium is visible (arrow); (**d**) Coronal image of the maxillary sinus and its ostium (arrow)

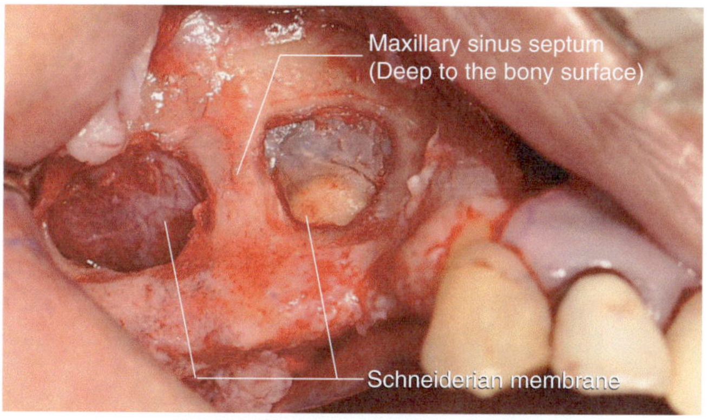

Fig. 3.13 Maxillary sinus septum during sinus lift (Courtesy of Dr. Ibaragi)

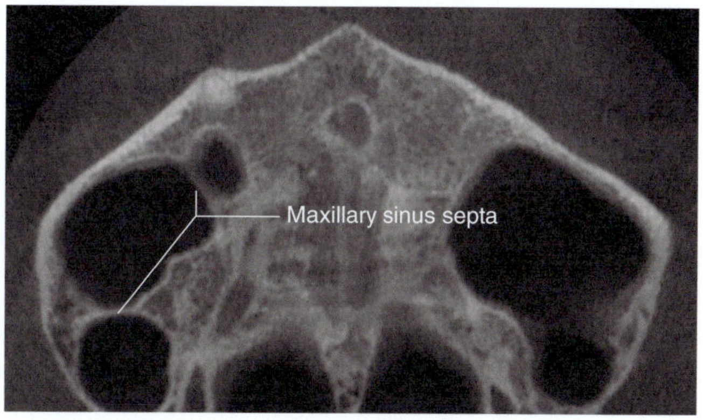

Fig. 3.15 CBCT axial image of maxillary sinus septa

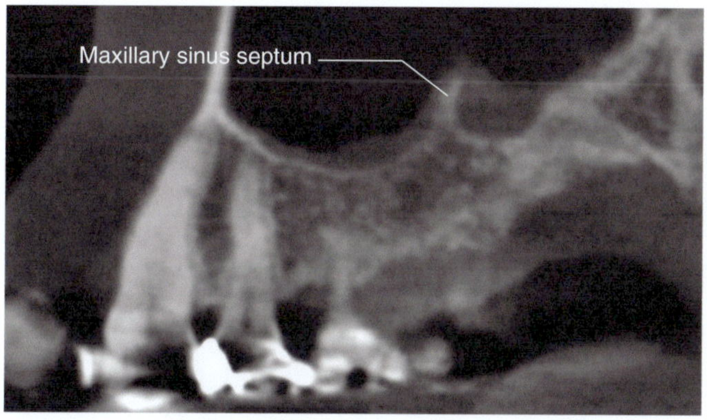

Fig. 3.14 CBCT sagittal image of the maxillary sinus septum

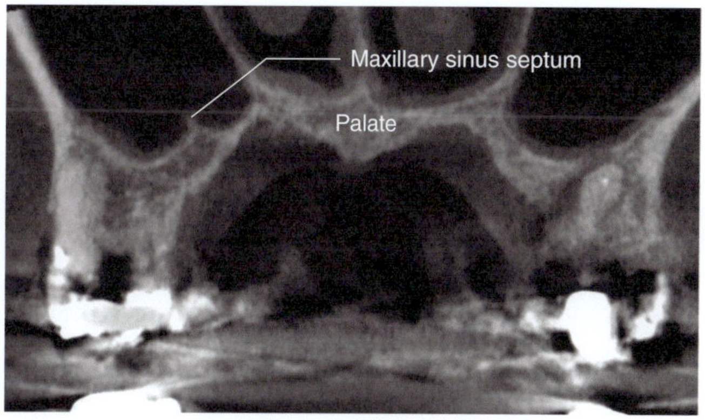

Fig. 3.16 CBCT coronal image of the maxillary sinus septum

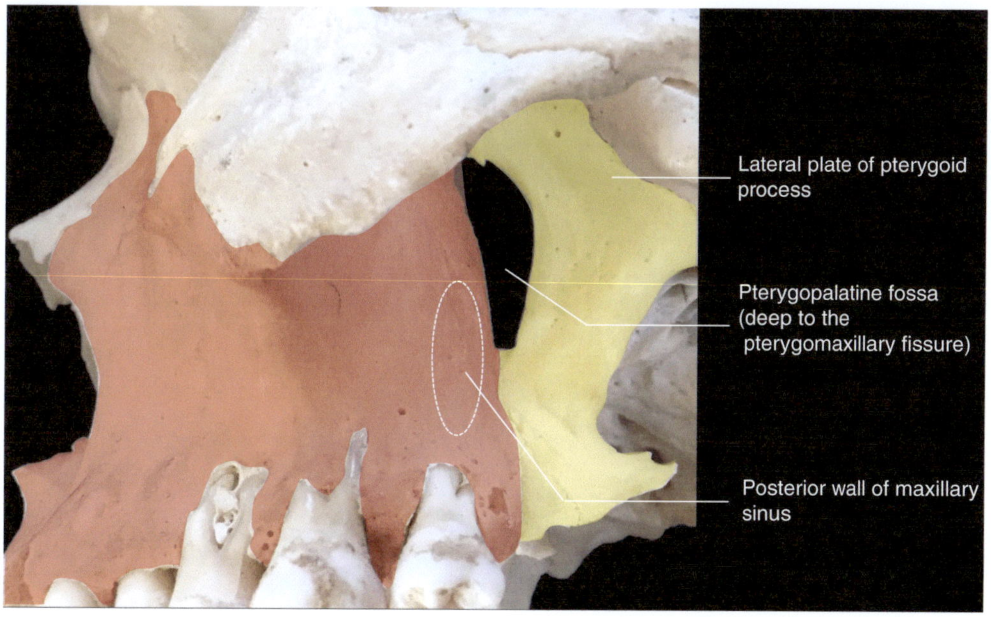

Fig. 3.17 Lateral view of the skull. The posterior superior alveolar nerve/vessels enter the posterior wall of the maxillary sinus (circle). Note that the pterygopalatine fossa deep to the pterygomaxillary fissure is formed between the posterior wall of the maxillary sinus and lateral plate of the pterygoid process of the sphenoid

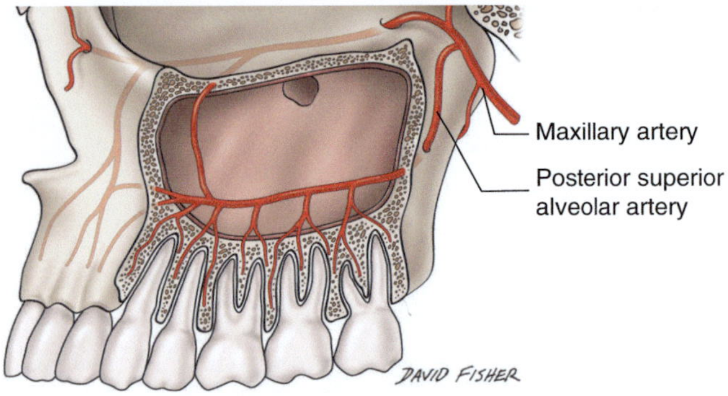

Fig. 3.18 Schematic drawing of the arterial supply of the maxilla. The posterior superior alveolar artery arises from the maxillary artery within and around the pterygopalatine fossa. It forms an arterial plexus with the anterior and middle superior alveolar arteries to supply the maxillary sinus and upper teeth. © Fisher/Tubbs 2020. All Rights Reserved

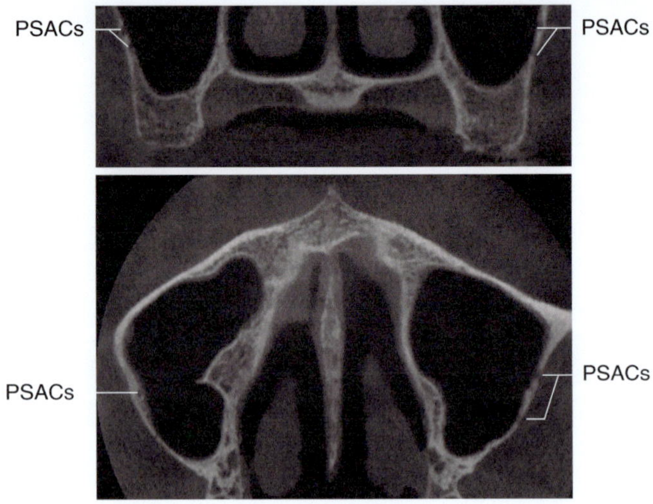

Fig. 3.20 Although reports in the literature on implant dentistry have referred to these canals as posterior superior alveolar arteries and have performed morphometric analysis such as the diameter and length of the "arteries," the only structures seen in the CT/CBCT images are bony canals or grooves, not the vessels or nerves. Here, we only refer to these structures as posterior superior alveolar canals (PSACs) in CBCT images

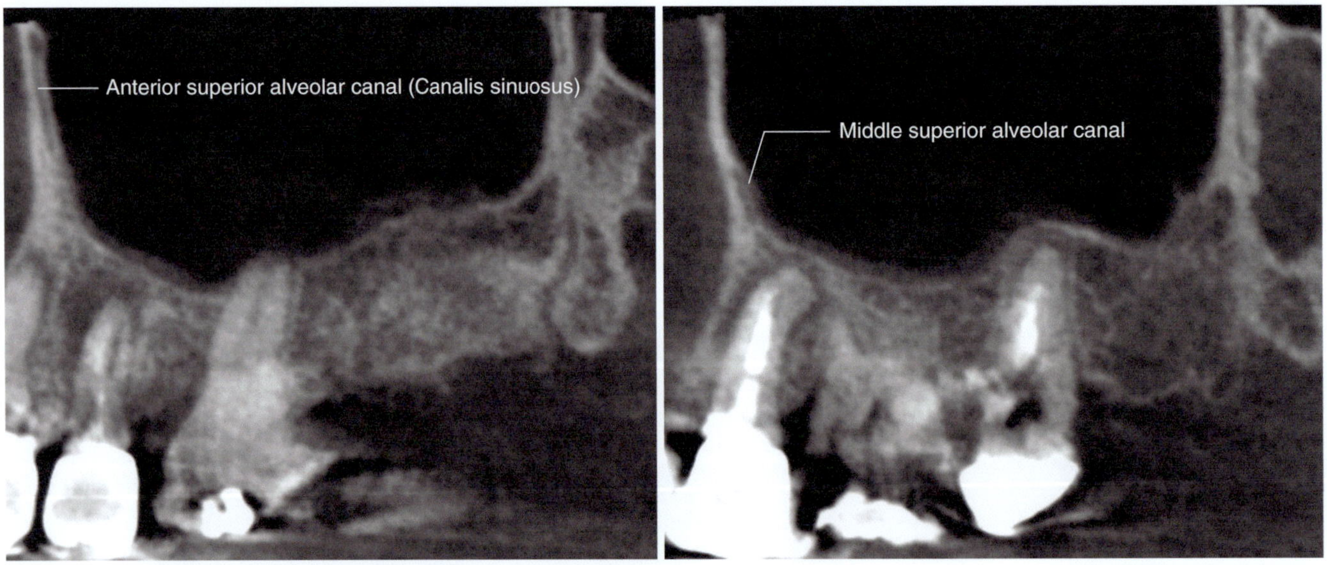

Fig. 3.19 Anterior and middle superior alveolar canals run within the anterior and lateral walls of the maxillary sinus, respectively

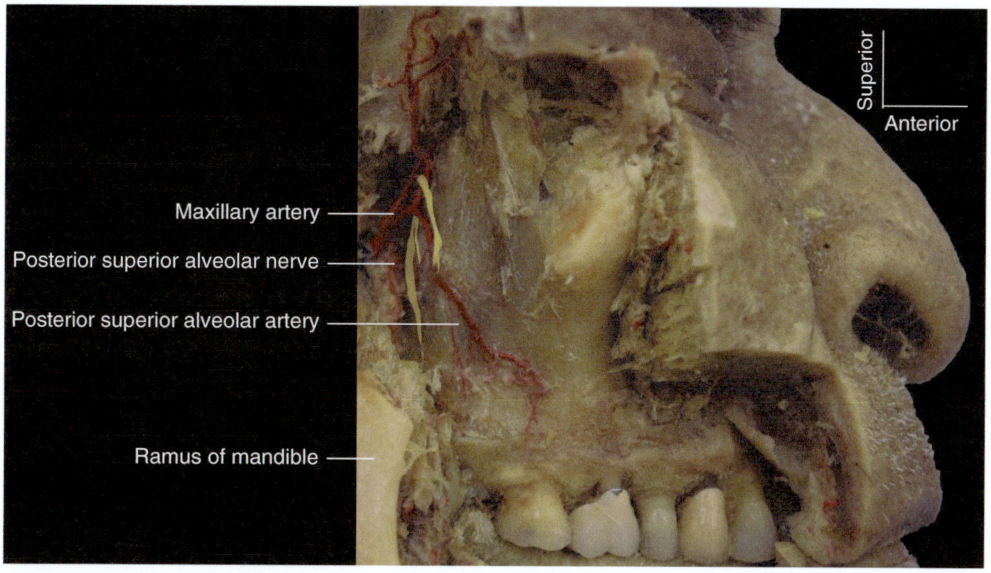

Fig. 3.21 Lateral cadaveric dissection of the face. Note that all of the soft tissues except the posterior superior alveolar artery and nerve (PSAA/PSAN) on the right lateral face have been removed to see the relationship between the PSAA/PSAN and bone. The PSAA arises from the maxillary artery and gives rise to multiple branches. The PSAN leaves the maxillary nerve (not shown here) in the pterygopalatine fossa

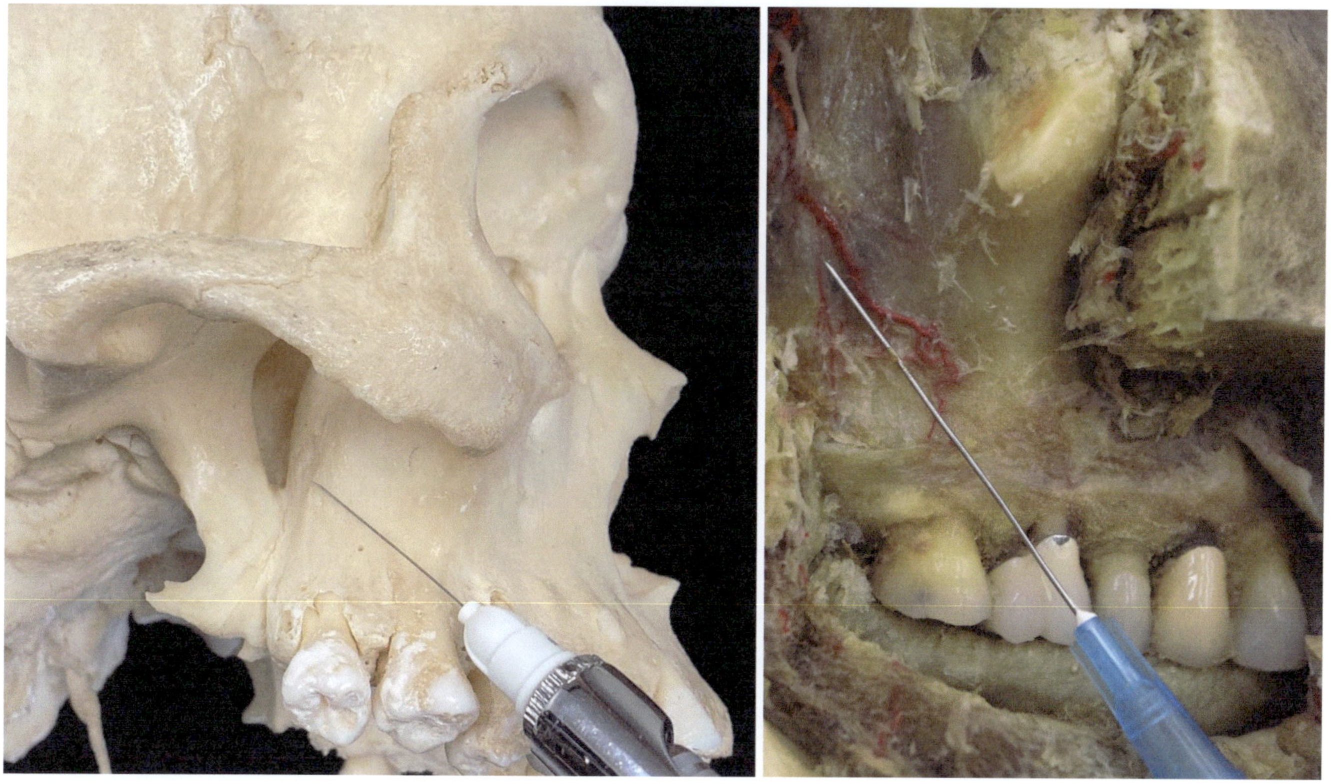

Fig. 3.22 Cadaveric demonstration of posterior superior alveolar nerve blockade. Blockade of the posterior superior alveolar nerve can damage the posterior superior alveolar artery due to its close relationship (right image)

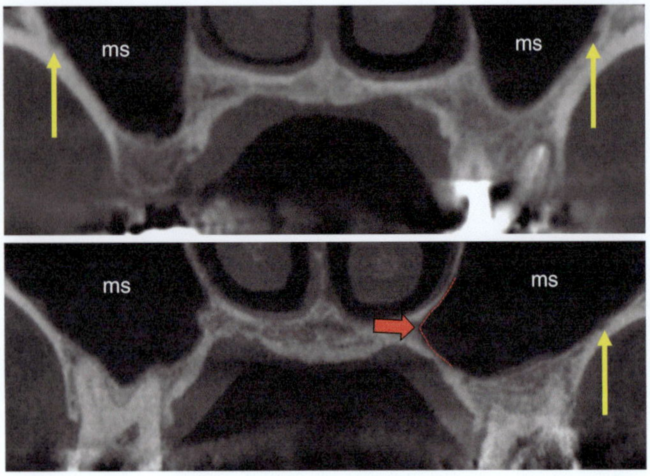

Fig. 3.23 Coronal CT image of the maxillary sinus. The intraosseus course of the posterior superior alveolar canals are shown (yellow arrows). Various studies reported that an intraosseus course, within the maxillary sinus, and a superficial course (external cortex) are seen in 47–71%, 13–47%, and 5–6%, respectively (Tehranchi et al. 2017; Chitsazi et al. 2017; Pandharbale et al. 2016; Danesh-sani et al. 2017). The red arrow indicates the concavity where periosteal elevation could be challenging during sinus lift due to its depth and angle

3.4 Mental Area

Summary

The mental area is often incised during oral surgery. The mental nerve and vessels pass through the mental foramen. In dentistry, some dentists believe that "touching the mental foramen" means results in paresthesia although this might be an exaggeration. However, as a terminal branch of V3, the mental nerve supplies the skin of the lower lip and chin areas, which are very sensitive. Therefore, even minimal damage to the mental nerve can potentially cause discomfort and affect a patients' quality of life. Except resection of malignant tumors or other large pathology of the mandible such as ameloblastoma, the mental nerve should be preserved, e.g., dental implant surgery, tooth removal, apicoectomy, and mandibular fracture surgery. Therefore, anatomical knowledge of this area should include not only the mental foramen but also the accessory mental foramen which could be overlooked on computed tomography if the interpreter is not familiar with this variation.

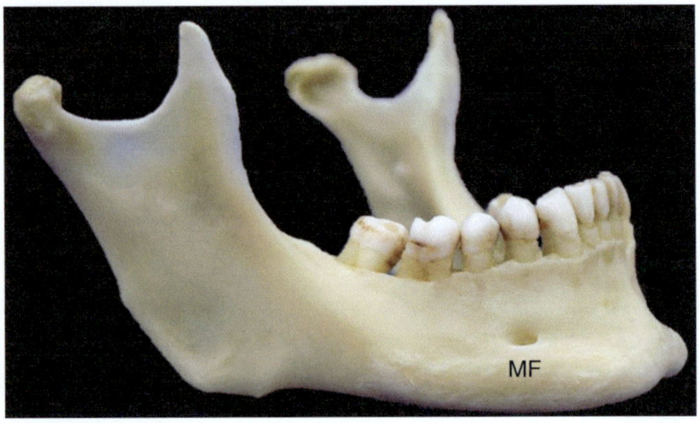

Fig. 3.24 In a dentulous mandible, the mental foramen (MF) is usually located in the middle of the mandibular body (between the alveolar ridge and inferior to the border of the mandible). In most cases, the MF is positioned below the second premolar or between the first and second premolars and opens posterosuperiorly and this is the so-called "anterior loop" of the mandibular canal

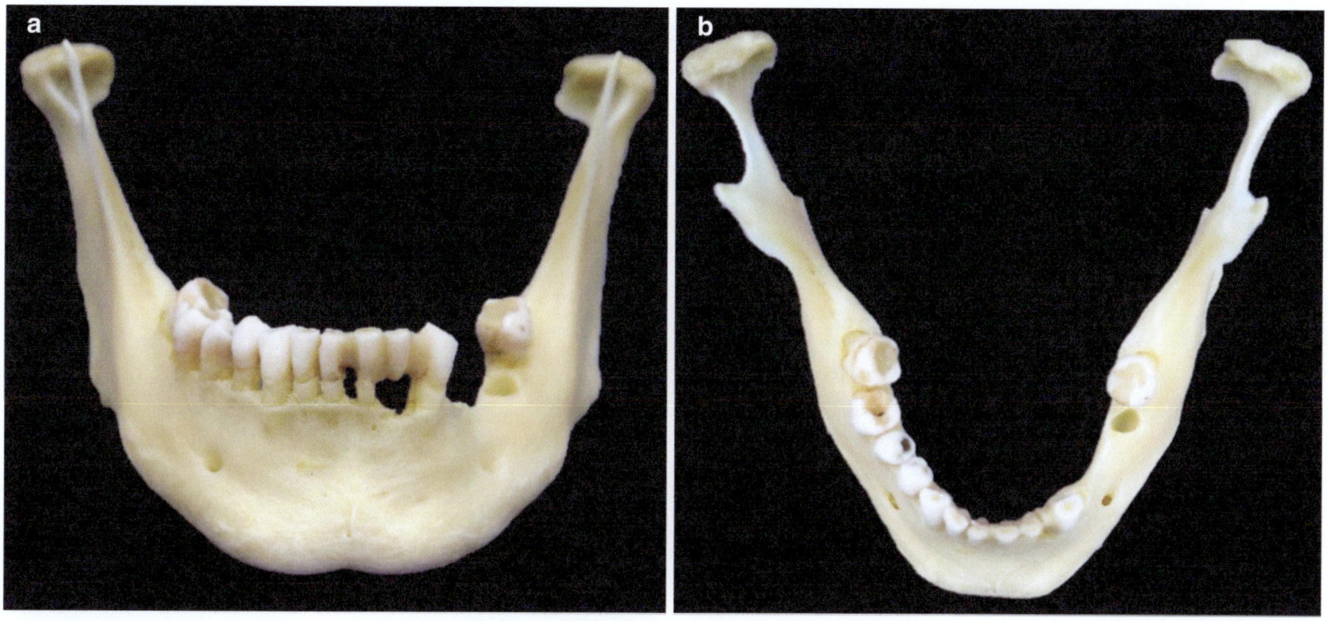

Fig. 3.25 Dentulous mandible. (**a**) anterior view; (**b**) superior view

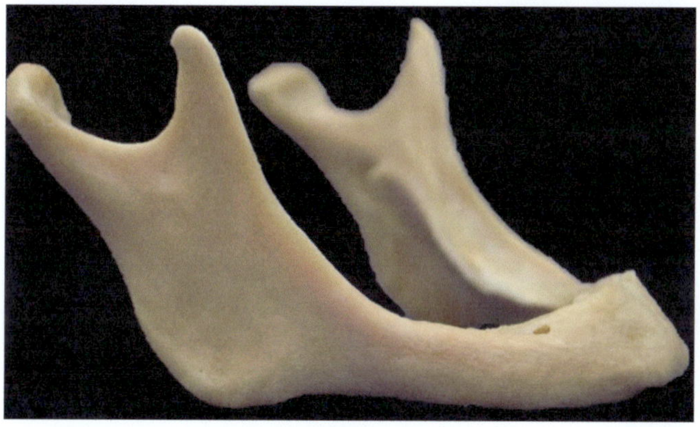

Fig. 3.26 In an edentulous mandible, especially a severely reduced mandible, the mental foramen is located on the superior surface of the mandibular body. Lateral view

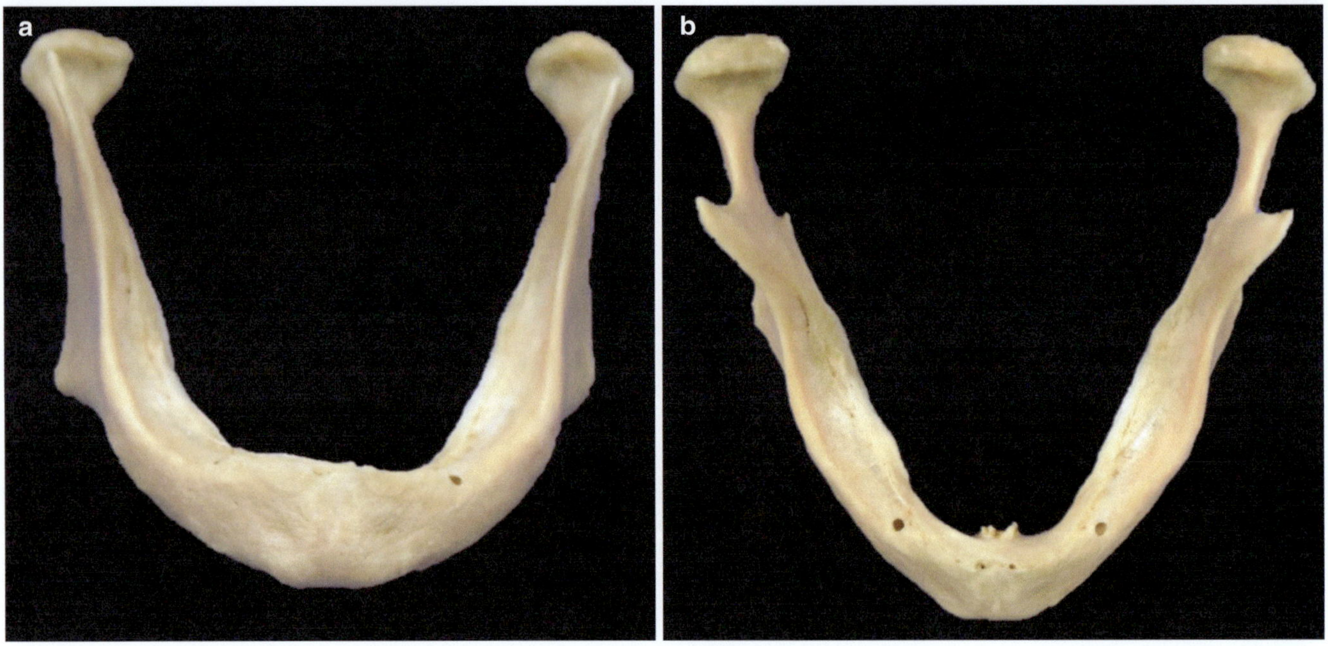

Fig. 3.27 Edentulous mandible. (**a**) Anterior view; (**b**) superior view

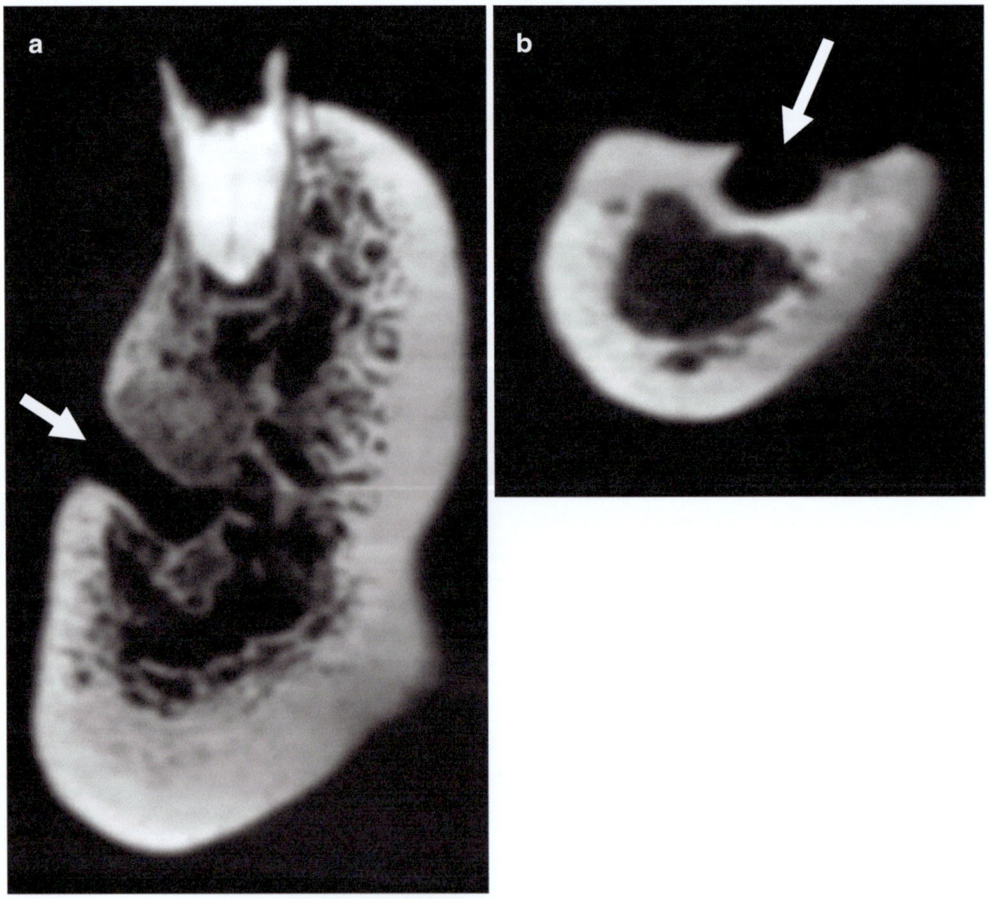

Fig. 3.28 Mental foramina (arrows) on coronal cone-beam computed tomography images. (**a**) dentulous; (**b**) edentulous

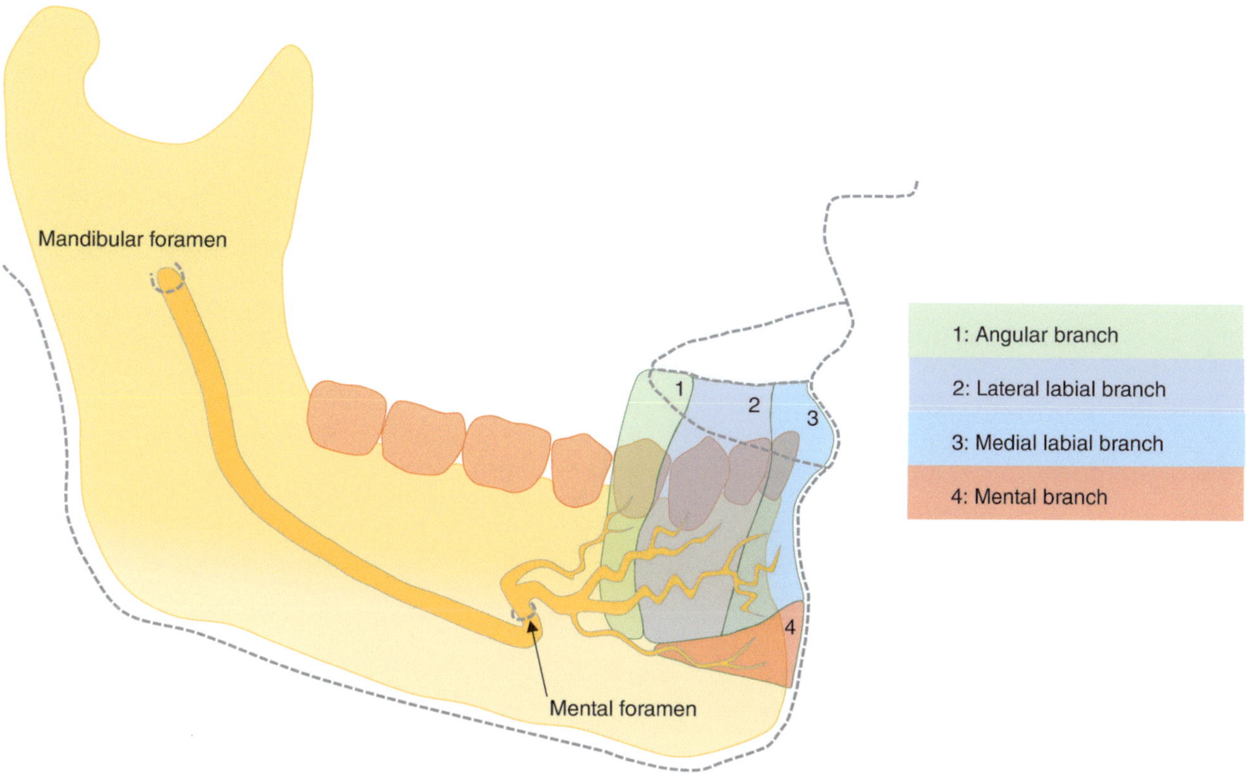

Fig. 3.29 Distribution of the mental nerve. The mental nerve arises from the mental foramen and divides into 3–4 branches. It supplies the angle, lower lip, mental area, and buccal (labial) gingiva and mucosa of from the incisors to the premolar area

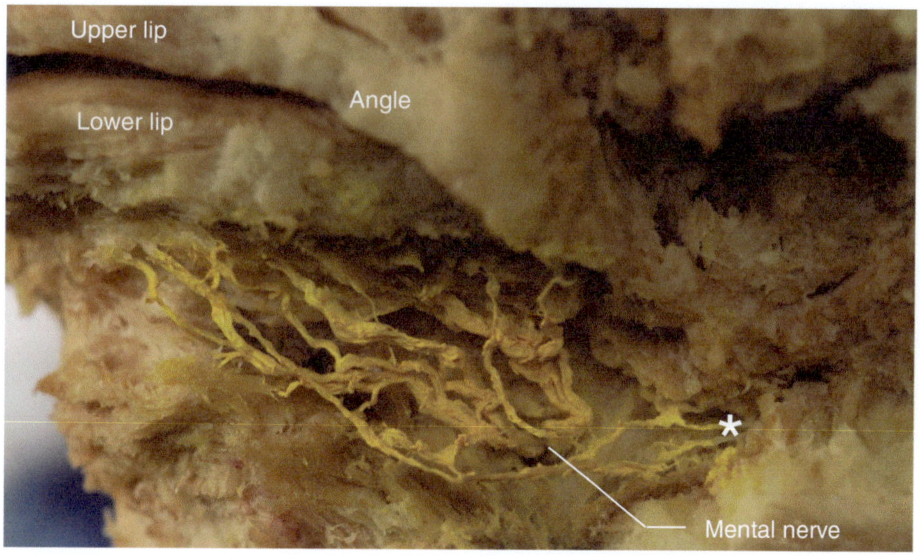

Fig. 3.30 The mental nerve arising from the mental foramen (left side). It innervates the lower lip, angle of the mouth, and mental area. Note the posterior branch (*) communicates with the marginal mandibular branch of CN VII

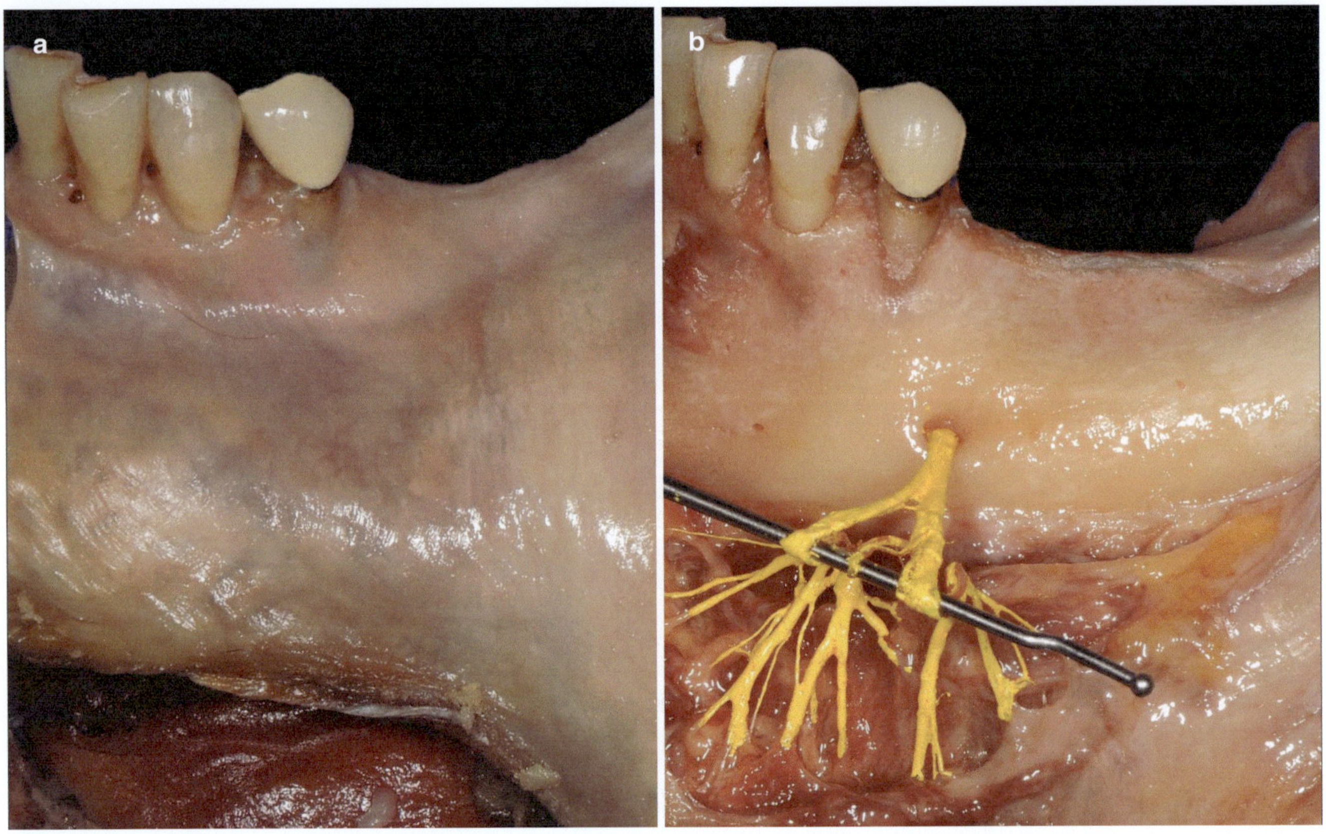

Fig. 3.31 Buccal mucosa in the premolar area and the mental nerve (left mandible). (**a**) Before dissection; (**b**) after dissection

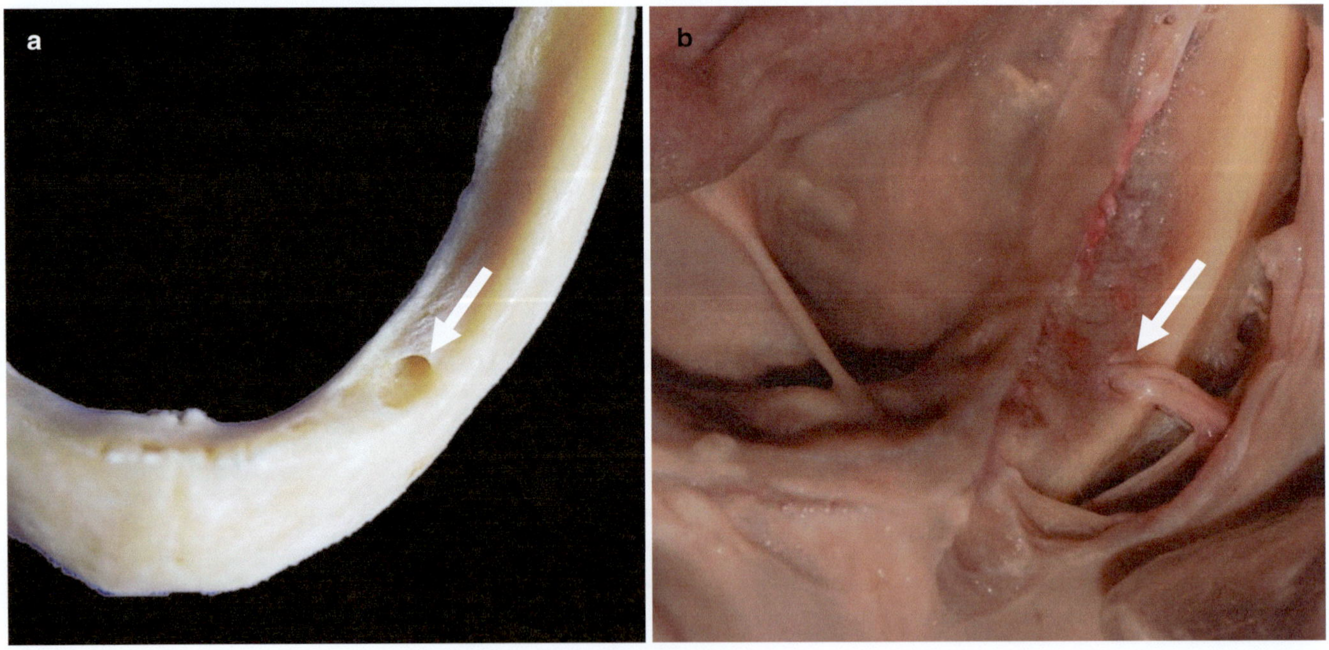

Fig. 3.32 Mental foramen located on the superior surface of the bone and mental nerve in an edentulous mandible (left mandible). (**a**) Dry mandible; (**b**) cadaveric dissection

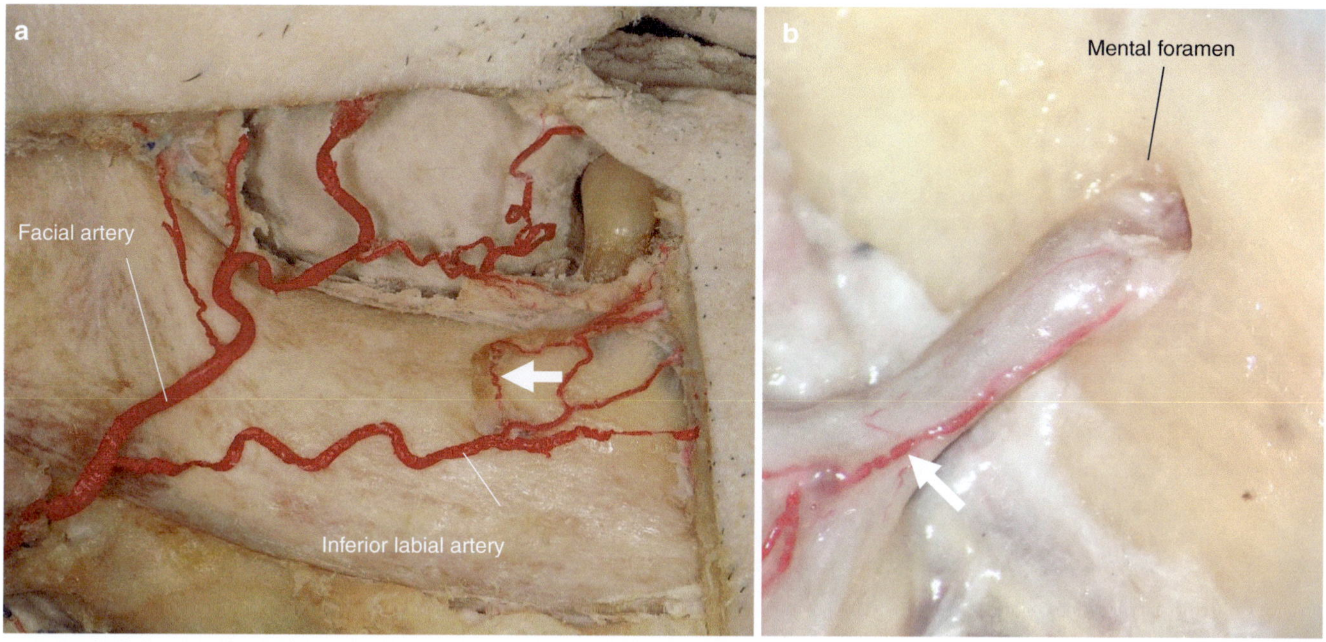

Fig. 3.33 Mental artery (arrows) running along with mental nerve. Its diameter is very small compared to the mental nerve. The mental artery usually anastomoses with branches of the submental and/or inferior labial artery (Kikuta et al. 2020). (**a**) Right mandible; (**b**) magnified picture

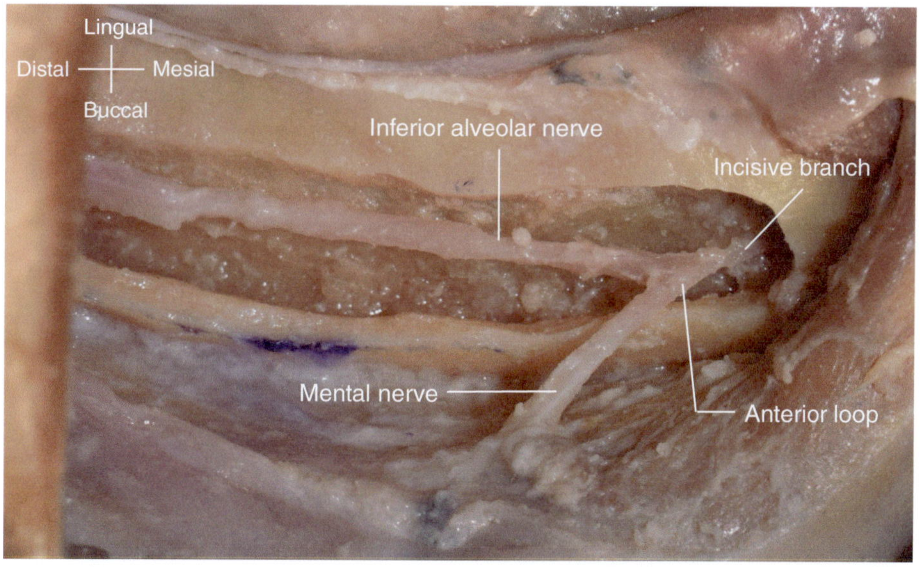

Fig. 3.34 The main trunk of inferior alveolar nerve turns posterosuperiorly to form an "anterior loop" and emerge from the mental foramen (superior view of right mandible). It is reported that anterior loop is observed in 28–94%. The longest loop was 11 mm reported by Neiva et al. (2004)

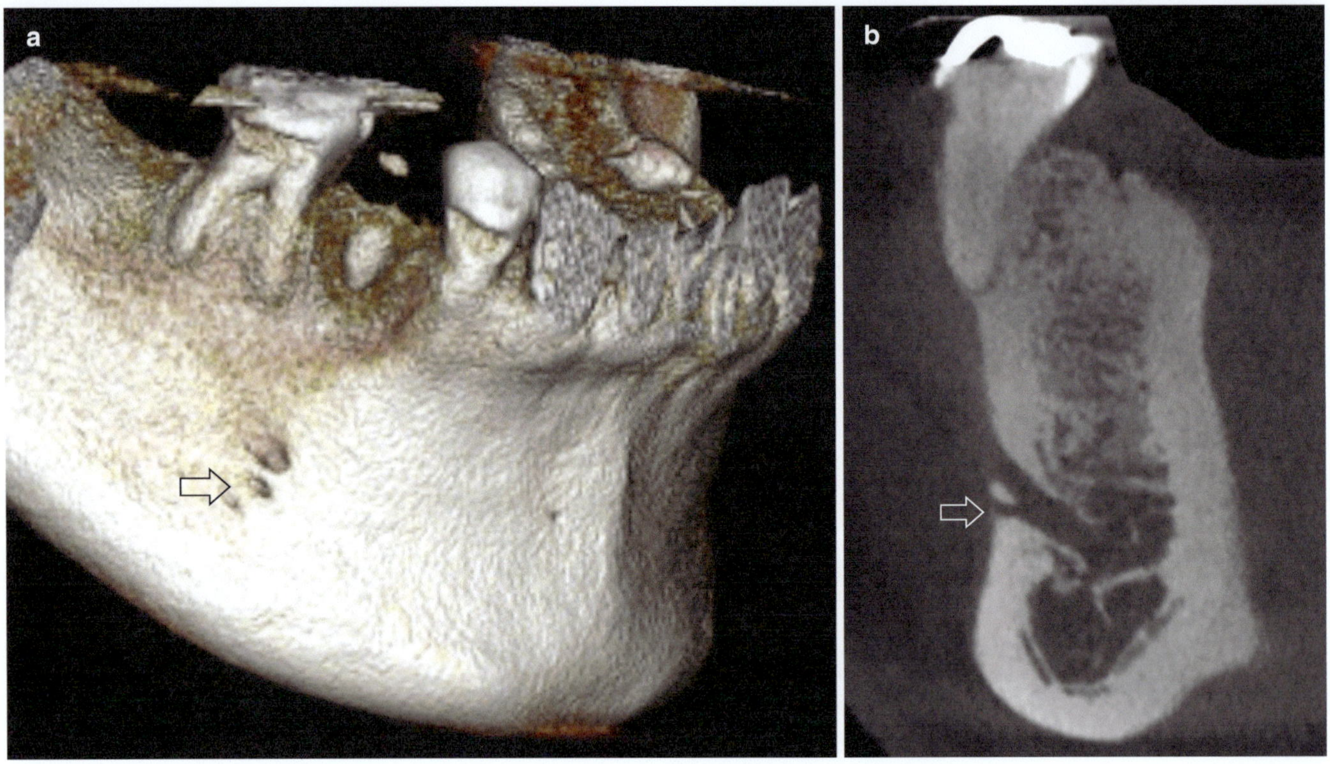

Fig. 3.35 Accessory mental foramina (AMFs, arrows). AMF is defined as a foramen located around but smaller than the mental foramen (MF) and displaying continuity with the mandibular canal by computed tomography (Naitoh et al. 2009a; Iwanaga et al. 2016). Accessory mental nerves and/or arteries travel through the AMF (Iwanaga et al. 2015). (**a**) Three-dimensionally reconstracted CT image; (**b**) Coronal CT image

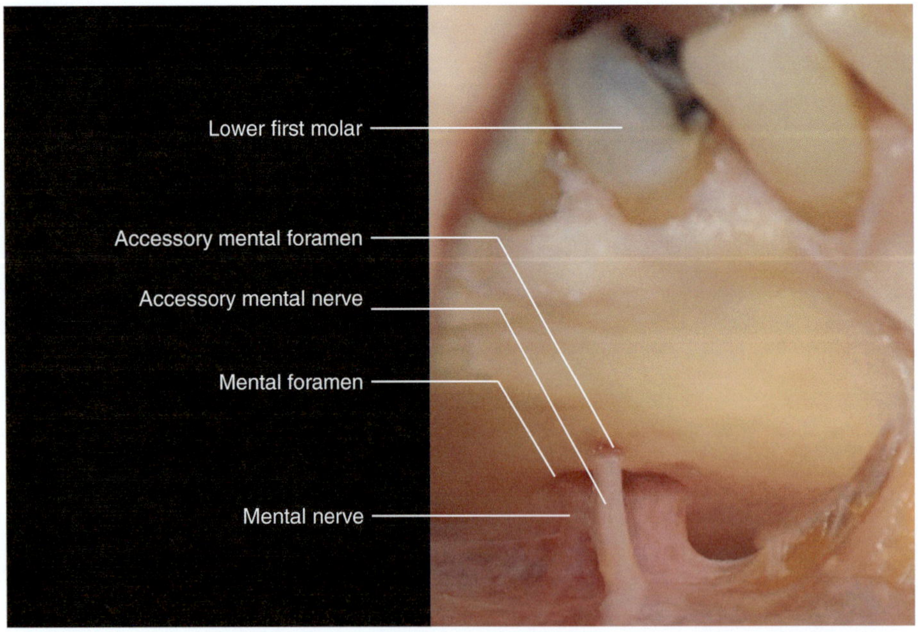

Fig. 3.36 Accessory mental nerve (AMN) arising from an accessory mental foramen (AMF) (right side). Large AMF tends to open near the mental foramen. Injury of AMF/AMN could lead to neurosensory disturbance of the lower lip/mental area. The area of numbness might depend on the foramen size and degree of injury (Iwanaga et al. 2016)

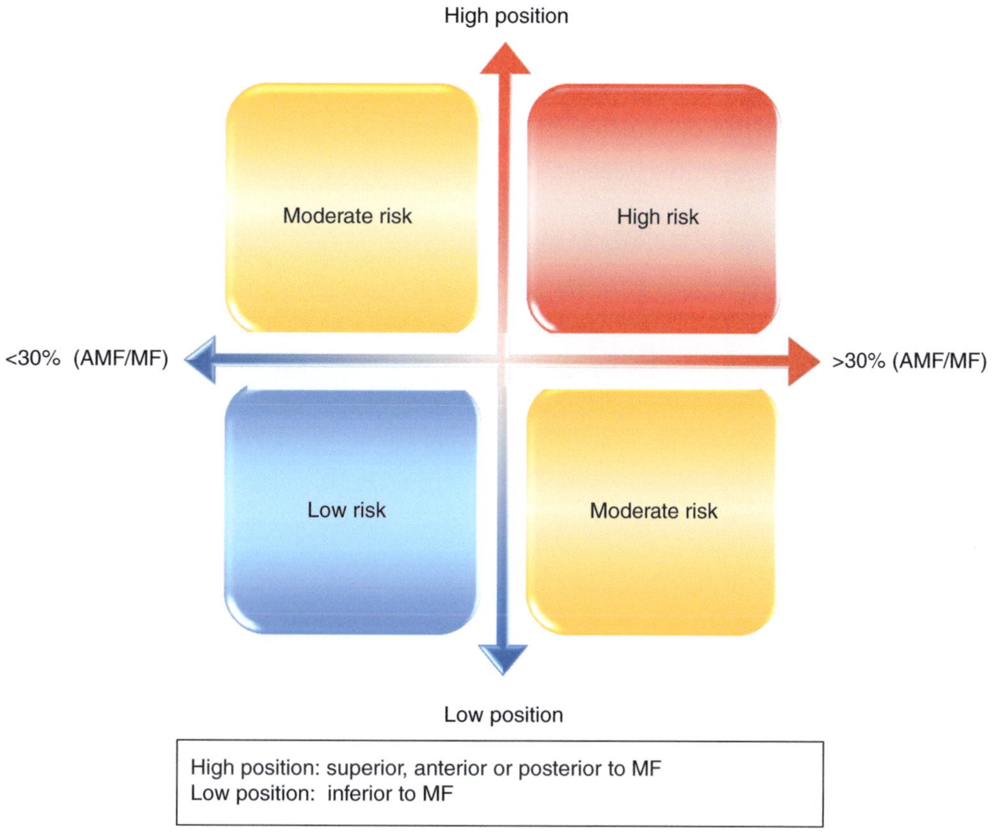

Fig. 3.37 A high-positioned AMF is more likely to be damaged and a large size AMF is more likely to cause neurosensory disturbance when damaged (Iwanaga et al. 2019a, 2019b)

3.5 Mandibular Canal

Summary
The mandibular canal is a bony canal coursing inside the mandible and it carries the inferior alveolar nerve and vessels. The mandibular foramen is the entrance of the canal with the lingula being located anteromedially and the ramus of the mandible laterally. The main component of the canal is the inferior alveolar nerve which is more than twice as large as the vessels. The structure of the superior wall of the mandibular canal can change with tooth loss. When teeth are present, the majority of the superior wall shows a trabecular or osteoporotic pattern, however, with tooth absence, a smooth-type wall is seen. After entering the mandibular foramen, the mandibular canal runs anteroinferiorly and gradually approaches the lingual cortical plate. When it reaches below the first molar, the canal becomes closest to the lingual plate and then suddenly changes its angle buccally and courses toward the mental foramen with/without an anterior loop. Anatomical variations of the mandibular canal will also be demonstrated.

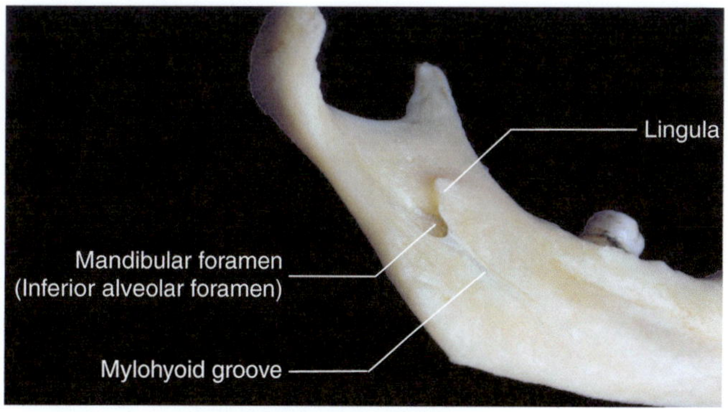

Fig. 3.38 The mandibular foramen, the entrance of the mandibular canal, is located almost at the center of the medial aspect of the ramus of the mandible. The lingula is a small tubercle/spine to which the sphenomandibular ligament attaches

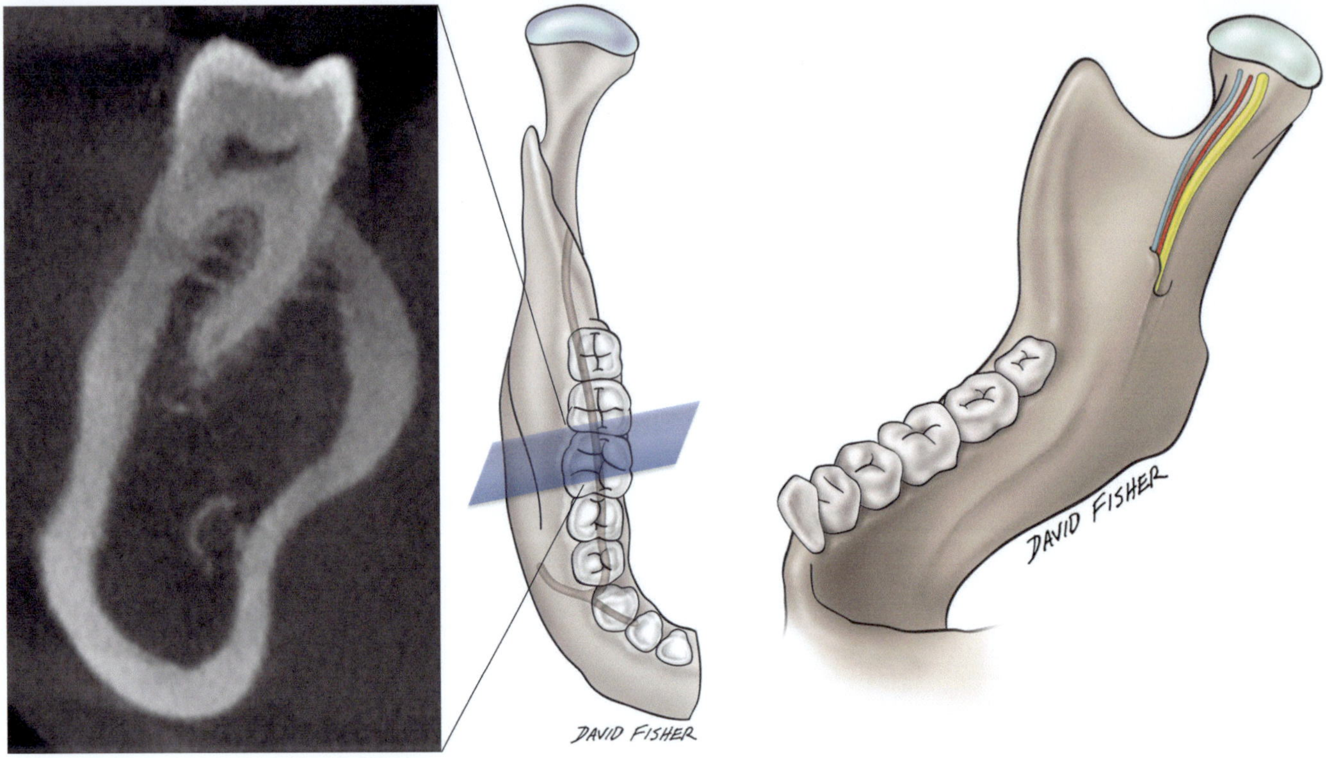

Fig. 3.39 The mandibular canal contains the inferior alveolar nerve/vessels. Entering the mandibular foramen, the mandibular canal runs anteroinferiorly and slightly medially to approach the lingual cortical plate. Below the first molar, the canal becomes closest to the lingual plate and then suddenly changes its angle buccally and courses toward the mental foramen with/without an anterior loop (Yu et al. 2016).

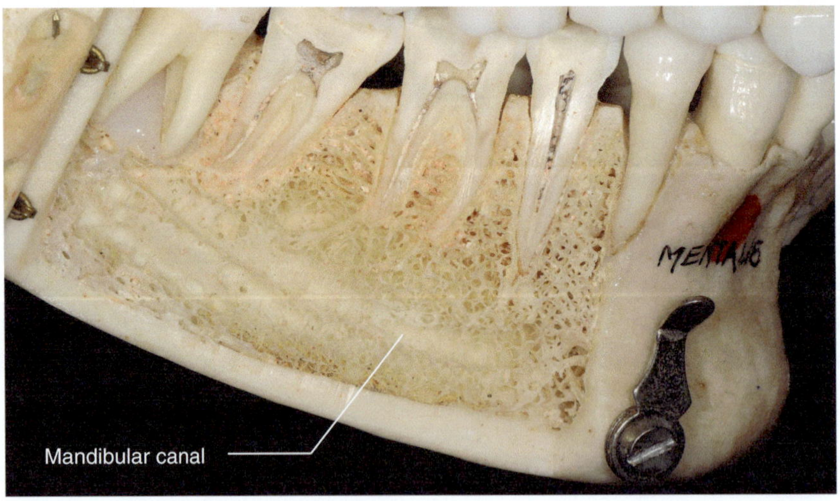

Fig. 3.40 Lateral view of the mandibular canal (right side). The mandibular canal courses inside the mandible. The inferior alveolar nerve/vessels give rise to branches to the retromolar area and molar and premolar teeth. The anterior teeth (central and lateral incisors) are supplied by incisive branches that leave the main trunk of the nerve

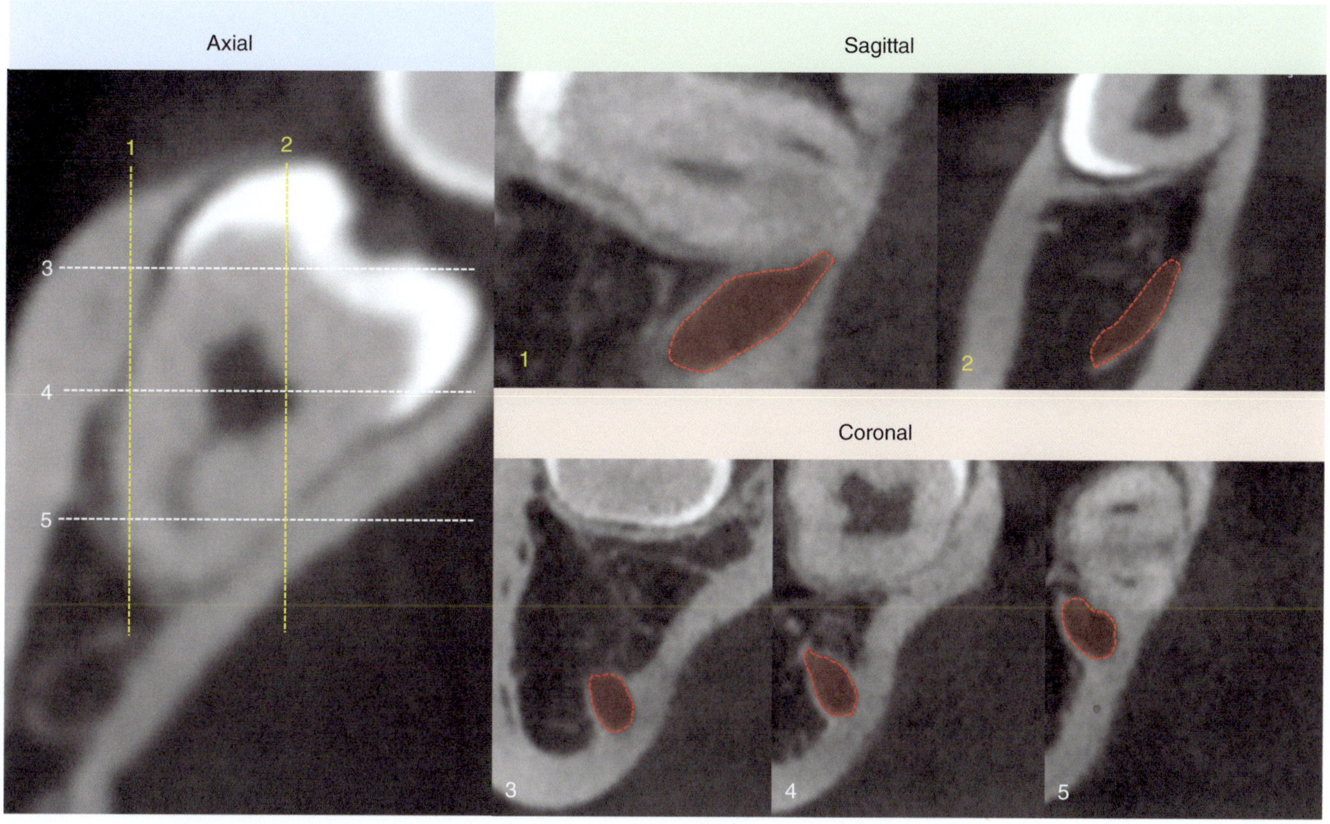

Fig. 3.41 Relationship between the root of the lower third molar and the mandibular canal (red dashed circles) in CBCT

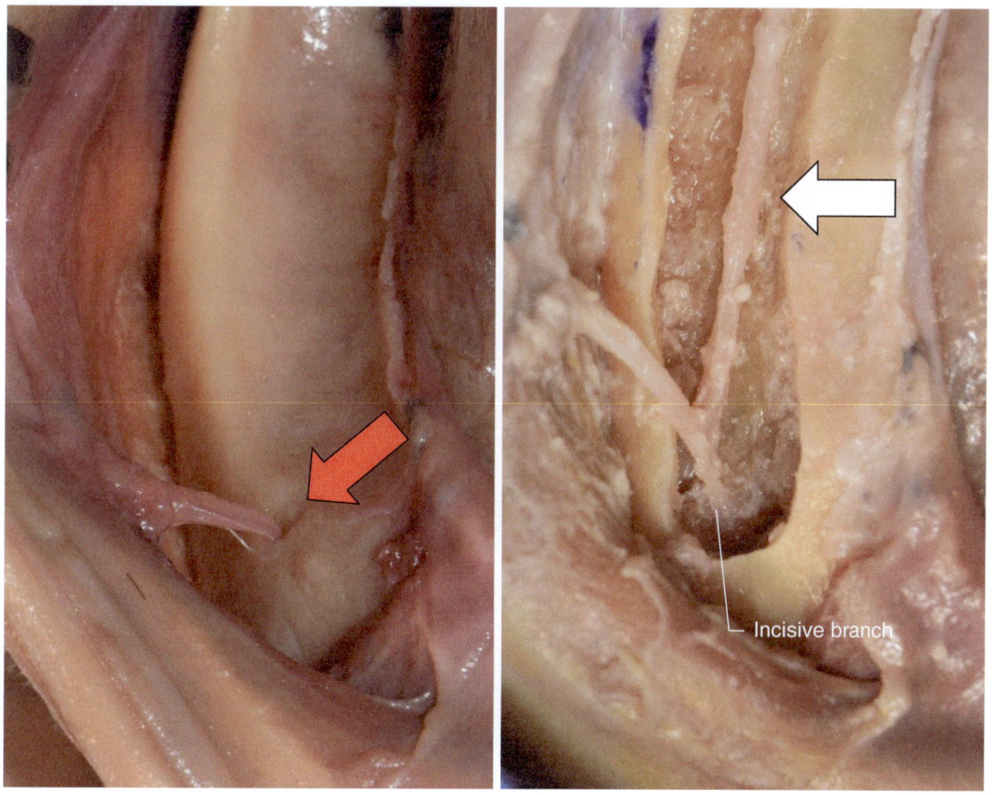

Fig. 3.42 Superior view of the mandibular canal and the anterior loop of the right mandible. The mental neurovascular bundles emerge from the mental foramen (red arrow in the left photo). The wall of the mandible is removed in the right photo to show the inferior alveolar neurovascular bundle (white arrow)

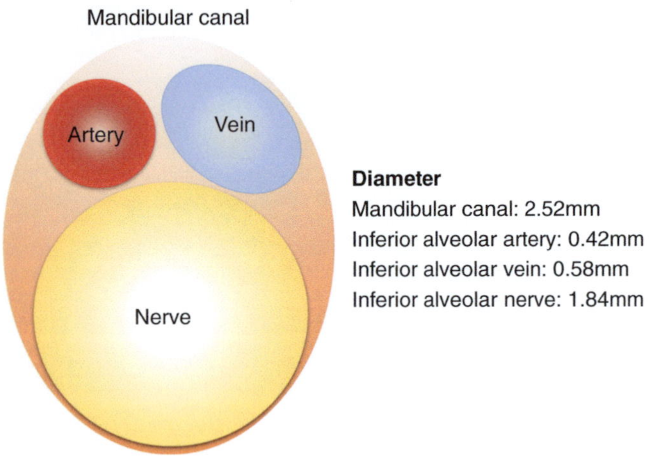

Fig. 3.43 Contents in the mandibular canal. The inferior alveolar nerve is usually the largest structure in the canal. Although the majority of the canal accommodates the nerve below the artery and vein, various positions in the canal have been reported (Kilic et al. 2010; Matani et al. 2014)

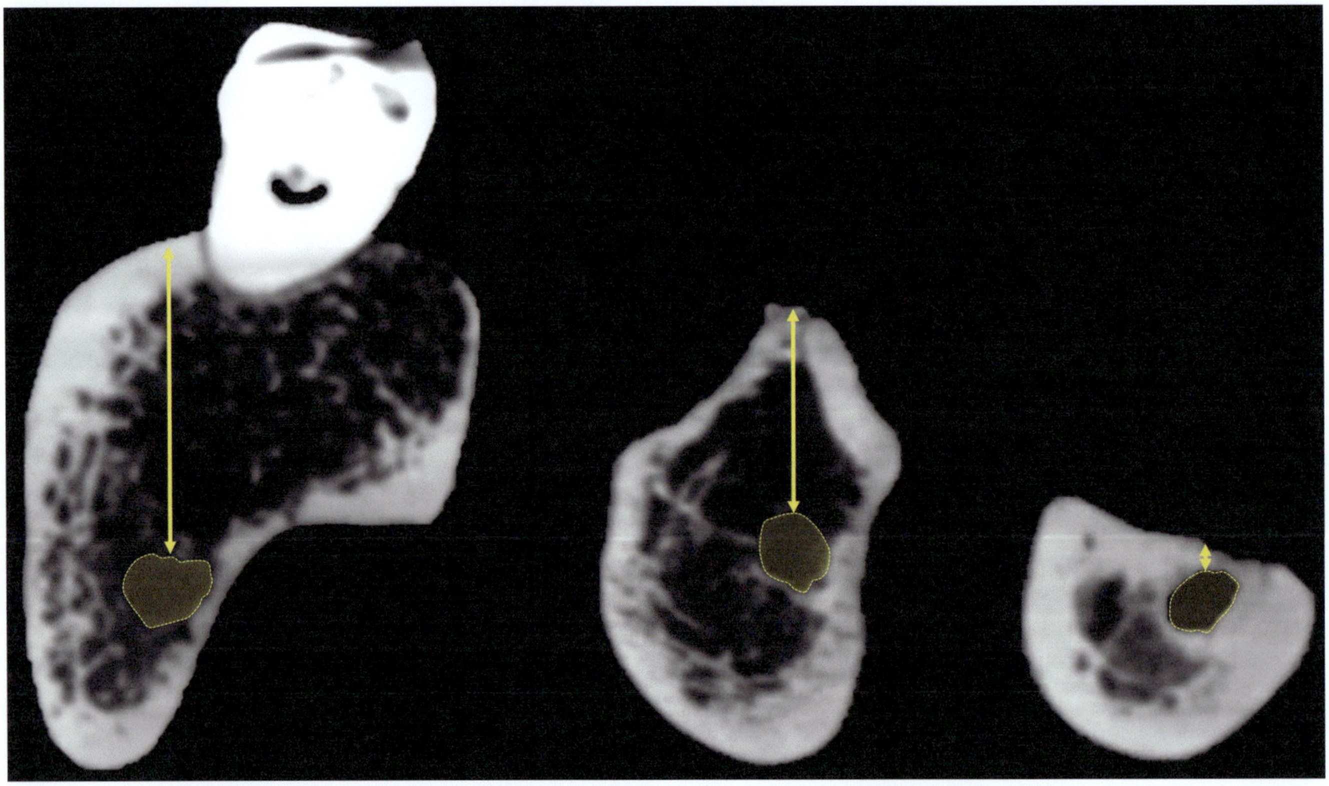

Fig. 3.44 Coronal CBCT images of different mandibles. The distance from the alveolar ridge to the mandibular canal decreases with tooth loss. This is extremely important when planning dental implant surgery. Also, complete/partial dentures can cause nerve compression when bony resorption is severe

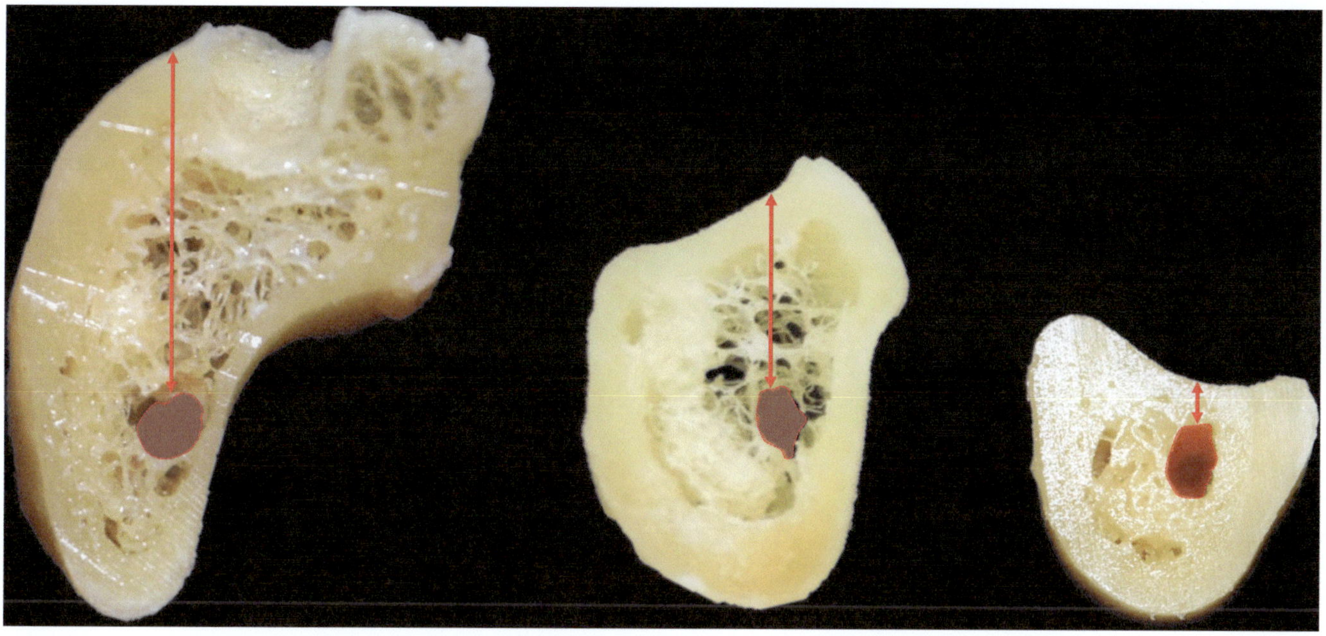

Fig. 3.45 Cadaveric coronal slices through different mandibles (same specimens as the CBCT images in Fig. 3.44). The distance from the alveolar ridge to the mandibular canal decreases with tooth loss. This fact is extremely important when planning dental implant surgery. Also complete/partial dentures can cause nerve compression when bony resorption is severe

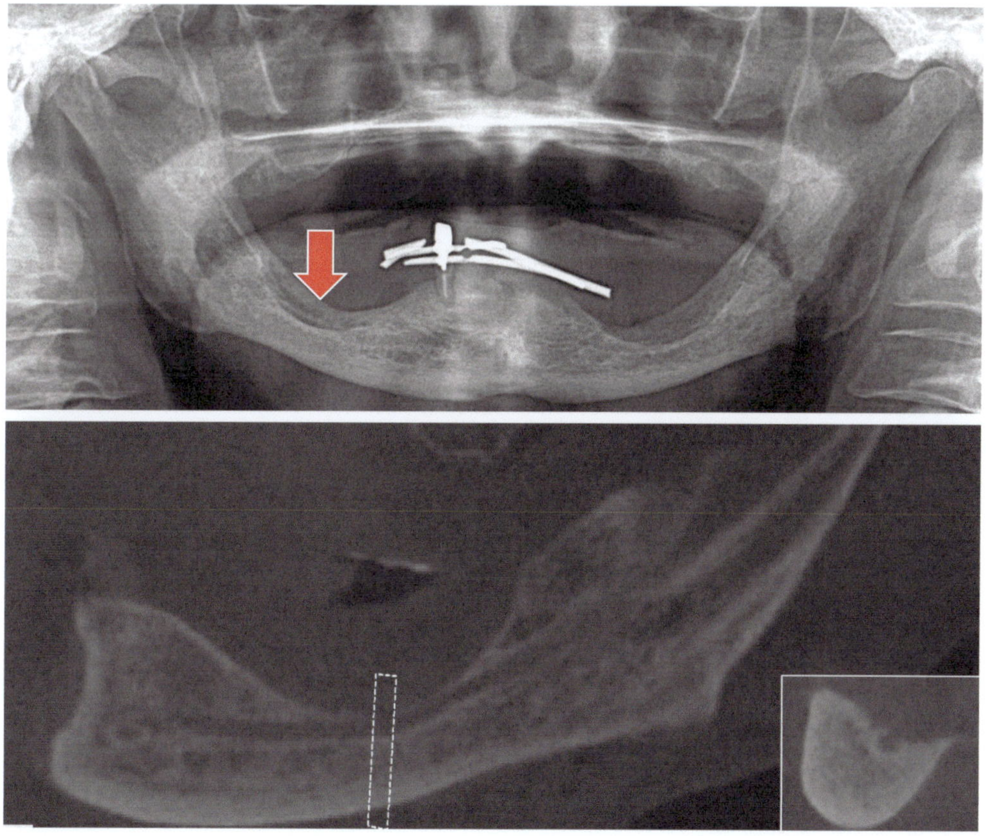

Fig. 3.46 A case of a severely resorbed mandible in a patient using a partial denture. The patient presented with severe pain in the right chin area when chewing (Courtesy of Dr. Keisuke Noridomi)

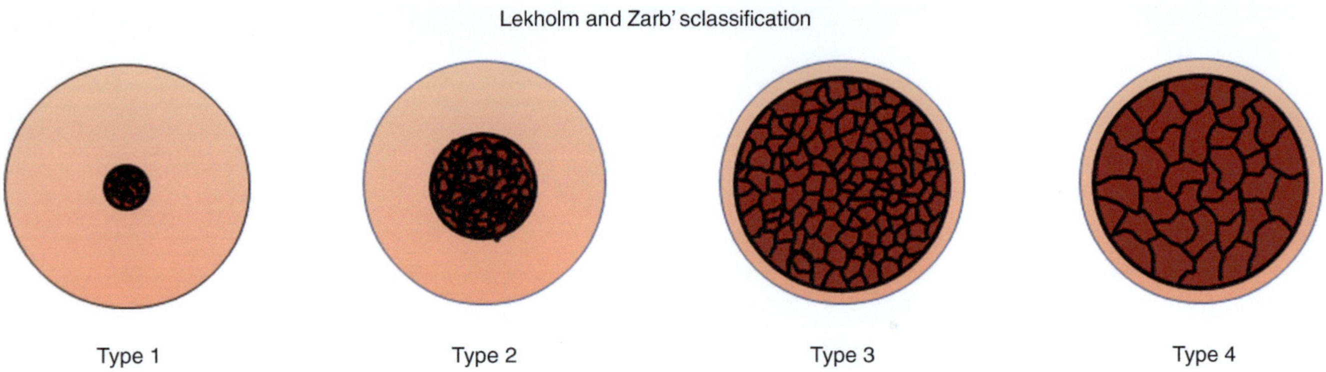

Fig. 3.47 Lekholm and Zarb's bone density classification for dental implants (Lekholm and Zarb 1985)

	Type 1	Type 2	Type 3	Type 4
Type of bone	Homogeneous cortical bone	Thick cortical bone with marrow cavity	Thin cortical bone with dense trabecular bone of good strength	Very thin cortical bone with low density trabecular bone of poor wtrength

Fig. 3.48 Lekholm and Zarb's bone density classification for dental implants (Lekholm and Zarb 1985). This classification is originally based on plain radiography and morphology

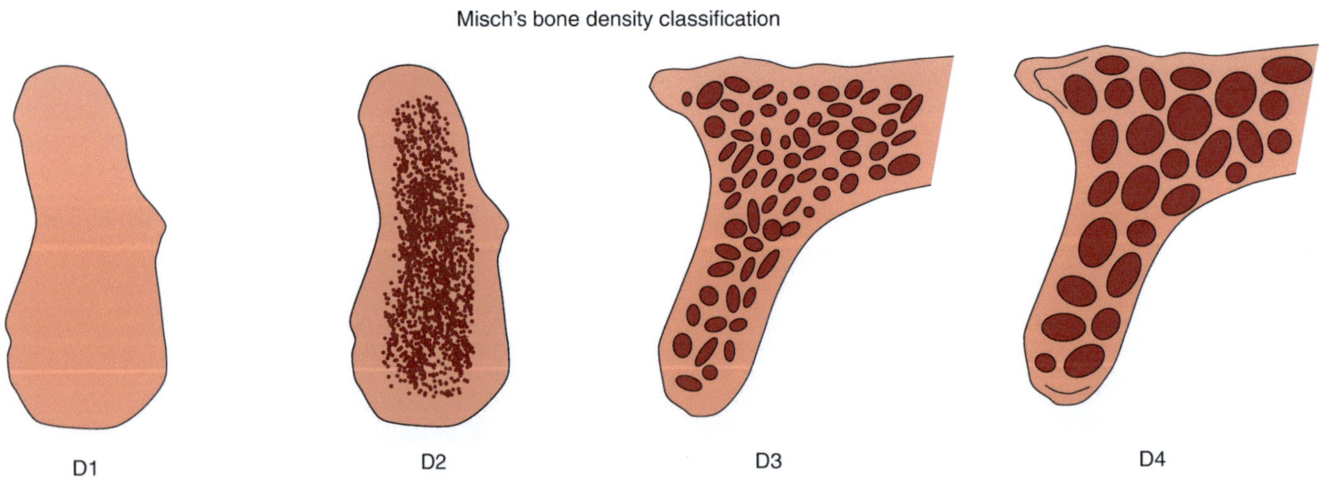

Fig. 3.49 Schema of Misch's bone density classification for dental implants (Misch 1988)

	D1	D2	D3	D4
Description	Dense cortical	Thick porous cortical and coarse trabecular	Thin porous cortical and fine trabecular	Fine trabecular
Type of bone	Oak-like bone	White pine wood	Balsa wood	Styrofoam
Typical anatomical location	Atrophic anterior mandible	Anterior mandible Posterior mandible Anterior maxilla	Anterior maxilla Posterior maxilla Posterior mandible Osteoplasty D2	Posterior maxilla Osteoplasty D3
Hounsfield units	>1250 HU	850-1250 HU	350-850 HU	150-350 HU

Fig. 3.50 Description of Misch's bone density classification for dental implants (Misch 1988, 1990, 1999). This classification was originally based on only the operator's perception (hand feel resistance). Related Hounsfield units were added later

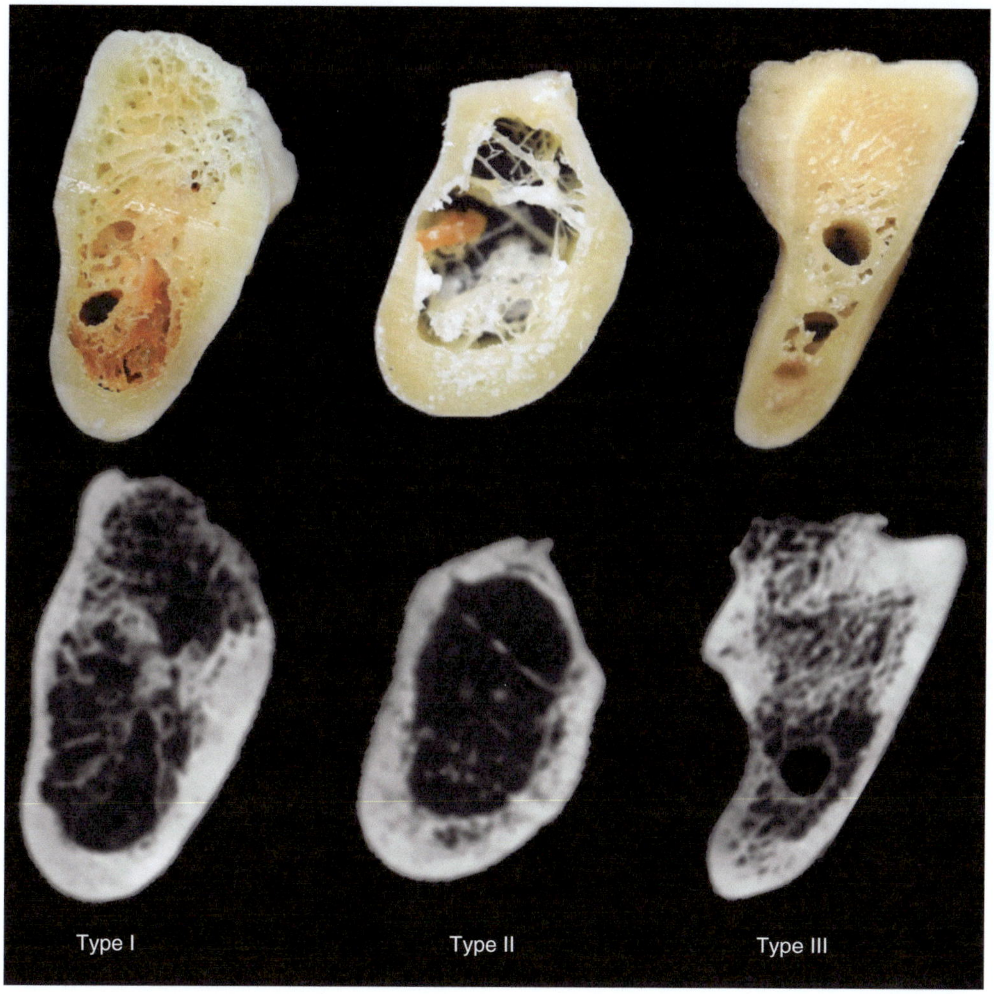

Fig. 3.51 Iwanaga's classification for dental implants (Iwanaga et al. 2019a, 2020a). The cancellous bone pattern of the mandible is classified into three different types based on microscopic and gross anatomical observations: type I, trabecular pattern; type II, osteoporotic; and type III, dense-irregular patterns

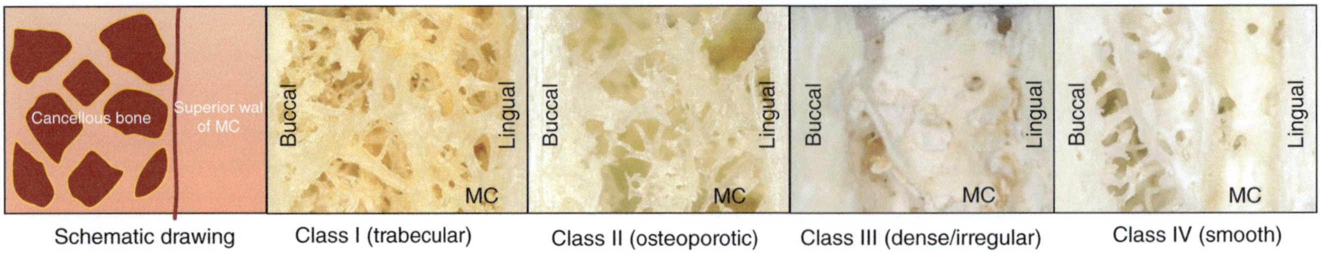

Fig. 3.52 Iwanaga's classification for dental implants (Iwanaga et al. 2019b, 2020b). The superior wall of the mandibular canal is classified into four classes based on microscopic and gross anatomical observations: class I, trabecular pattern; class II, osteoporotic; class III, dense-irregular; and class IV, smooth

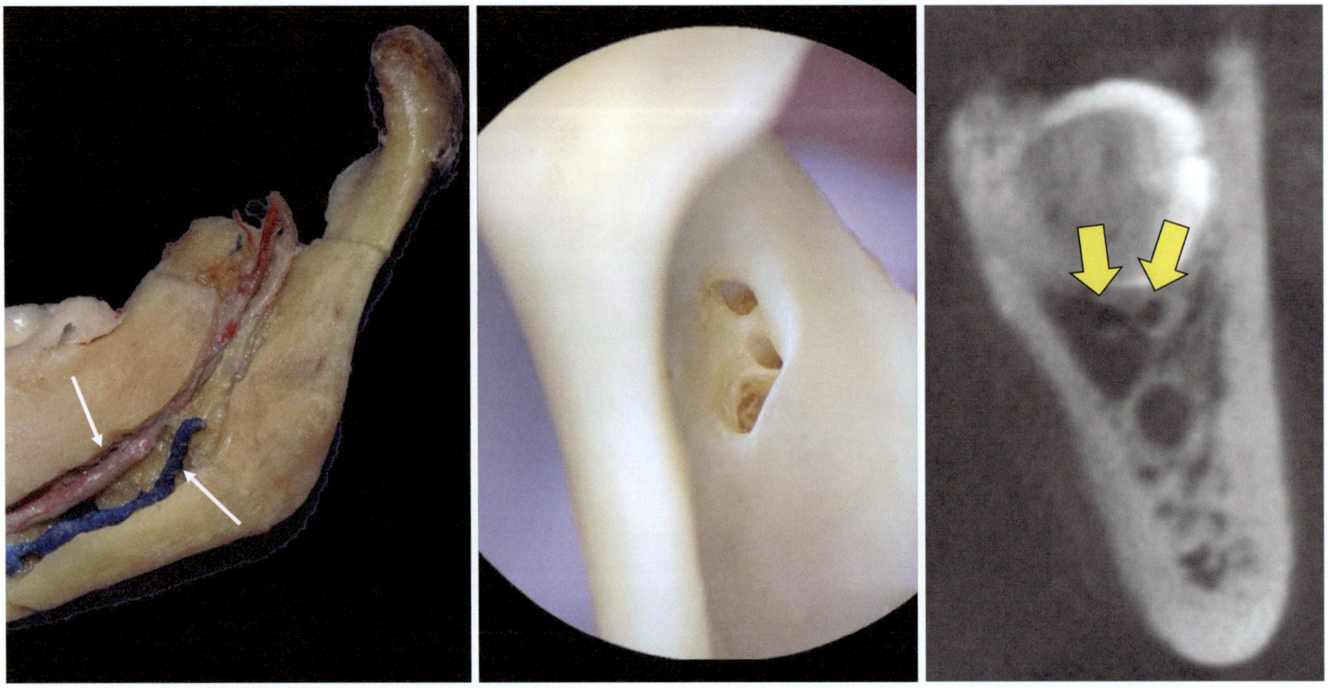

Fig. 3.53 Bifid/trifid mandibular canal. Left cadaveric photo shows a bifid mandibular canal (superior and inferior). The superior mandibular canal includes the nerve and artery and the inferior one the vein. The cadaveric photo in the center focuses on a trifid mandibular canal (posterior view of the mandibular foramen). The right coronal CBCT image shows branches of the mandibular canal (yellow arrows). It can be very confusing to differentiate the branches of the canal and multiple mandibular canals

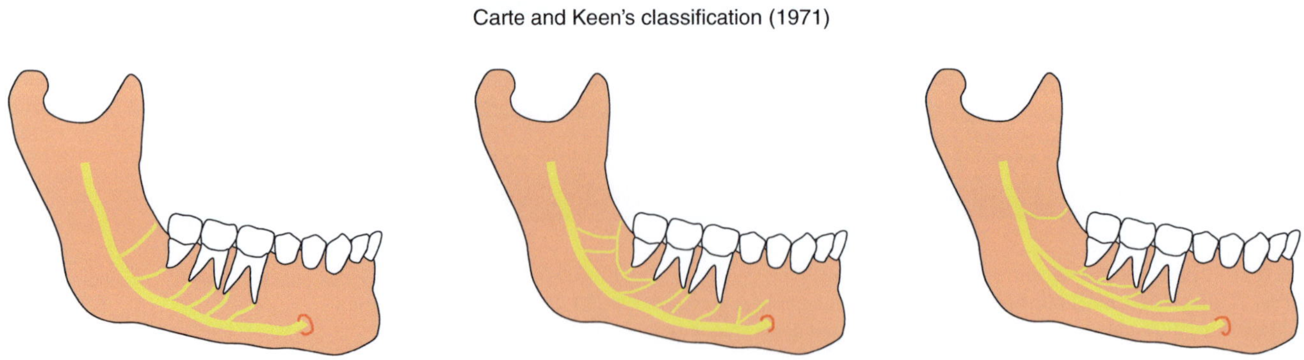

Fig. 3.54 Carter and Keen (1971) classified the mandibular canal into three different types

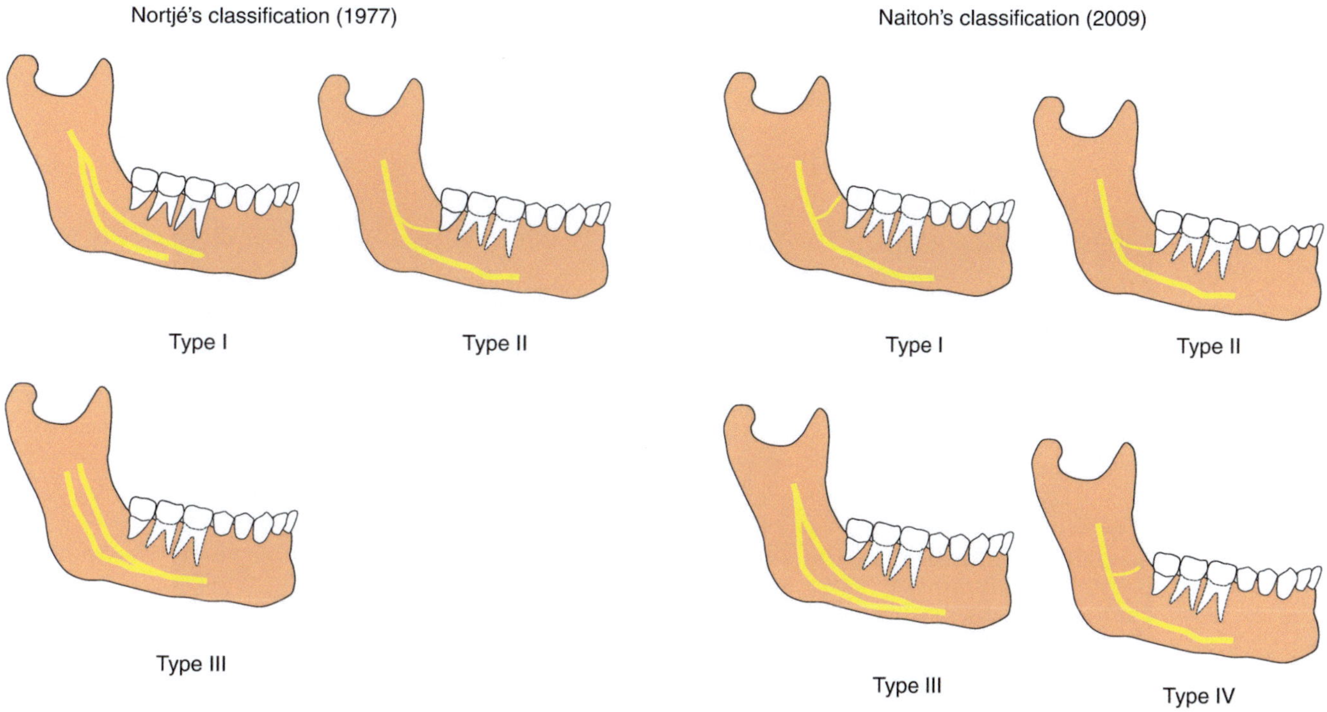

Fig. 3.55 Bifid/trifid mandibular canal. Nortjé (1977) and Naitoh et al. (2009b) proposed different classifications for the bifid mandibular canal. The retromolar canal is categorized as one type of bifid mandibular canal

3.6 Pterygomandibular Space and Retromolar Area

Summary

The pterygomandibular space is bordered by the ramus of the mandible laterally and the medial pterygoid muscle medially where the mandibular foramen, the target of the inferior alveolar nerve block, is located.

The retromolar area is situated posterior to the molar teeth and is surrounded by the pterygomandibular and parapharyngeal spaces posteriorly and by the floor of the oral cavity inferomedially. Regardless of its small area, several important structures exist in the retromolar area, e.g., lingual nerve, retromolar gland, buccinator muscle, buccal nerve, retromolar pad. Some of these are not well discussed in the literature despite their potential clinical importance. In this section, anatomical structures in the retromolar area will be shown as well as anatomical variations such as the retromolar canal/foramen, which was discussed in the mandibular canal section as one of the subtypes of the bifid mandibular canal. In dentistry and oral surgery, the course of the lingual nerve in the retromolar area is important when the mucosal incision is made for wisdom tooth extraction.

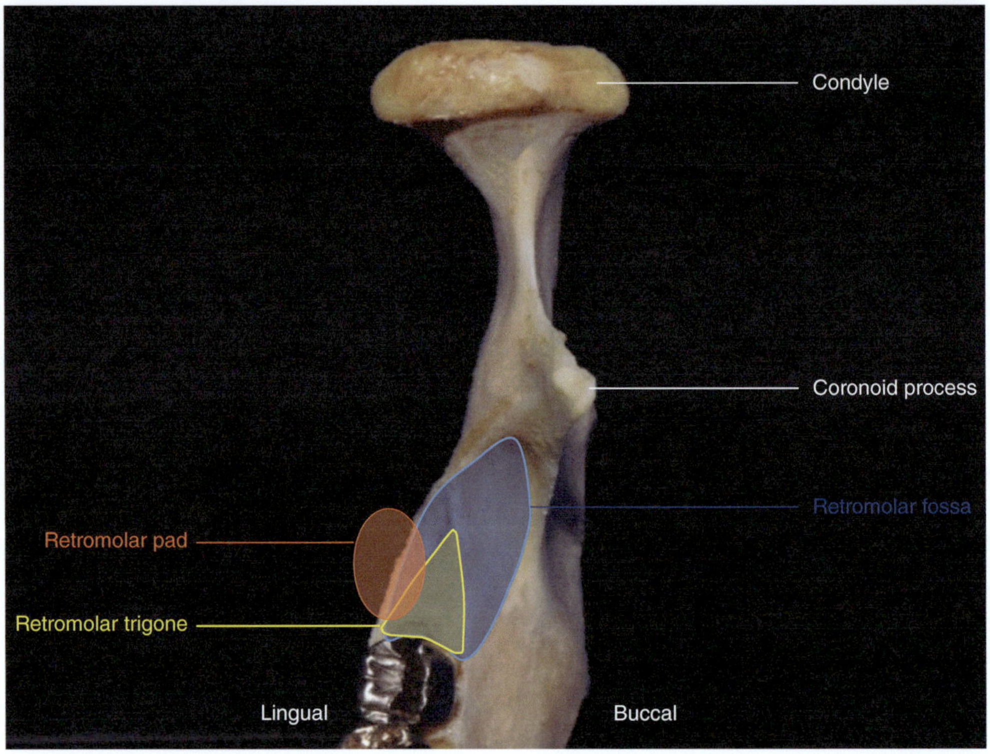

Fig. 3.56 The retromolar fossa is the concavity of the retromolar area that extends to the anterior border of the ramus of the mandible. The retromolar trigone is a smaller triangular-shaped, flat area. Both structures are on the surface of the mandible. The retromolar pad is a soft tissue structure and does not attach to the mandible

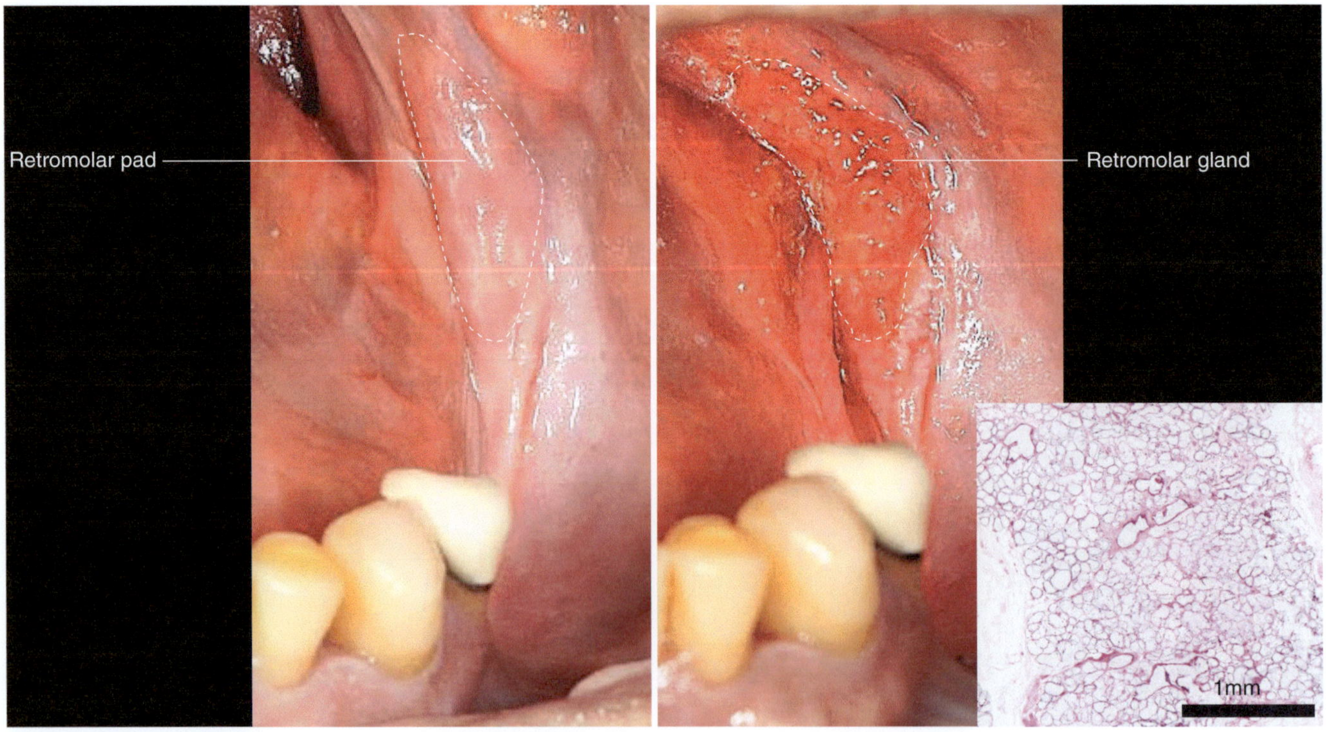

Fig. 3.57 Intraoral dissection of the left retromolar area in a fresh cadaver. Note that the retromolar gland and overlying mucosa form the retromolar pad. The retromolar gland is a mucinous gland and is innervated by a branch of the lingual nerve (Iwanaga et al. 2018)

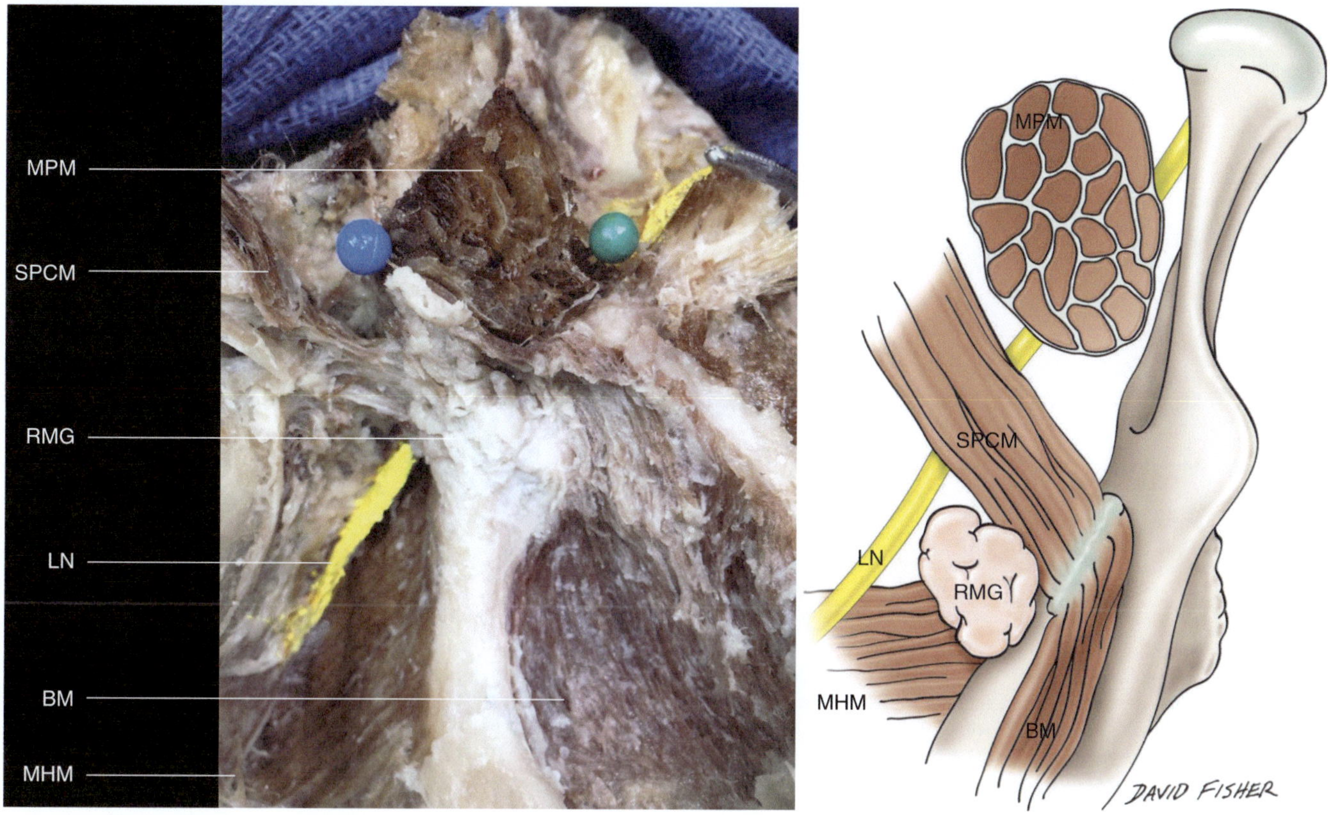

Fig. 3.58 Various structures in and around the retromolar area, floor of the oral cavity, and pterygomandibular space. *BM* buccinator muscle, *LN* lingual nerve, *MHM* mylohyoid muscle, *MPM* medial pterygoid muscle, *RMG* retromolar gland, *SPCM* superior pharyngeal constrictor muscle (Iwanaga et al. 2018).

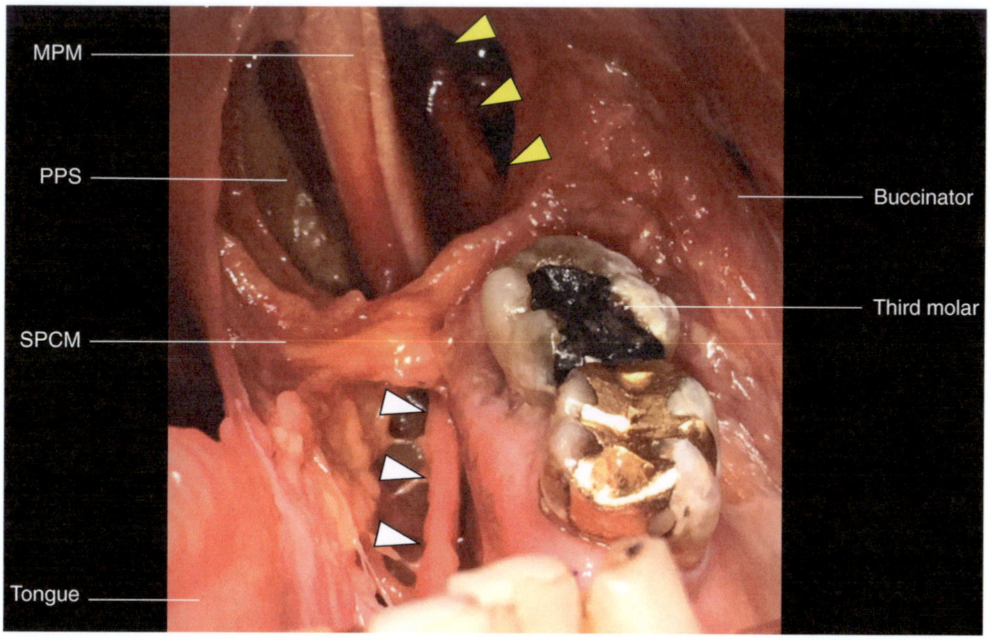

Fig. 3.59 The lingual nerve traveling through pterygomandibular space (yellow arrowheads) runs below the inferior border of the superior pharyngeal constrictor muscle and appears in the floor of the mouth (white arrowheads). Note the medial pterygoid muscle is located between the pterygomandibular and parapharyngeal spaces. *MPM* medial pterygoid muscle, *PPS* parapharyngeal space, *SPCM* superior pharyngeal constrictor muscle

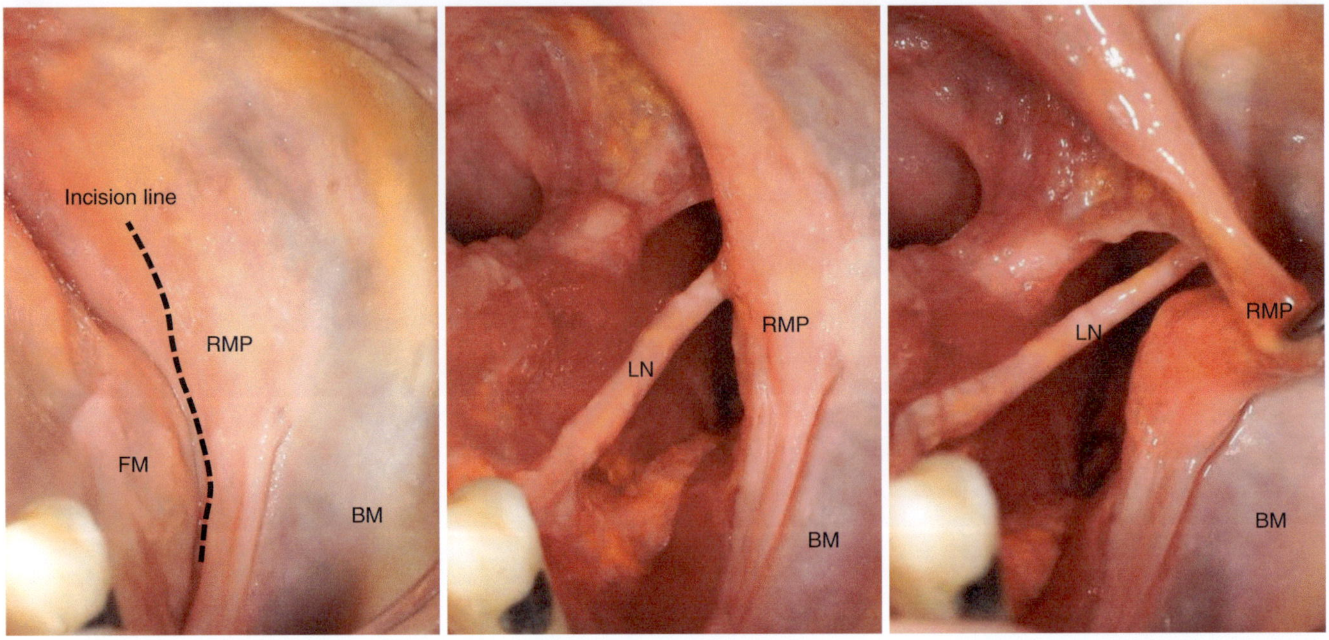

Fig. 3.60 When looking into the retromolar area from a dentist's point of view, the lingual nerve runs from and travels posterior to the retromolar pad and appears medial to the retromolar pad (gland). Therefore, if a mucosal incision is made medial to the retromolar pad deep enough, the lingual nerve might be damaged. The lingual nerve does not "pierce" the retromolar gland/pad. *BM* buccal mucosa, FM floor of mouth, *RMP* retromolar pad (Iwanaga et al. 2020a)

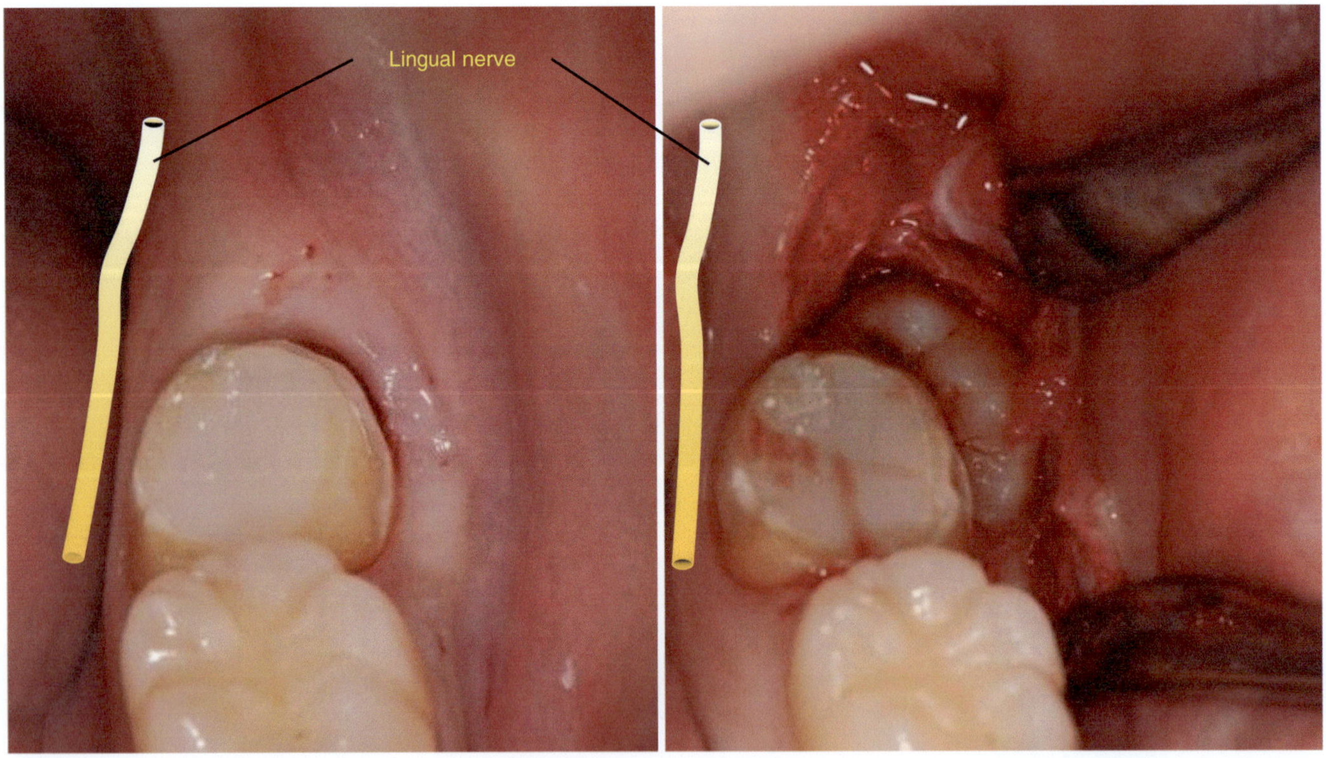

Fig. 3.61 Removal of the impacted lower third molar often requires distal mucosal incision, which can damage the lingual nerve if the incision is too medial (lingually)

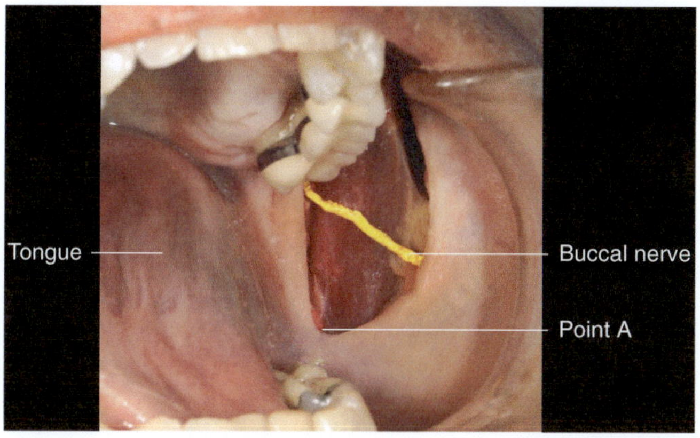

Fig. 3.62 Recommended injection site for buccal nerve blockade is seen at Point A (on the anterior border of the ramus of the mandible and 1 mm lateral to the third molar tooth). However, two recent anatomical studies have shown that the buccal nerve is not adjacent to Point A (mean distance of 12–13 mm) (Iwanaga et al. 2019a; Takezawa et al. 2018)

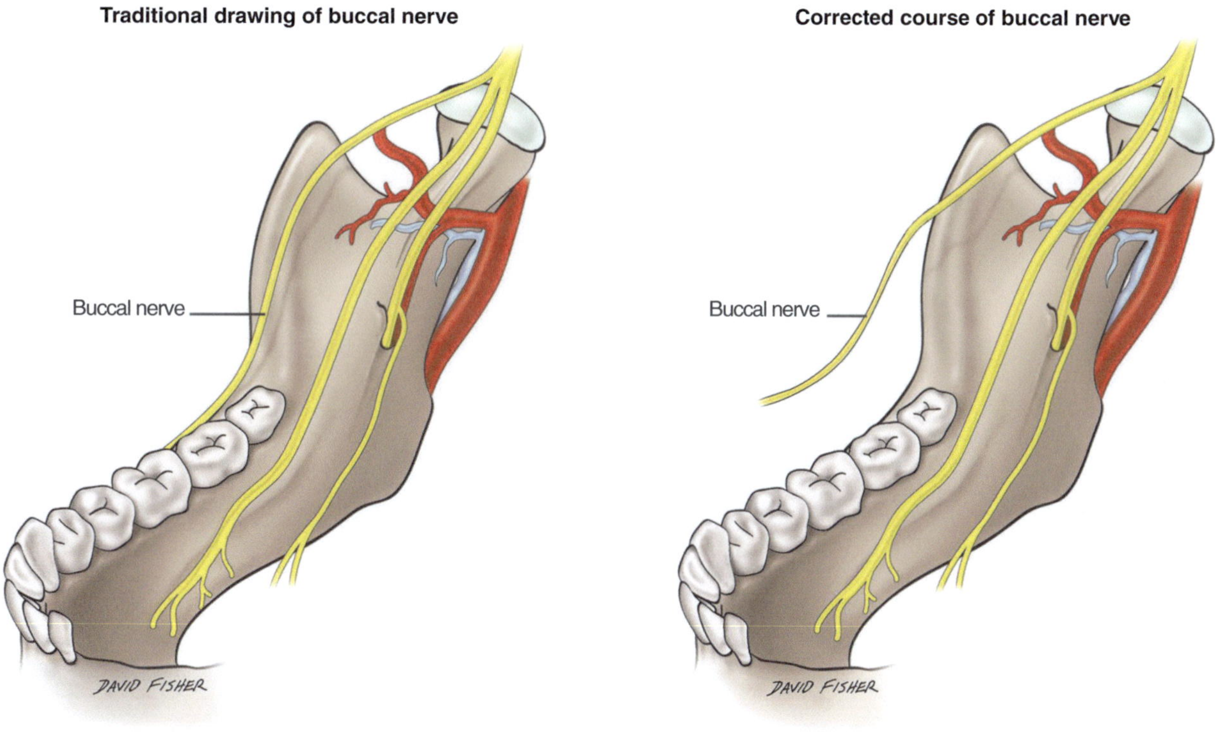

Fig. 3.63 Many dental textbooks have shown an incorrect course of the main trunk of the buccal nerve due to a lack of evidence via intraoral dissection (left). This traditional concept has been the reason that injection of Point A is called "buccal nerve block." However, the main trunk of the buccal nerve is not blocked with injection at Point A. The corrected course of the buccal nerve based on the result of intraoral dissection is shown on the right (Iwanaga et al. 2019b).

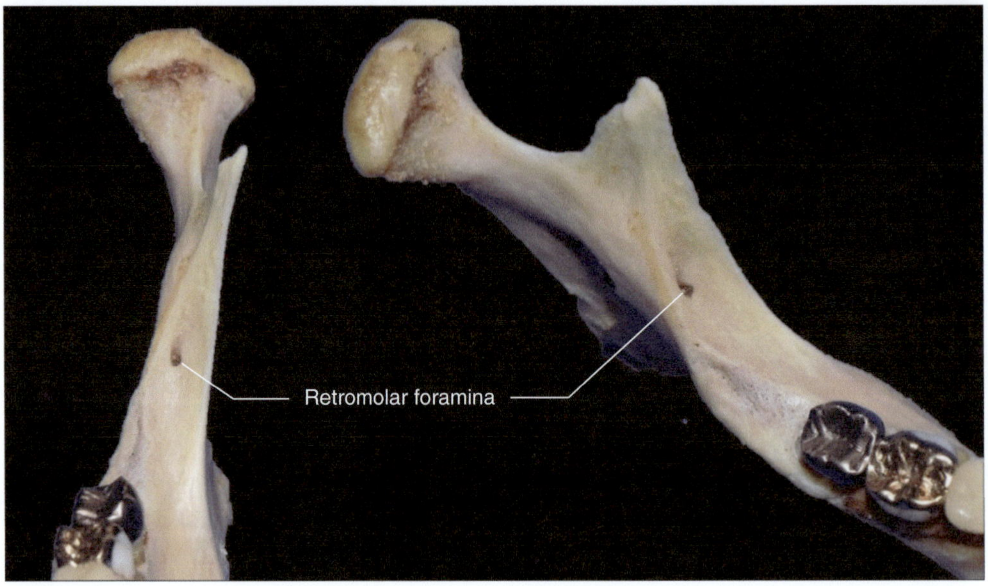

Fig. 3.64 In this mandible, the retromolar foramen is located in the retromolar fossa. The retromolar foramen accommodates a part of the inferior alveolar nerve/vessels. However, the nerve from this foramen innervates the buccal gingiva of the lower molars and is the area where the branch of the buccal nerve usually travels (Motamedi et al. 2016)

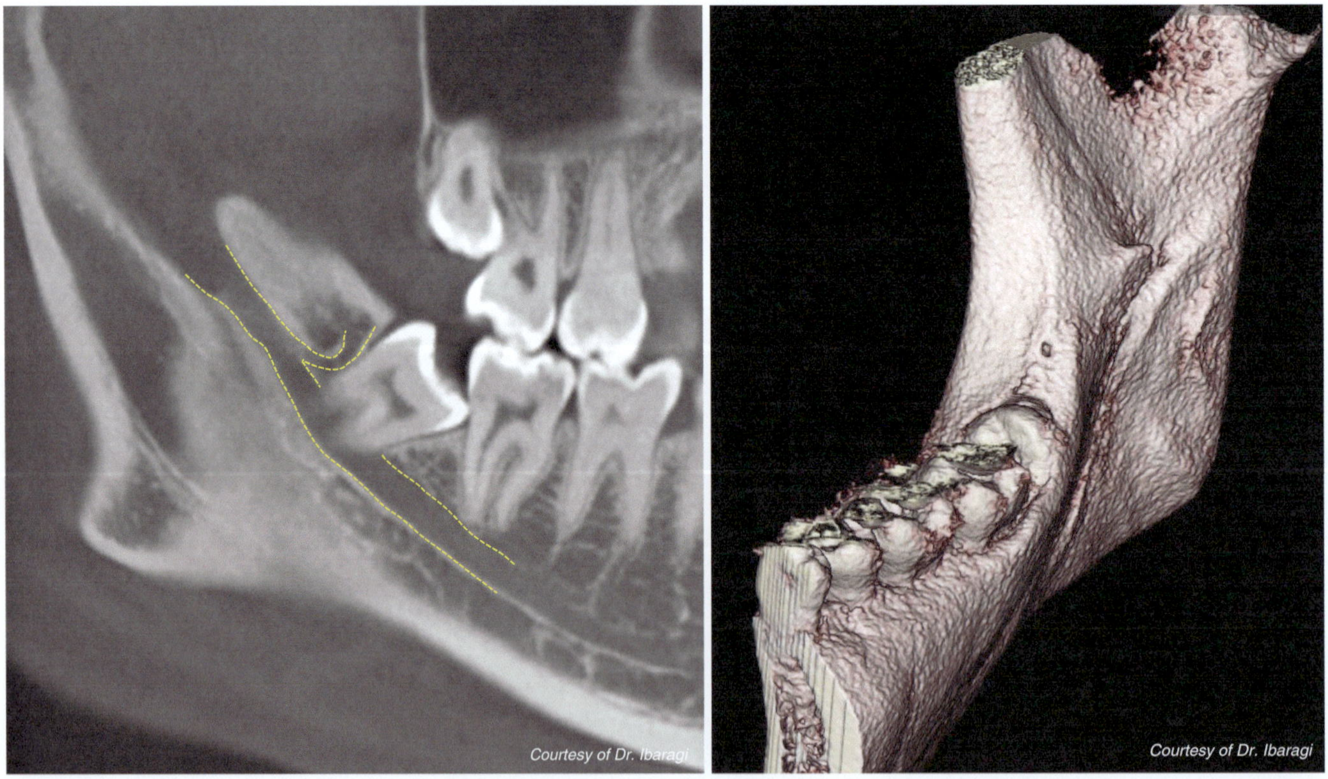

Fig. 3.65 Retromolar foramen and canal. According to Naitoh et al. (2009b), the retromolar canal is one of the subtypes of a bifid mandibular canal. In this case, the opening of the retromolar foramen is located in the retromolar triangle

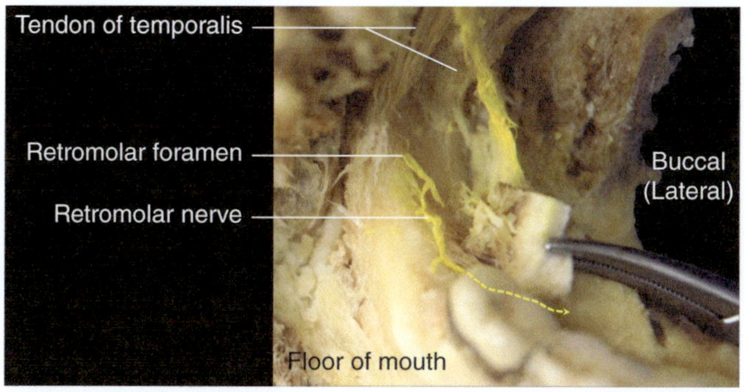

Fig. 3.66 The retromolar nerve, arising from the retromolar foramen, innervates the buccal gingiva and mucosa of the lower molars

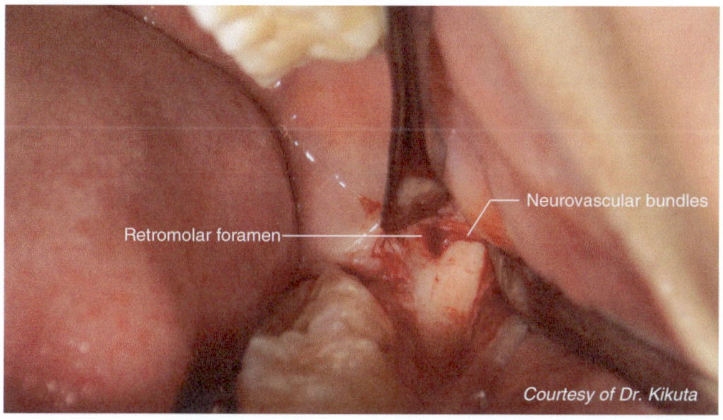

Fig. 3.67 Retromolar neurovascular bundles arising from the retromolar foramen. One clinical study showed that injury of the large retromolar foramen during removal of the lower third molar resulted in paresthesia of the buccal gingiva of the lower molar (Kikuta et al. 2018)

3.7 Palate

Summary

The palate forms the roof of the oral cavity and is divided into hard and soft palates. The hard palate is lined with keratinized and immobile mucosa. The soft palate is lined by non-keratinized and mobile mucosa which forms the entrance for the fauces between the oral cavity and oropharynx. The depth of the palatal mucosa, maxilla and palatine bone forms the bony palate.

The palate is supplied by the greater and lesser palatine arteries posteriorly, and sphenopalatine artery anteriorly. Sensory and parasympathetic fibers are carried by the greater and lesser palatine nerves posteriorly and the nasopalatine nerve anteriorly. The palatine glands are minor salivary glands that are mostly located bilaterally in the posterior palate. Greater palatine nerve blockade and other surgical techniques require detailed knowledge of the palatal area.

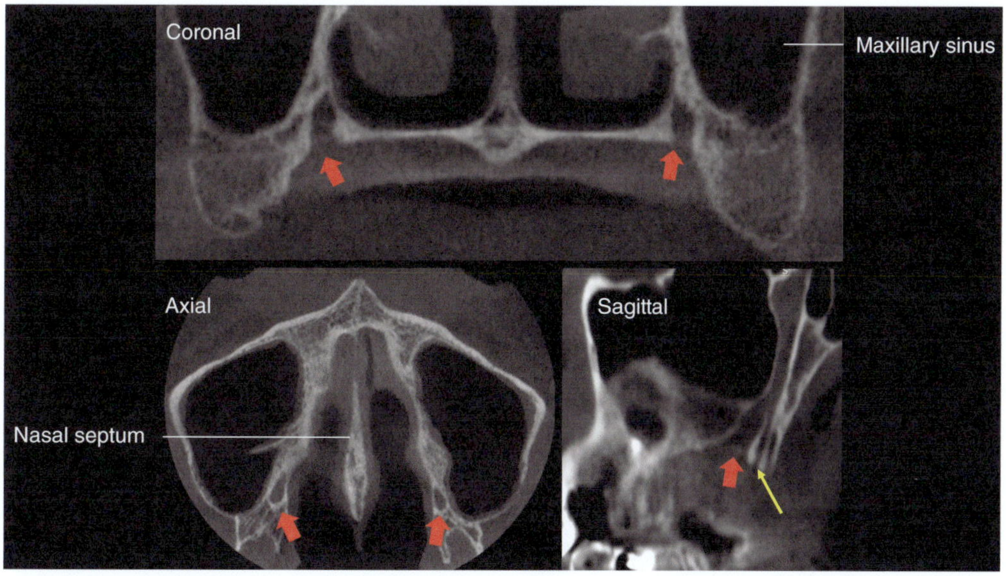

Fig. 3.68 The greater palatine foramina (red arrows) are intraoral exits of the greater palatine canals which contain the greater palatine nerve and vessels. The greater palatine foramina usually open in an inferior-anterior-medial direction. Posterior to the greater palatine foramina, there are lesser palatine foramina (yellow arrow) which accommodate the lesser palatine nerve and vessels. The greater and lesser palatine nerves and vessels supply the hard and soft palates, respectively

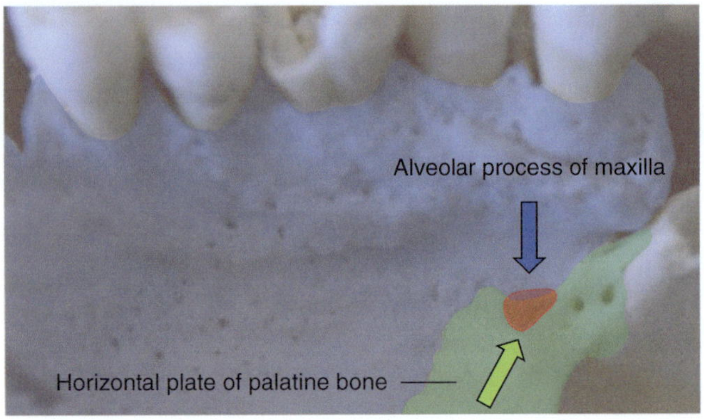

Fig. 3.69 The greater palatine foramen (red area) is located near the posterior edge of the bony palate and formed at the junction of the alveolar process of the maxilla and the horizontal plate of the palatine bone. Therefore, the greater palatine foramen can be located by tracing the base of the alveolar process from anteriorly to posteriorly with the edge of the dental mirror or Q-tip

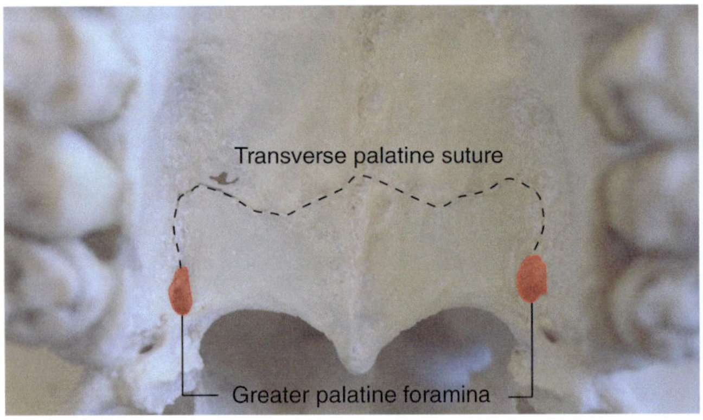

Fig. 3.70 Inferior view of the greater palatine foramina (red areas). The course of the greater palatine nerve and vessels can be predicted by following the junction of the two bones, the alveolar process of the maxilla and the horizontal plate of the palatine bone, where the greater palatine foramen is formed

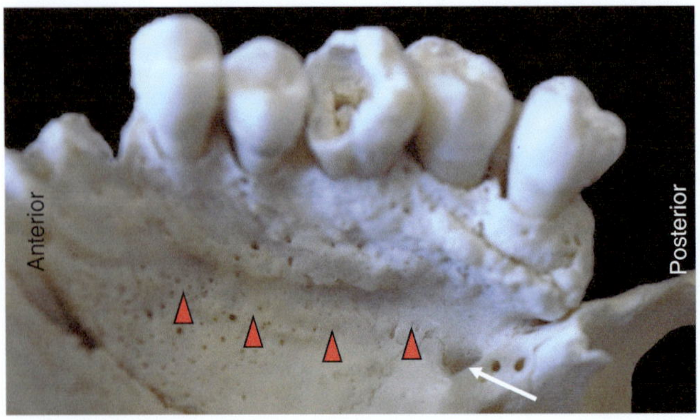

Fig. 3.71 Greater palatine groove (arrowheads) for the greater palatine nerve/vessels extending from the greater palatine foramen (arrow)

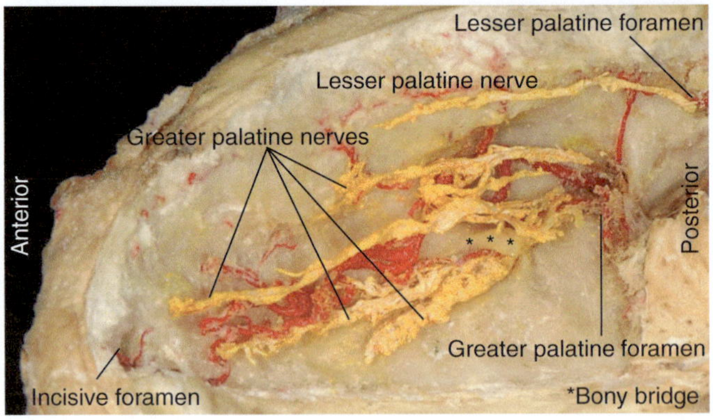

Fig. 3.72 Inferior view of the left palate in an edentulous maxilla. The greater palatine foramen (dashed line) gives rise to the greater palatine artery (red) and nerve (yellow). The nerve usually splits into two to four branches (Hafeez et al. 2015). The artery is also highly branched along its course over the palate (Klosek and Rungruang 2009) . Note that the lesser palatine nerve arises from the lesser palatine foramen and innervates the lateral part of the hard palate (anatomical variation)

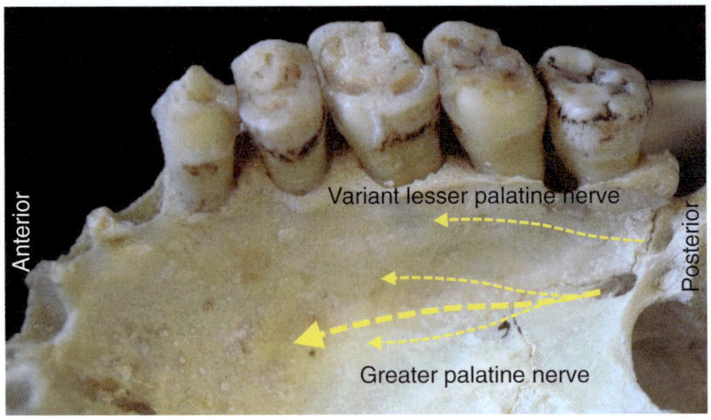

Fig. 3.73 Inferior view of the left palate in a partially dentulous dry maxilla. The variant lesser palatine nerve shown in the earlier figure is seen as a dashed arrow. In this variation, the branches of the greater palatine nerve mainly supply the hard palate and the variant nerve supplies the palatal gingiva of the maxilla

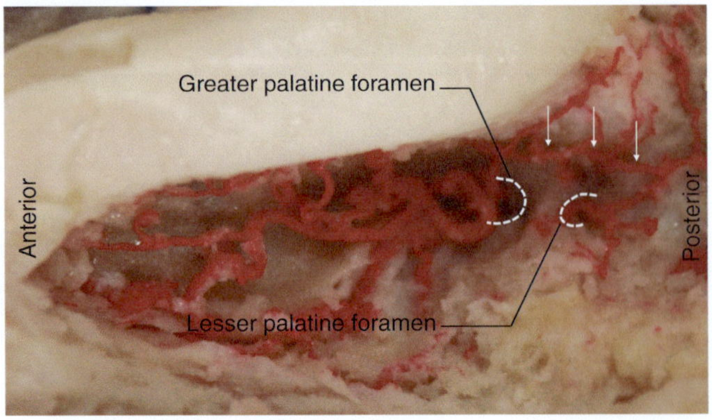

Fig. 3.74 Inferior view of the left palate in an edentulous maxilla. The greater palatine foramen gives rise to the greater palatine artery. Note that the artery from the lesser palatine foramen has an anastomosis (arrows) with the greater palatine artery that originates from the greater palatine foramen

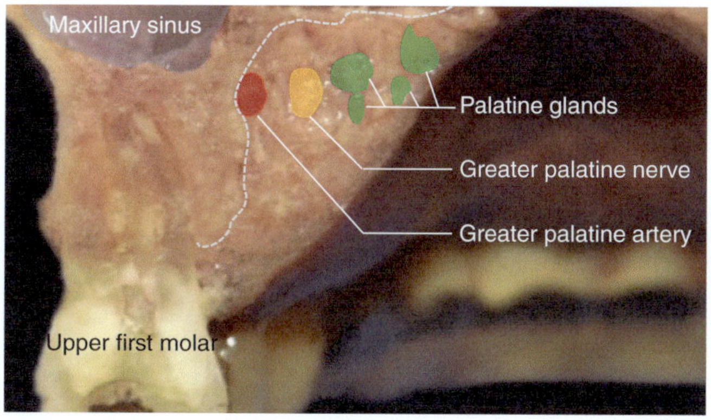

Fig. 3.75 Posterior view of a coronal section of the left palate at the first molar level. Note that the palatal mucosa is thick. In this case, the greater palatine artery runs on the surface of the base of the alveolar process of the maxilla

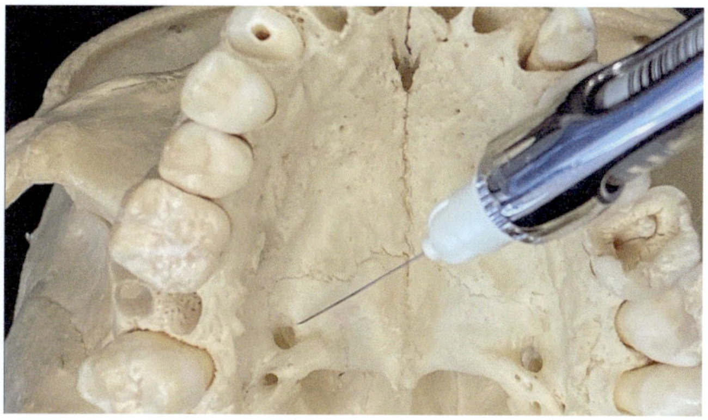

Fig. 3.77 Example of the greater palatine nerve block. After locating the greater palatine foramen using the Q-tip method as shown in the following two figures, the needle is inserted into the mucosa approximately 5-mm deep

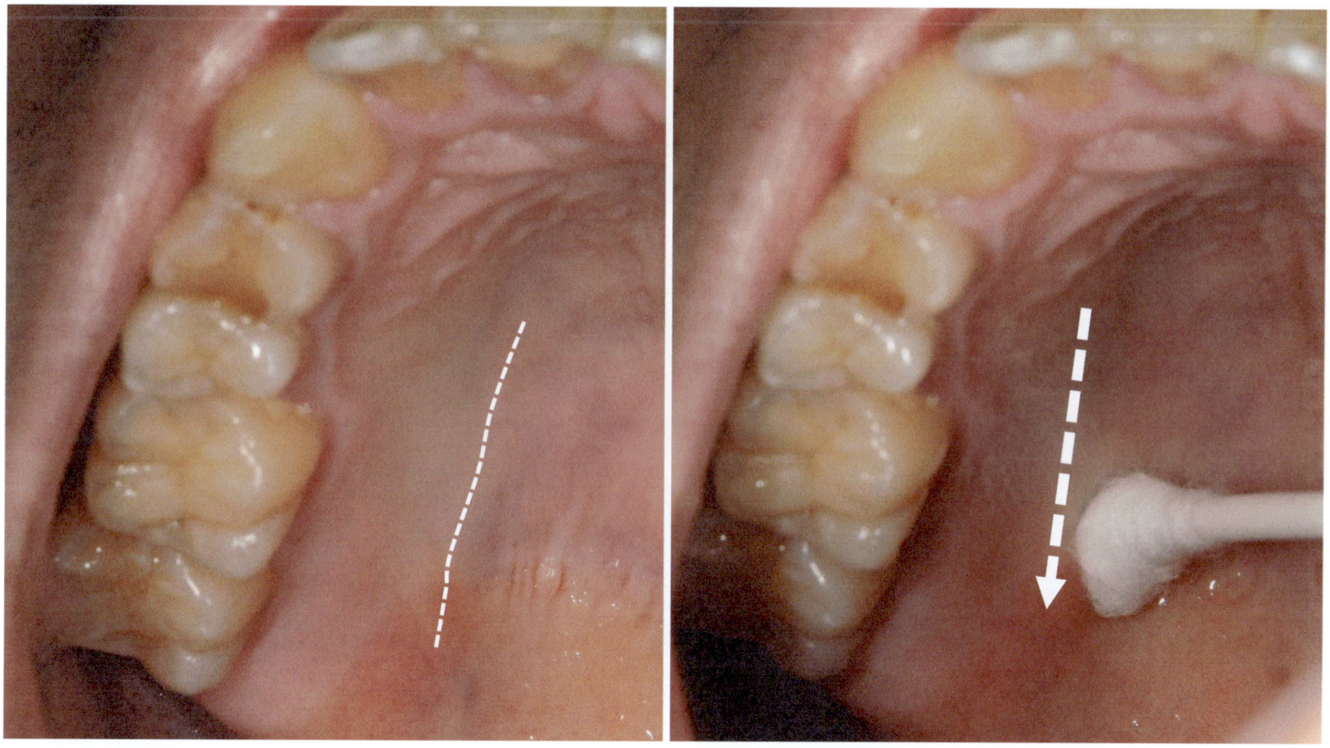

Fig. 3.76 Example of how to detect the greater palatine foramen in a patient. The dashed line in the left figure shows the junction of the horizontal and alveolar parts. A Q-tip or the edge of a dental mirror is gently slid anteriorly to posteriorly to find the depression on the surface of the mucosa near the last molar region. This is where the greater palatine foramen is located deep to the mucosa

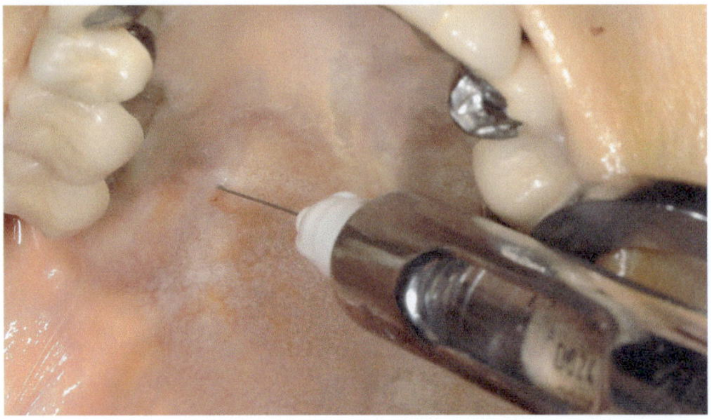

Fig. 3.78 Greater palatine nerve block. The needle is aimed slightly anterior to the depression located with a Q-tip from the corner of the contralateral side of the mouth. As the target is the greater palatine nerve, the needle should not be inserted too deeply into the foramen. In case the needle enters too deeply e.g., 30 mm, the pterygopalatine ganglion can be blocked as the ganglion is situated in the pterygopalatine fossa which is approximately 30 mm from the foramen

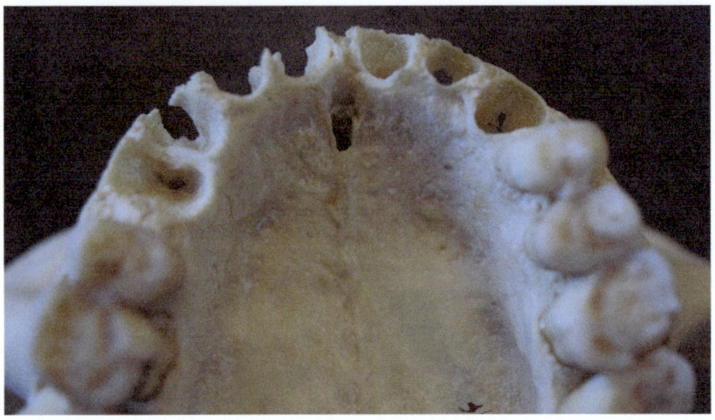

Fig. 3.79 The incisive foramen is seen posterior to the central incisors. The incisive canal, running in the depth of the foramen, connecting the oral and nasal cavities, is where the greater palatine and sphenopalatine arteries anastomose. The nasopalatine nerve leaves the incisive foramen to innervate the anterior palate

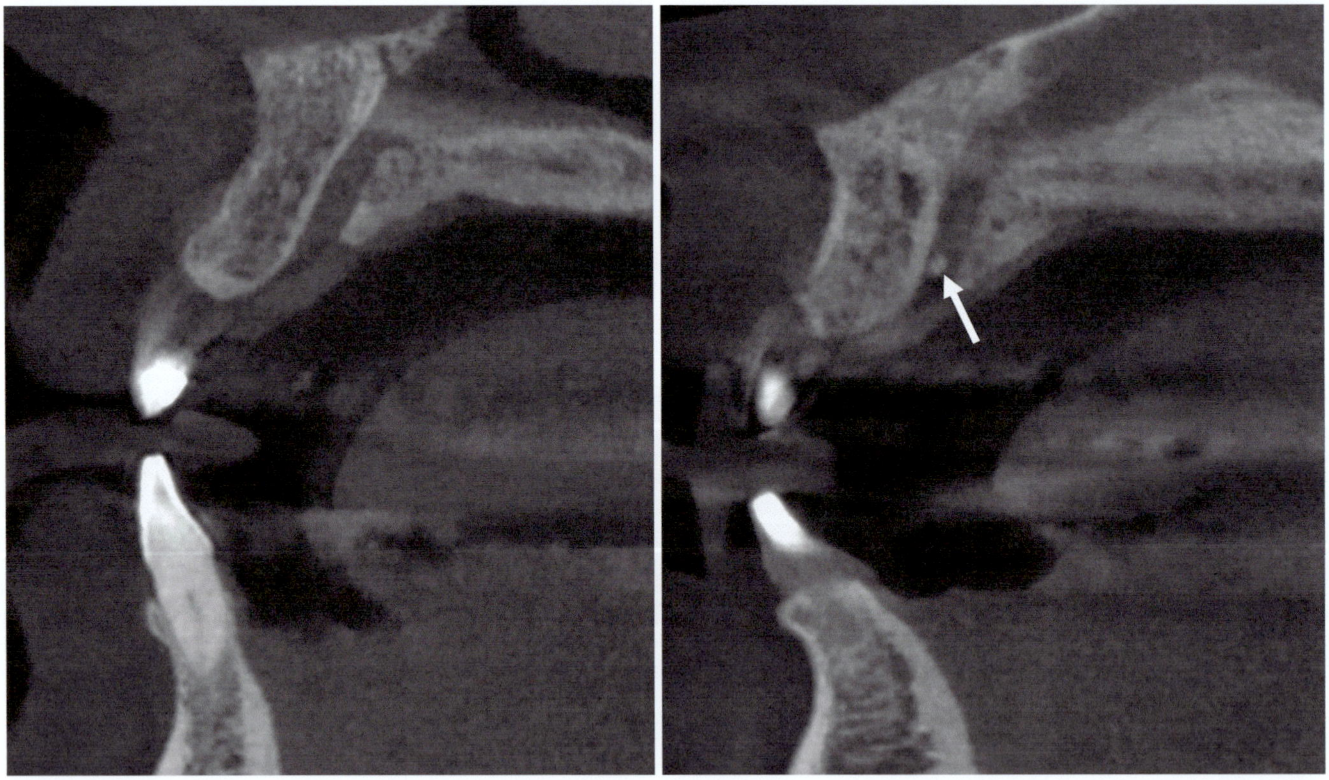

Fig. 3.80 Midsagittal CBCT images showing incisive canals. The arrow points to a septum in the canal

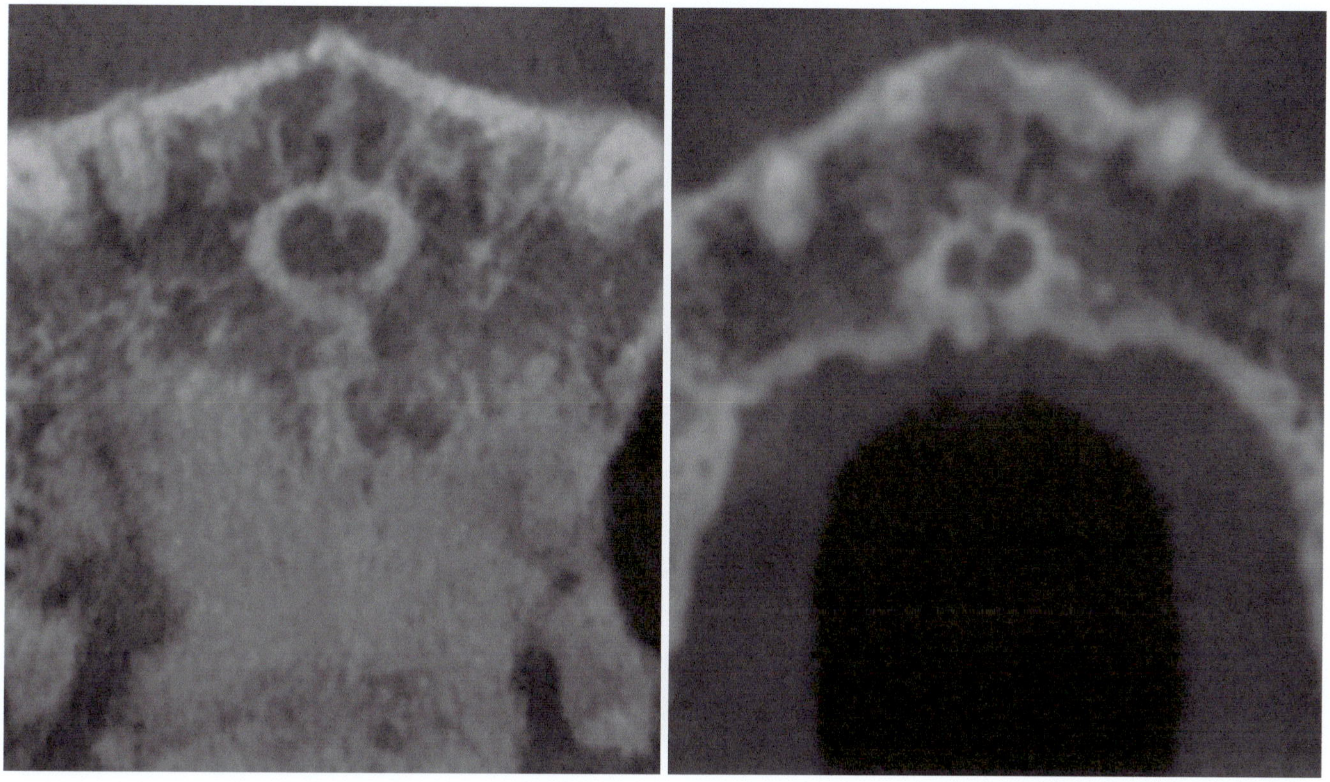

Fig. 3.81 Axial CBCT image showing incisive canals. Inside the canal, a septum/septa are often observed. It is either an incomplete septum (left figure) or a complete septum (right figure)

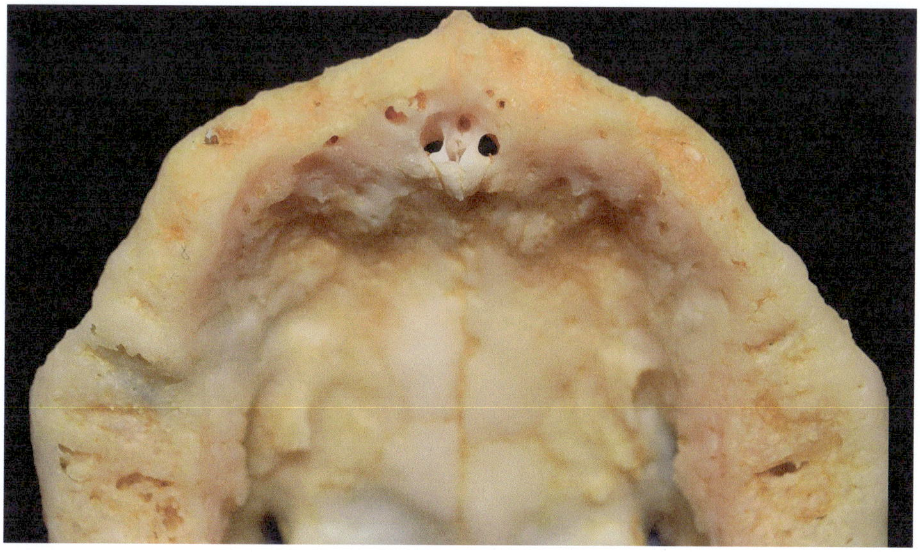

Fig. 3.82 A cadaveric image of the incisive canals in the depth of the incisive foramen. Note the multiple septa inside the canal

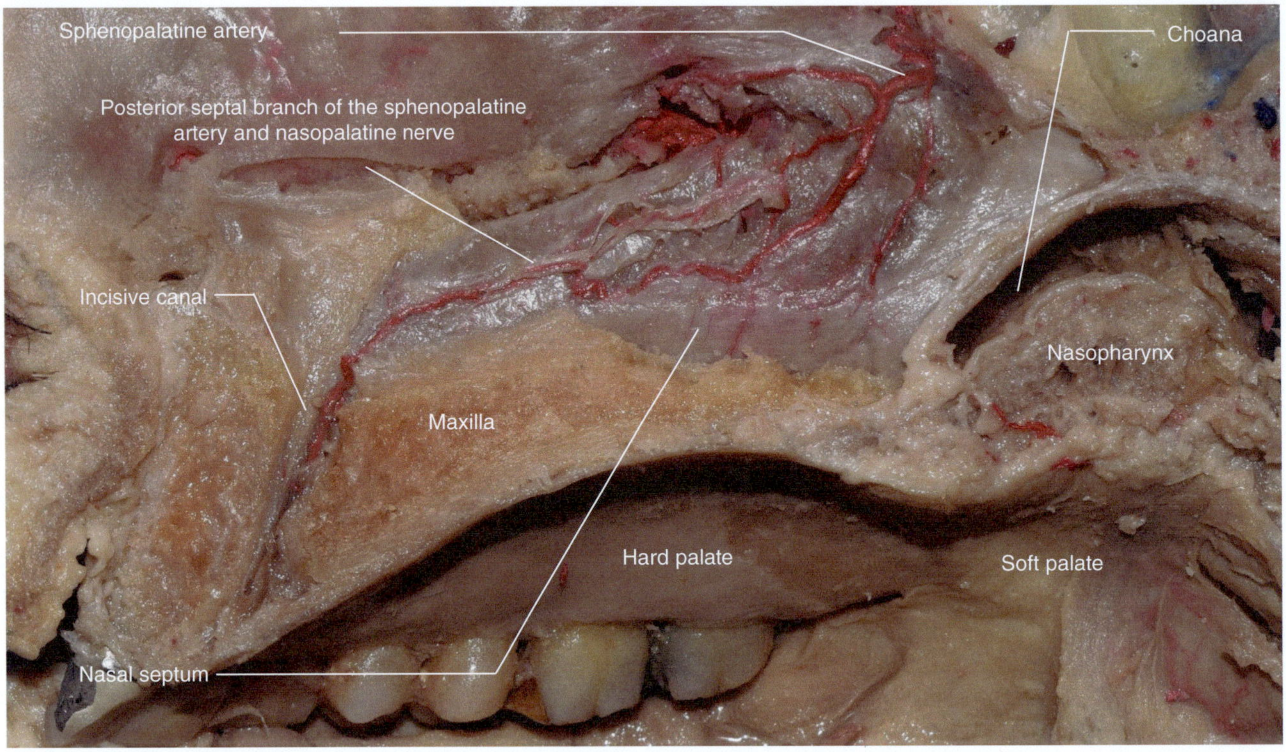

Fig. 3.83 A midsagittal cadaveric view of the nasal septum. Posterior septal branch of the sphenopalatine artery and nasopalatine nerve course together and enter the incisive canal

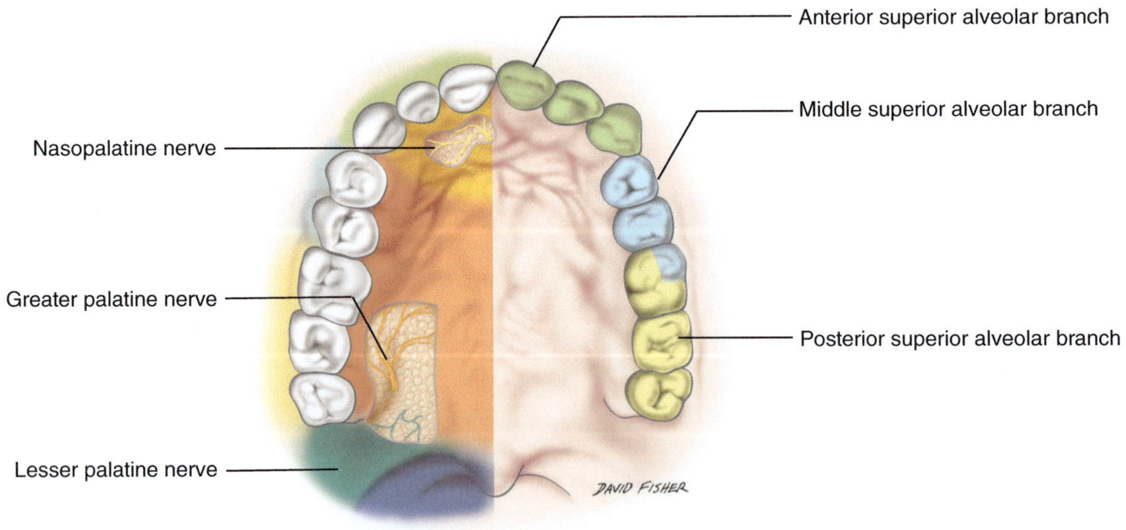

Fig. 3.84 Innervation of the palate. Anterior palate (from central incisor to canine) is innervated by the nasopalatine nerve and the posterior part is by the greater palatine nerve. Both nerves are branches of the maxillary nerve.

3.8 Tongue

Summary
The tongue is a muscular organ located in the oral cavity. The functions of the tongue include gustation, support of mastication and digestion, deglutition, and speech. Thus, the sensory and motor nerves contributing to the function of the tongue via cranial nerves V, VII, IX, and XII are important. The tongue muscles consist of intrinsic and extrinsic muscles. The anterior two-thirds and posterior one-third of the tongue have varied innervations.

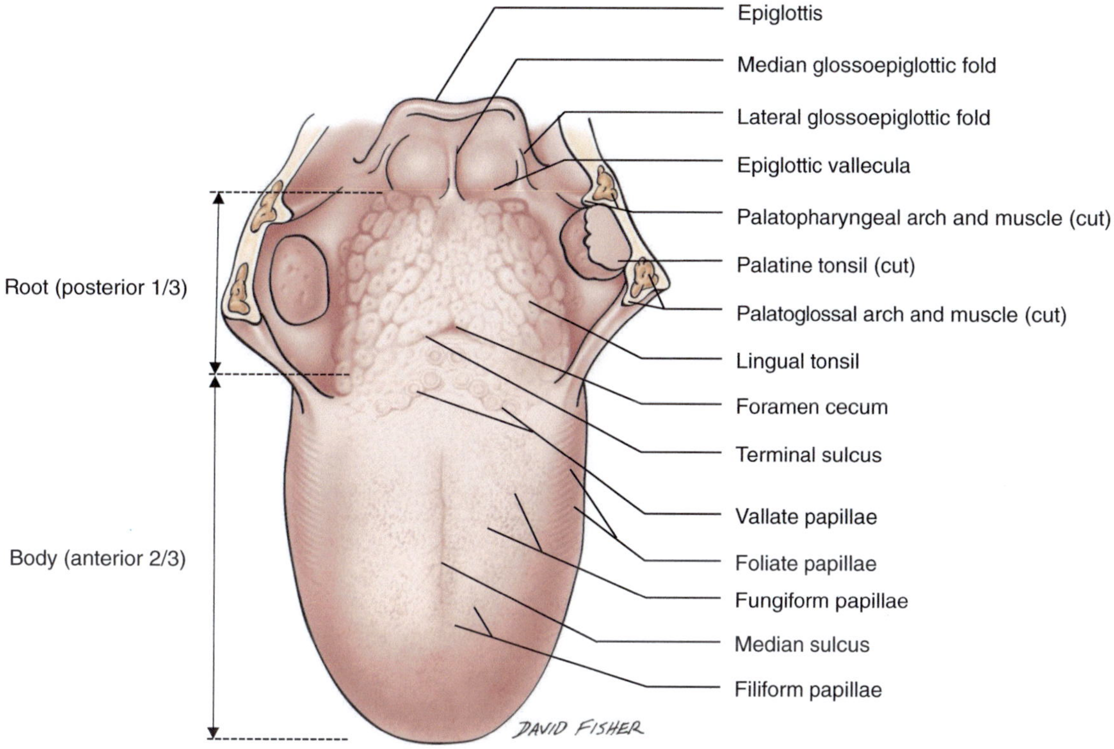

Fig. 3.85 The body (anterior two-thirds) and root (posterior one-third) of the tongue. There is a collection of lymphoid tissue on the surface of the root of the tongue (lingual tonsil). Also, the palatine tonsils are located in the tonsillar fossae between the palatoglossal and palatopharyngeal arches. There are four papillae of the tongue, i.e., circumvallate papillae, foliate papillae (leaf-like), filiform papillae (thread-like), and fungiform papillae (mushroom-like).

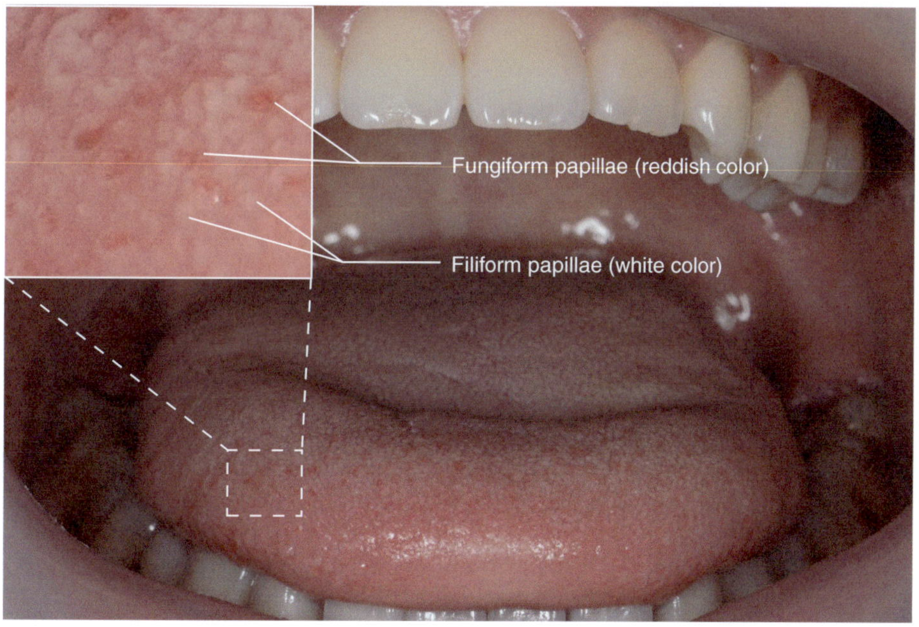

Fig. 3.86 Surface anatomy of the anterior tongue

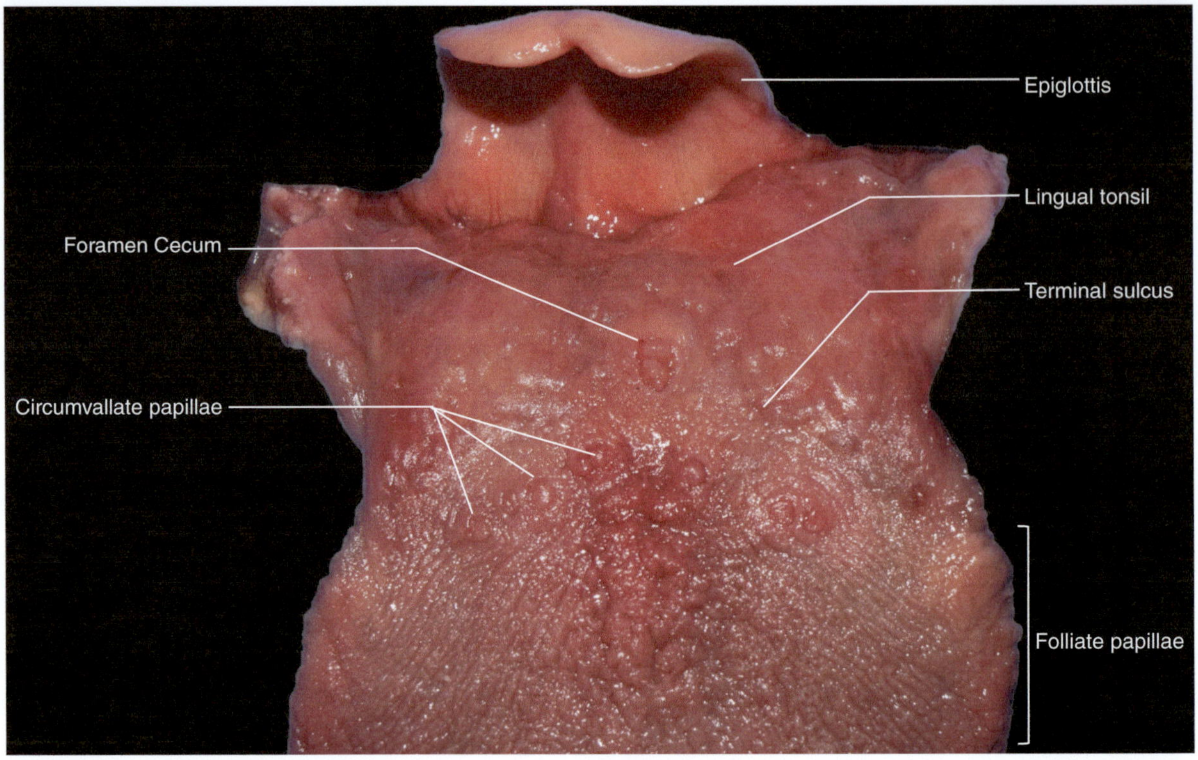

Fig. 3.87 Surface anatomy of the posterior tongue

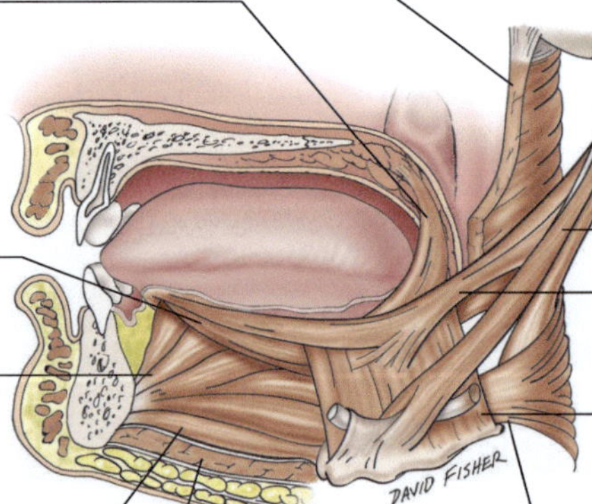

Fig. 3.88 Lateral view of the tongue and its related muscles. The tongue is formed mostly by muscles, i.e., intrinsic and extrinsic tongue muscles. They are all innervated by the hypoglossal nerve (CN XII) with the exception of the palatoglossus muscle which is innervated by the vagus nerve (CN X).

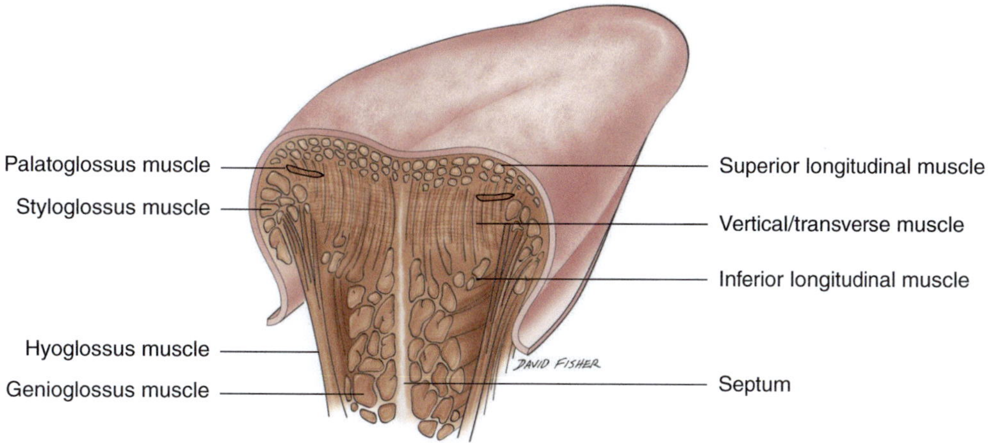

Fig. 3.89 Posterior view of the tongue and its related muscles. © Fisher/Tubbs 2020. All Rights Reserved

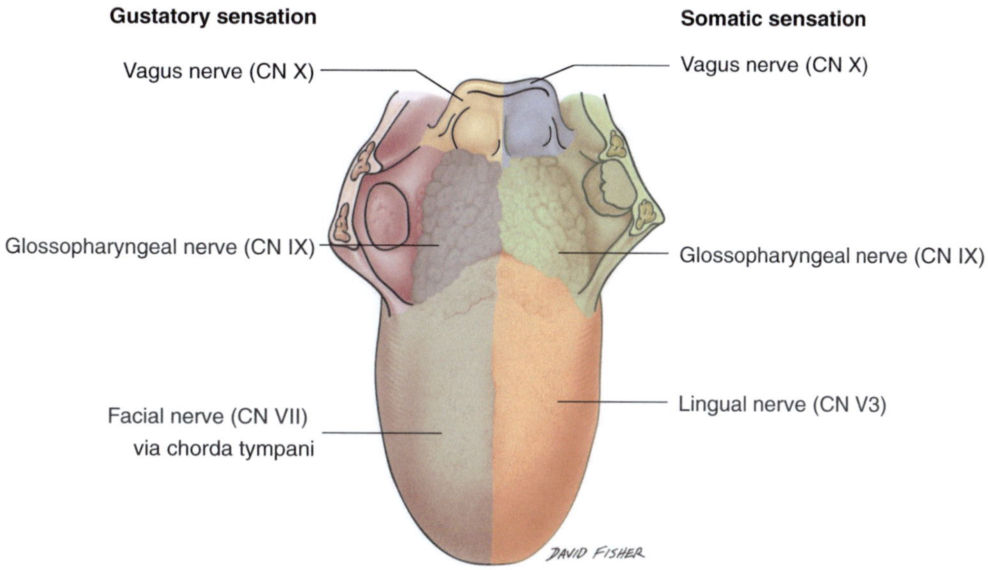

Fig. 3.90 The tongue is innervated by different cranial nerves including the trigeminal (CN V), facial (CN VII), glossopharyngeal (CN IX), and hypoglossal (CN XII) nerves. © Fisher/Tubbs 2020. All Rights Reserved

3.9 Floor of the Mouth (Sublingual and Submandibular Spaces)

Summary

The floor of the mouth is considered a "dangerous" area for dentists as it contains nerves and vessels which are not visible even on cone-beam computed tomography (CBCT). Also, non-malignant surgeries or even surgeries for cosmetic/functional reasons such as dental implant surgeries can damage structures in the floor of the mouth. These iatrogenic injuries can potentially lead to life-threatening hemorrhage and permanent injury to sensory nerves. To avoid these, a three-dimensional understanding of the anatomy of the floor is necessary. In this section, the general anatomy of the floor will be demonstrated. The course of many of these nerves that are not visible on CBCT images can be predicted if the anatomical relationships between the nerves and other landmarks are well understood.

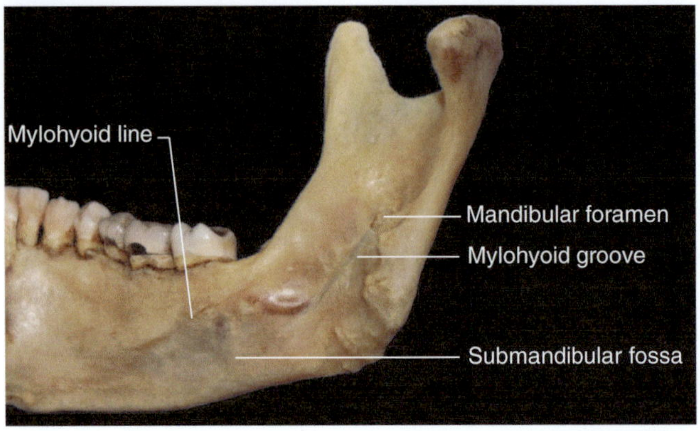

Fig. 3.91 The floor of the mouth is bound by the mylohyoid muscle inferiorly. The bony attachment of the muscle to the mandible is the mylohyoid line. Below the line, there is a concavity which is called the submandibular fossa

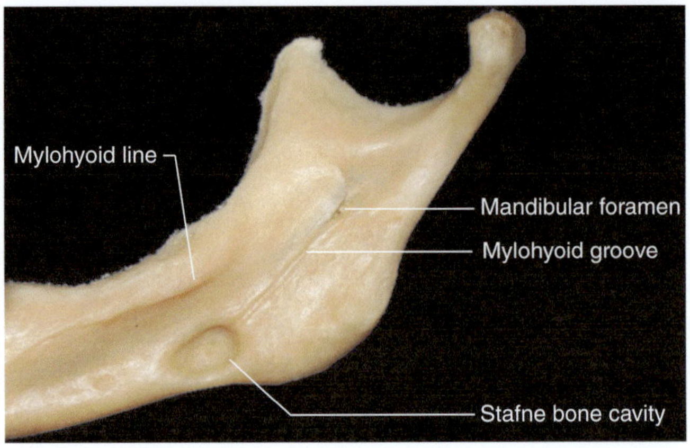

Fig. 3.93 The Stafne bone cavity is generally located slightly above the inferior border of the mandible and inferior to the mandibular canal with a reported incidence of 0.1–6.06%. The submandibular gland, connective tissue, fat tissue, muscle, lymphatic tissue or vessels have all been considered potential contents of the cavity. It is also called a salivary inclusion cyst, static bone cavity, lingual bone defect, and latent cyst (Iwanaga et al. 2019a)

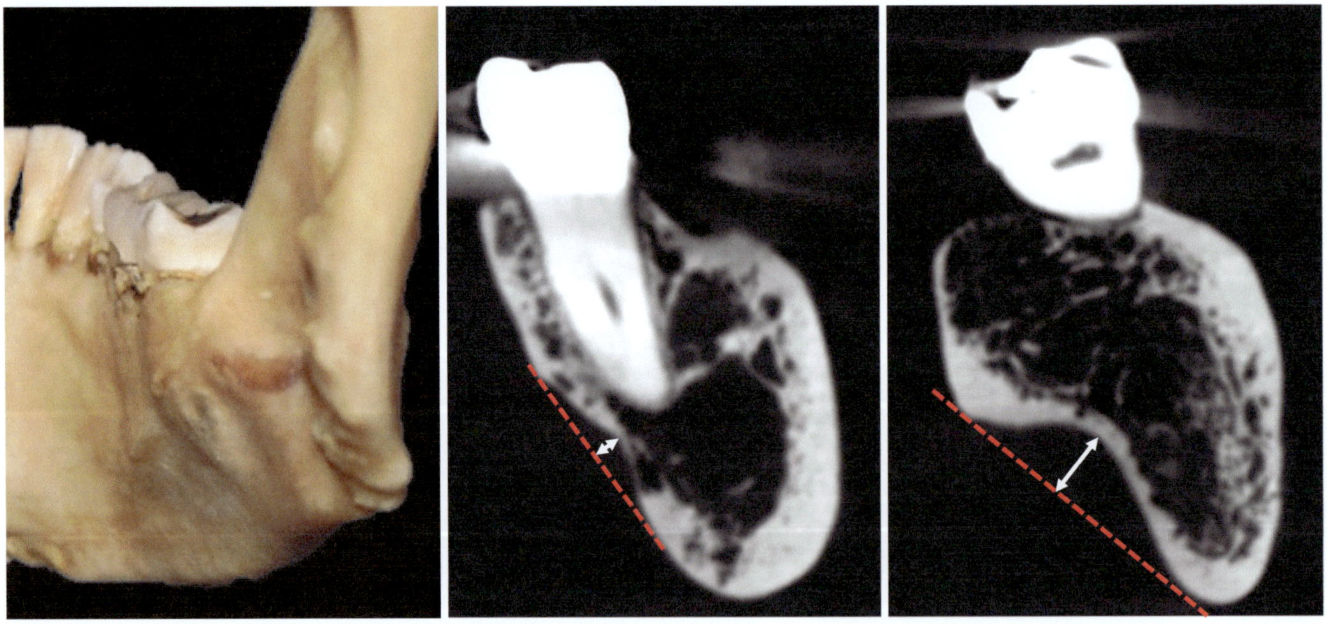

Fig. 3.92 The submandibular fossa is seen at the inferior part of the mandible in the lower molar area. The depth of the fossa varies in each individual or each tooth

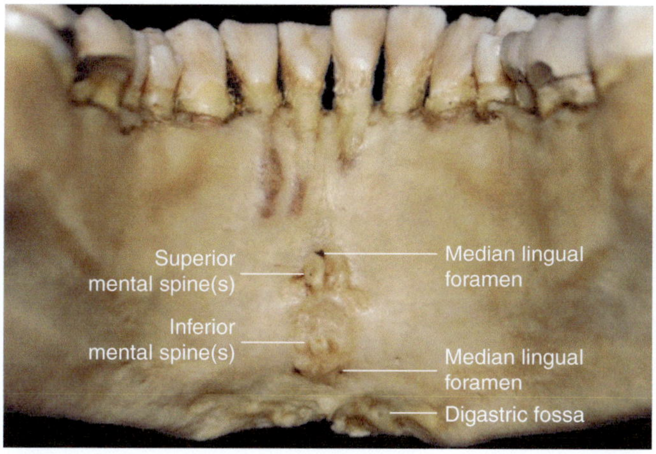

Fig. 3.94 Posterior view of the mandible. The superior and inferior mental spines are the origins of the genioglossus and geniohyoid muscles, respectively. The digastric fossa is the bony attachment of the anterior belly of the digastric muscle. The median lingual foramen is located in the midline on the lingual surface of the mandible and is considered the entrance for a branch of the submental/sublingual artery or nerve to mylohyoid

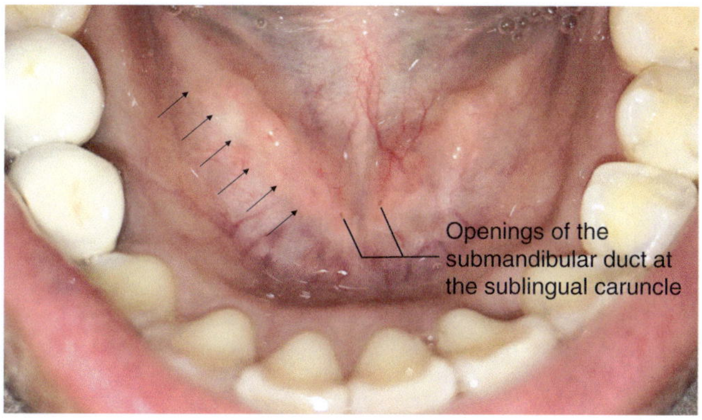

Fig. 3.96 The sublingual fold (white arrows) is formed along the openings of the minor sublingual ducts (Rivinus's ducts)

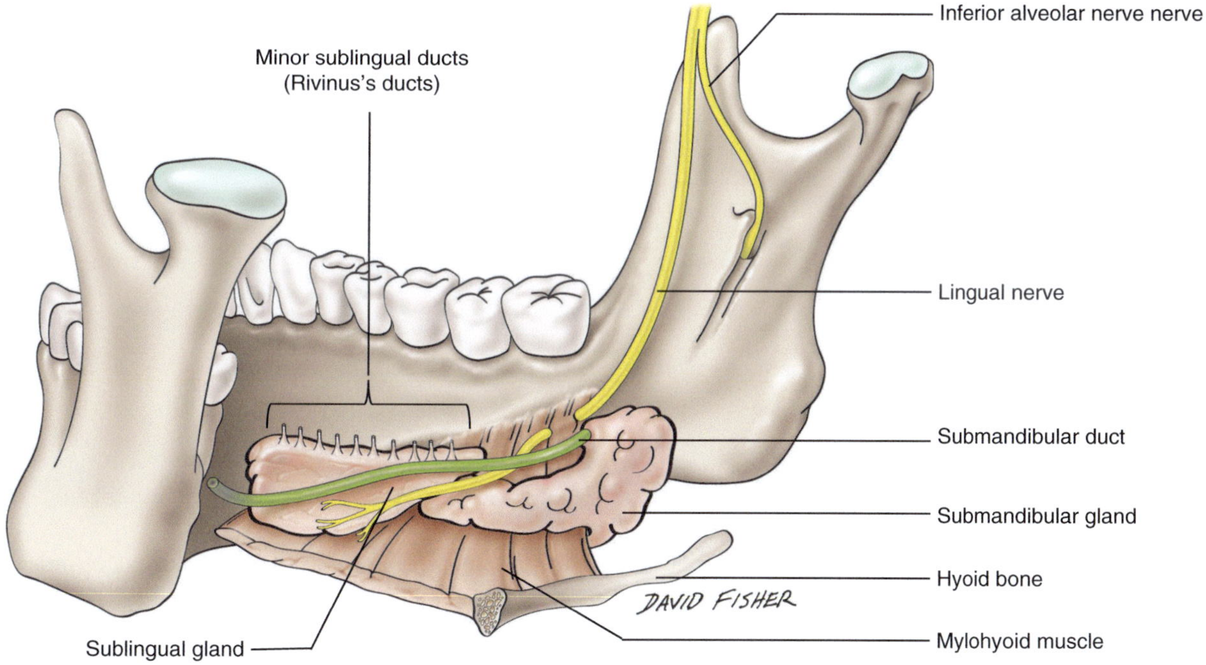

Fig. 3.95 The floor of the mouth is bound by the mylohyoid muscle inferiorly. The lingual nerve runs on the superior surface of the mylohyoid muscle and never runs inferior to the muscle. This means the position (height) of the mylohyoid muscle is one landmark for identifying the course of the lingual nerve.

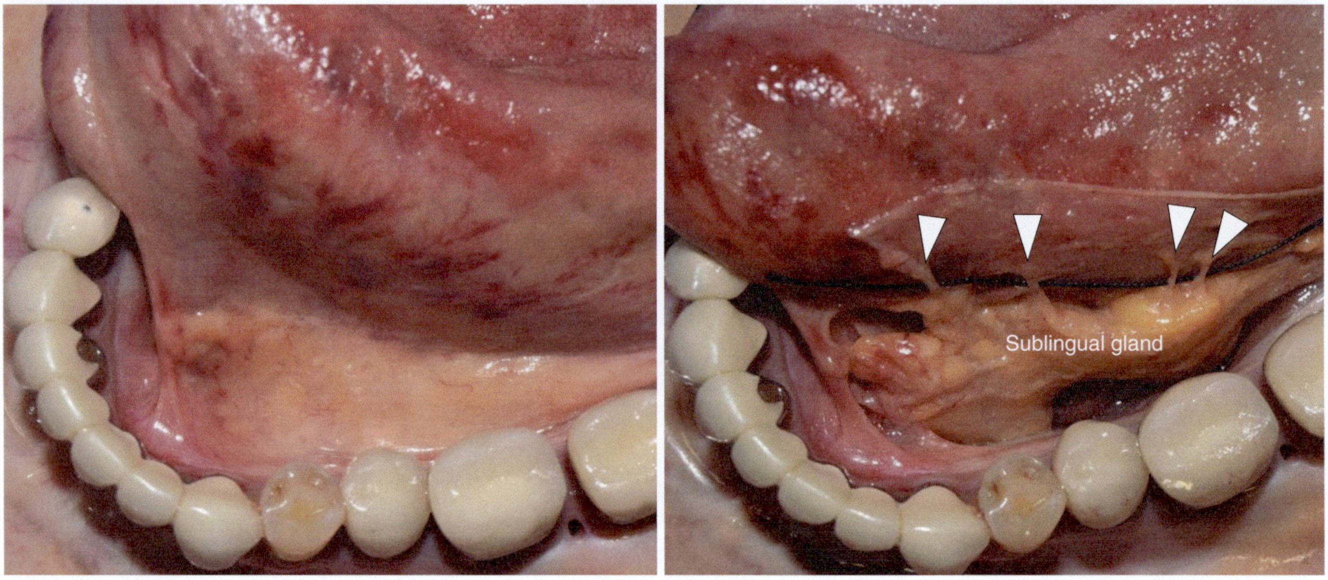

Fig. 3.97 Before (left) and after (right) the mucosa of the floor is reflected. Note that the minor sublingual ducts (Rivinus's ducts) are nearer the mucosa (arrowheads) over the sublingual gland and form the sublingual fold

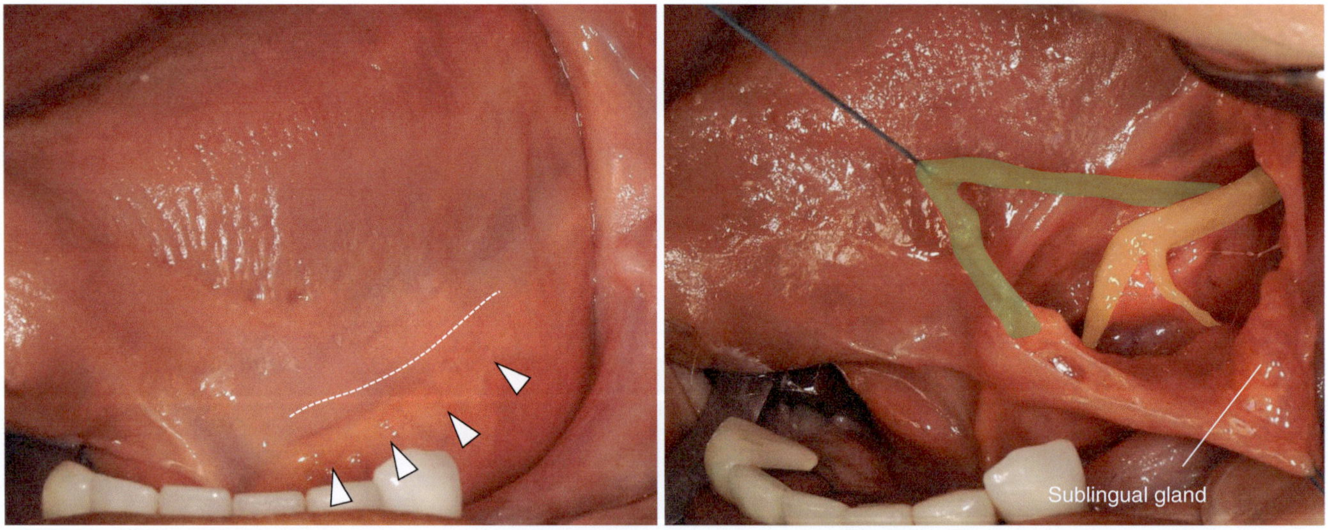

Fig. 3.98 Before (left) and after (right) mucous incision (dashed line) in the floor medial to the sublingual fold (arrowheads). Note that the incision leads to direct access to the submandibular duct (green, retracted superiorly) and lingual nerve (yellow). This shows that an incision lateral to the sublingual fold is less likely to injure the lingual nerve unless it is too deep

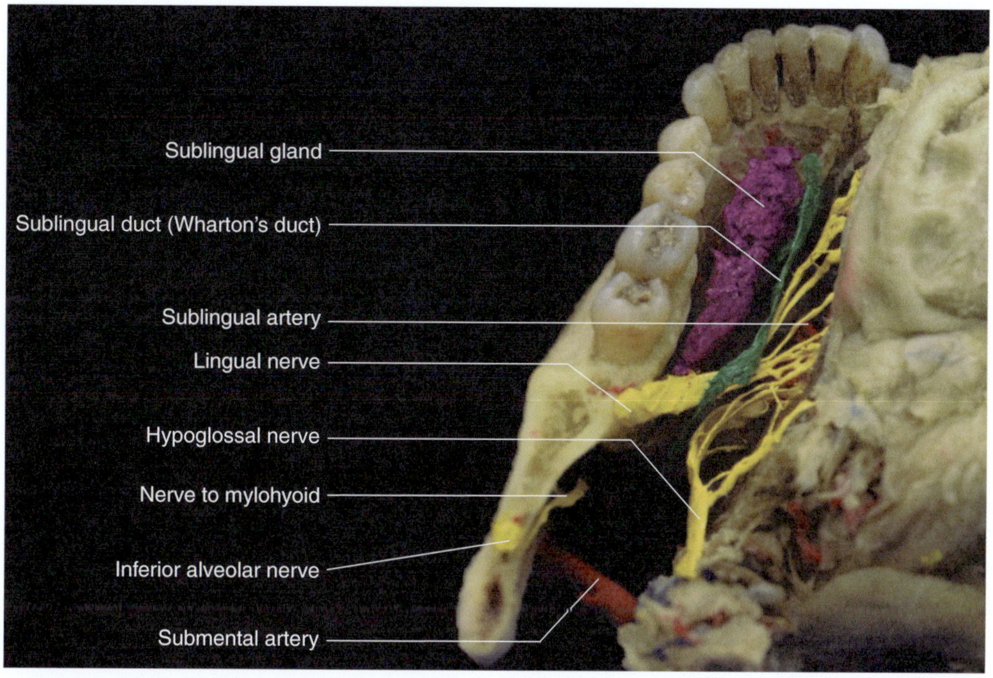

Fig. 3.99 Superior view of the floor. The mucosa and connective tissue of the floor of the mouth have been removed

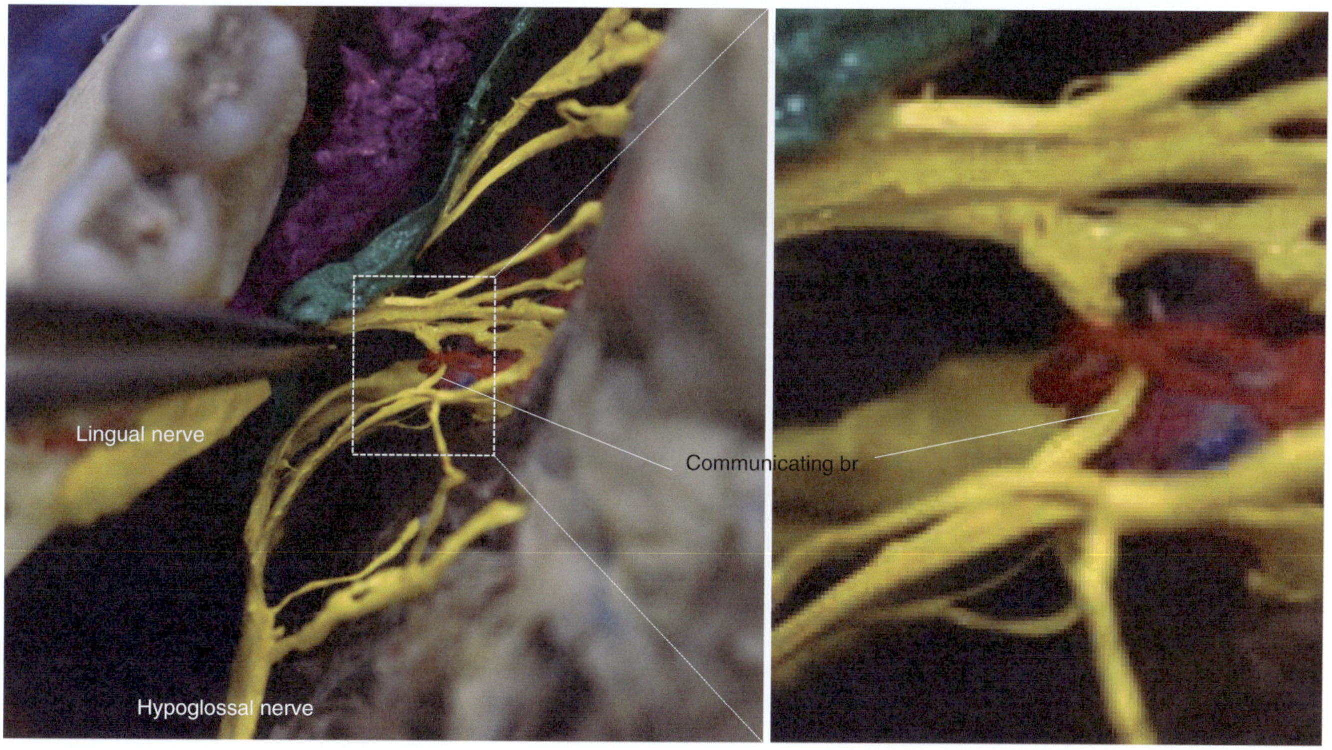

Fig. 3.100 Magnified view of the last figure. Note that a communicating branch between the lingual nerve and hypoglossal nerve is observed

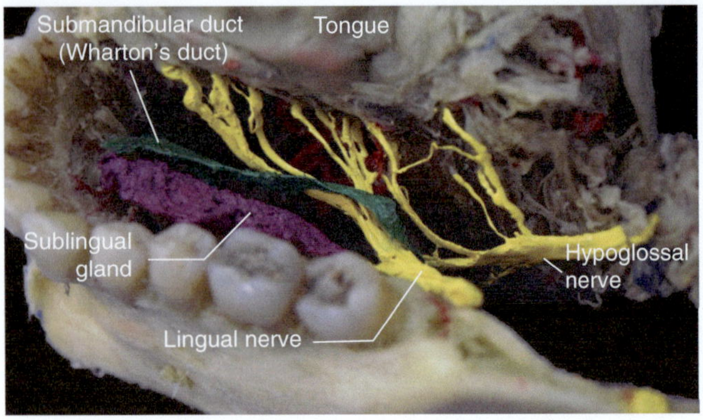

Fig. 3.101 Superolateral view of the floor of the oral cavity

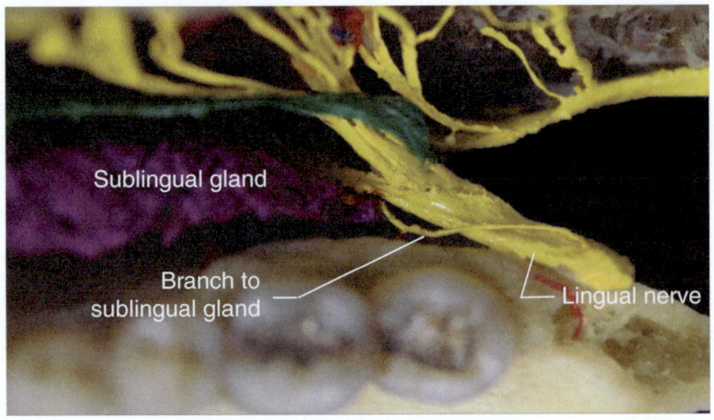

Fig. 3.102 A branch to the sublingual gland arising from the lingual nerve is shown. The postganglionic parasympathetic fibers in this branch originate from the submandibular ganglion via the chorda tympani

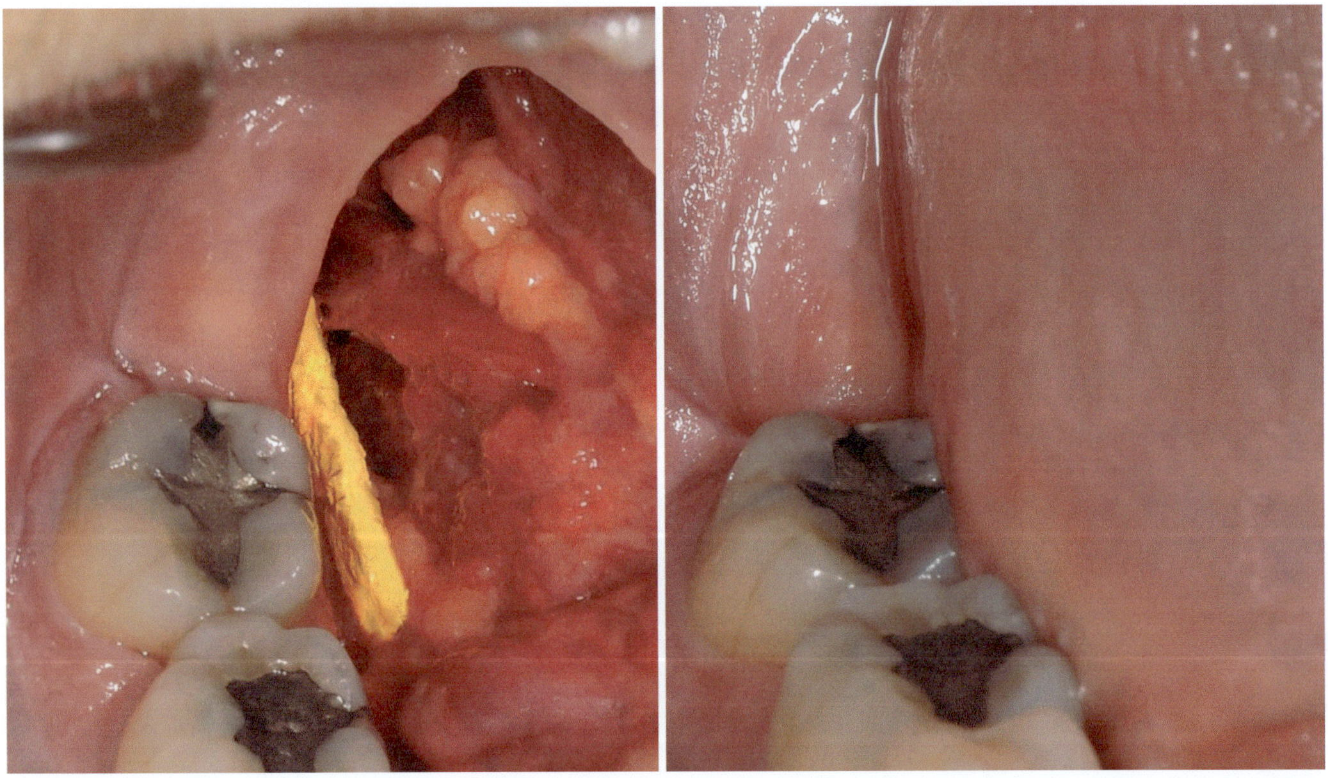

Fig. 3.103 Course of the lingual nerve. At its entry into the floor of the mouth, the lingual nerve runs next to the lingual cortical plate. This is the area where the lingual nerve is most likely to be damaged

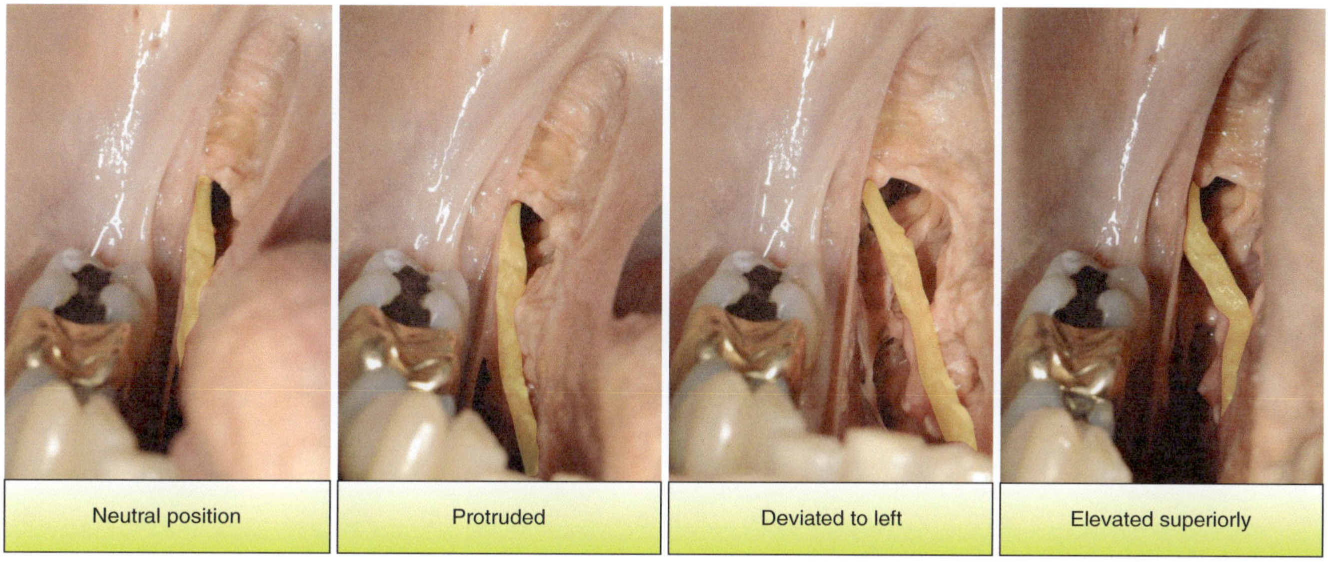

Fig. 3.104 The lingual nerve terminates at the anterior two-thirds of the tongue. So the lingual nerve always changes its course with various tongue positions. When the tongue is protruded, the course can be very close to the lingual plate. Again, the lingual nerve always runs above the mylohyoid muscle

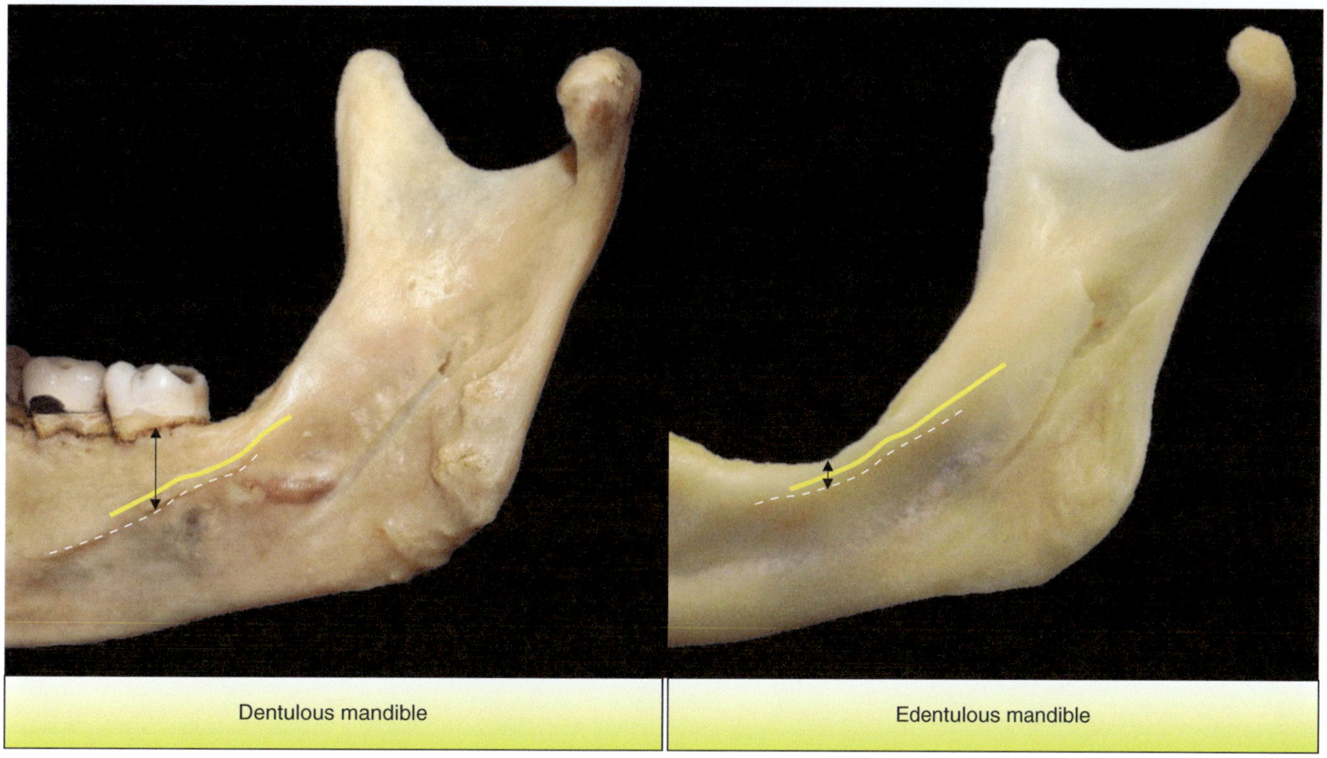

Fig. 3.105 The relative distance from the surface of the floor to the mylohyoid line (dashed lines) becomes closer when the alveolar bone is severely reduced (e.g., after tooth loss). The mylohyoid line (dashed lines) in the retromolar area is a good landmark for estimating the course of the lingual nerve (yellow lines) along the surface of the floor

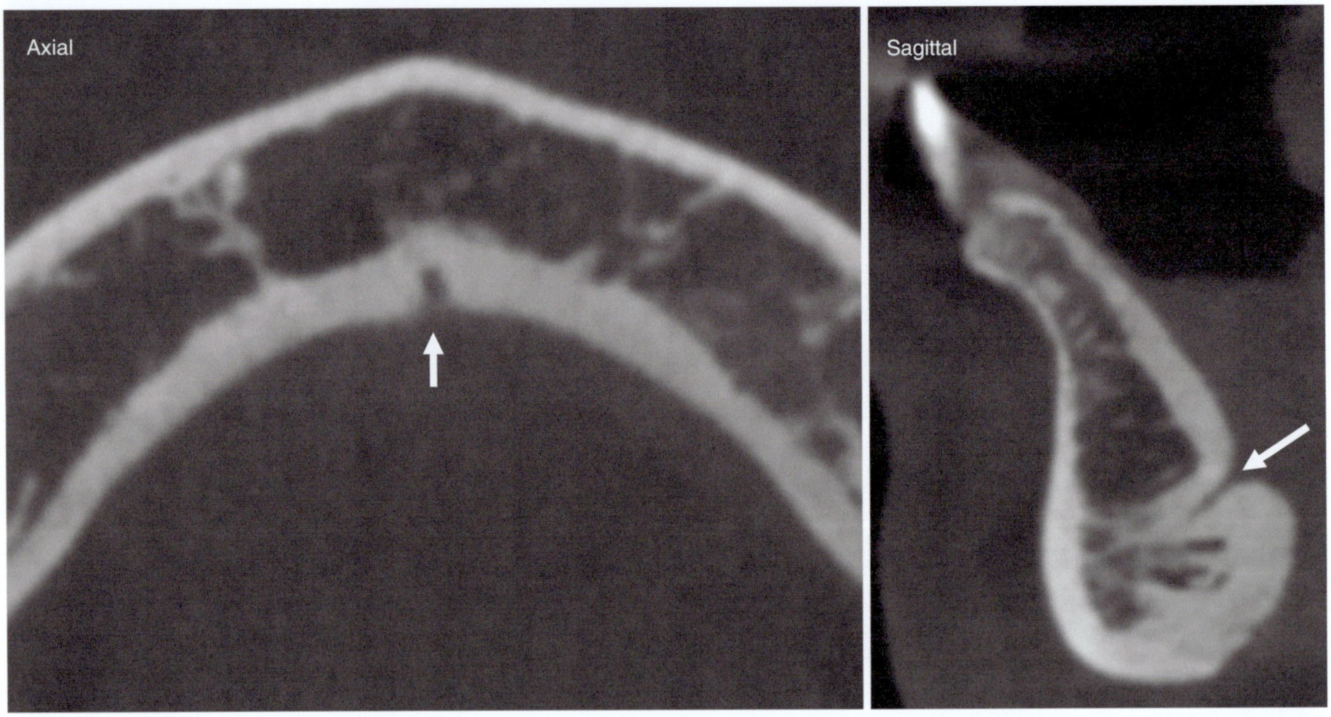

Fig. 3.106 A median lingual foramen (arrows)

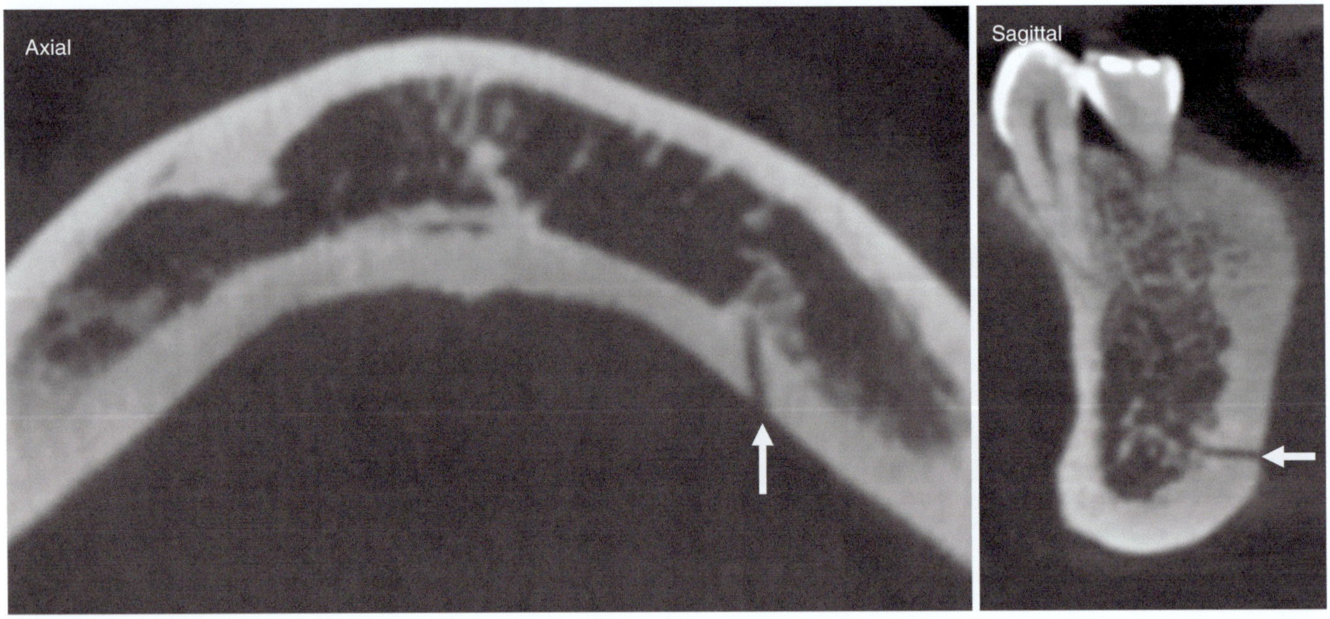

Fig. 3.107 A lateral lingual foramen (arrows)

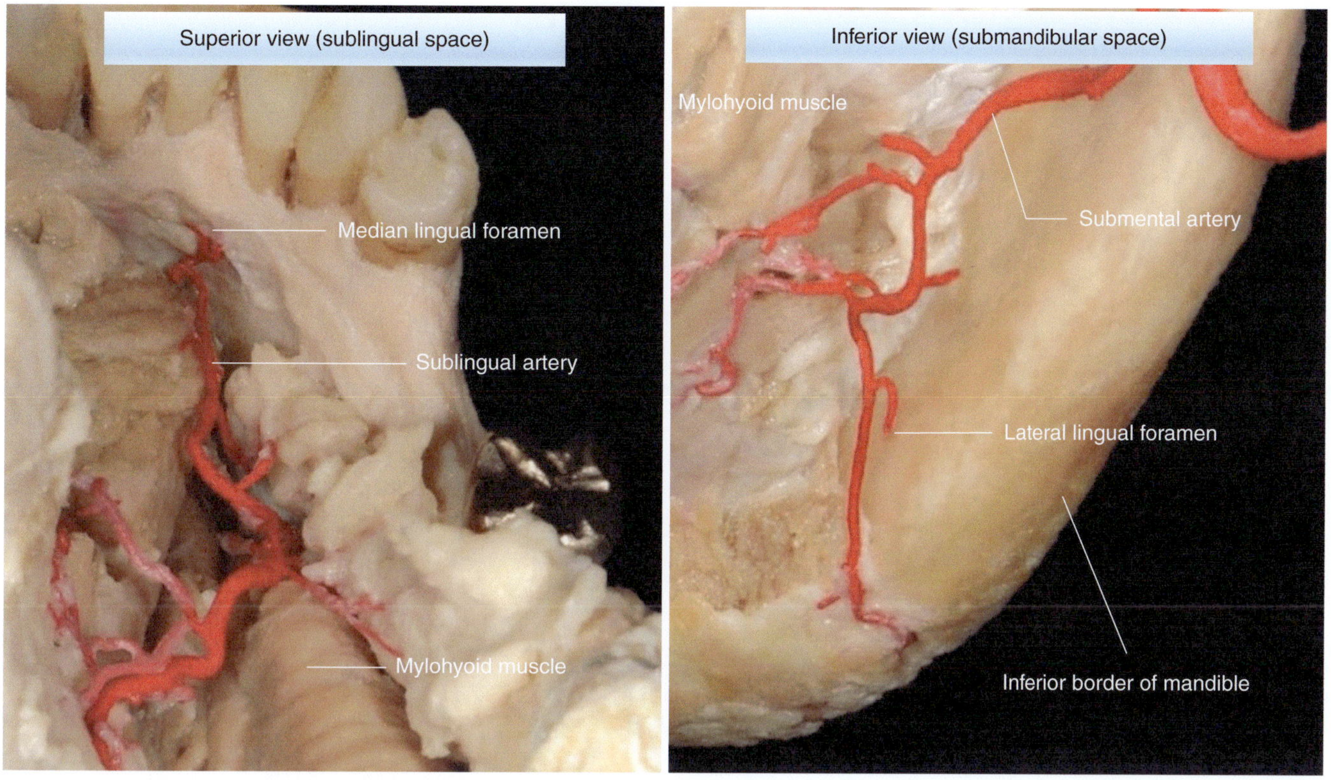

Fig. 3.108 The sublingual artery runs within the sublingual space (above the mylohyoid muscle) and gives rise to multiple branches in the floor. Some of the branches enter median/lateral lingual foramina. The submental artery runs within the submandibular space (below the mylohyoid muscle). The median/lateral lingual foramina receive the branches of the submental artery

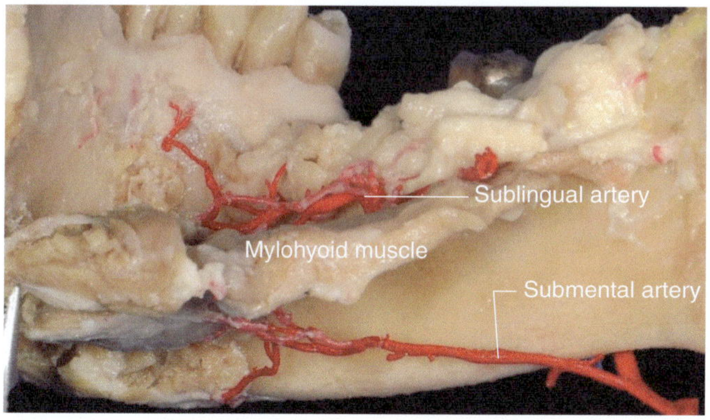

Fig. 3.109 Posterior view of the sublingual and submandibular spaces. Note that the mylohyoid muscle is a border of the oral cavity and submandibular area

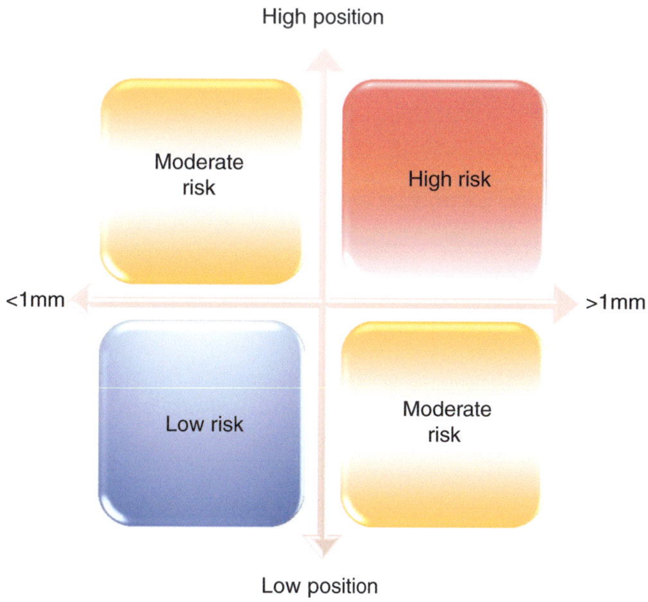

High position: superior to mental spine (MLF)/mylohyoid line (LLF)
Low position: inferior to mental spine (MLF)/mylohyoid line (LLF)

Fig. 3.110 Risk assessment chart for the lingual foramina (Iwanaga et al. 2019a). *MLF* median lingual foramen, *LLF* lateral lingual foramen

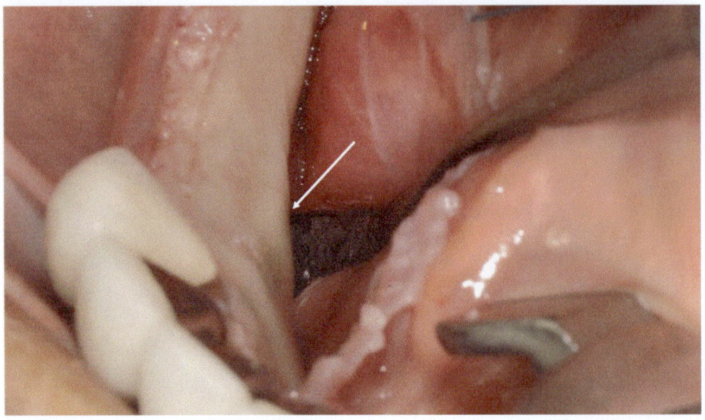

Fig. 3.111 The submandibular fossa is occasionally a deep concavity (arrow) so that the periosteal elevator might slip and tear the periosteum and lead to injury of the lingual foramina and lingual nerve. Most dentists are aware of the concavity, however, they should still be very careful not to perforate the periosteum especially if a CBCT is not taken prior to the surgery

3.10 Lip

Summary

The lips are two folds that surround the oral orifice. On each side, a labial commissure forms the angle (corner) of the mouth, usually near the first premolar tooth. The center of the upper lip has a shallow vertical groove, i.e., the philtrum, which is bounded by the columella of the nose superiorly. The lower lip has a small depression in the midline that corresponds to the tubercle. The junction between the hair bearing external skin and the hairless red surface of the upper lip usually forms the so-called Cupid's bow (Standring 2015). The blood supply of the lip is provided mainly by the facial artery and its branches. Skin sensation is provided by the trigeminal nerve and the cervical plexus. Histologically, the free external surface of the lips is covered by a thin keratinized epidermis, which is continuous with the mucosa at the vermilion (red) zone (Standring 2015). General knowledge of lip anatomy is necessary for surgeries in and around the lip such as cosmetic and reconstructive surgeries.

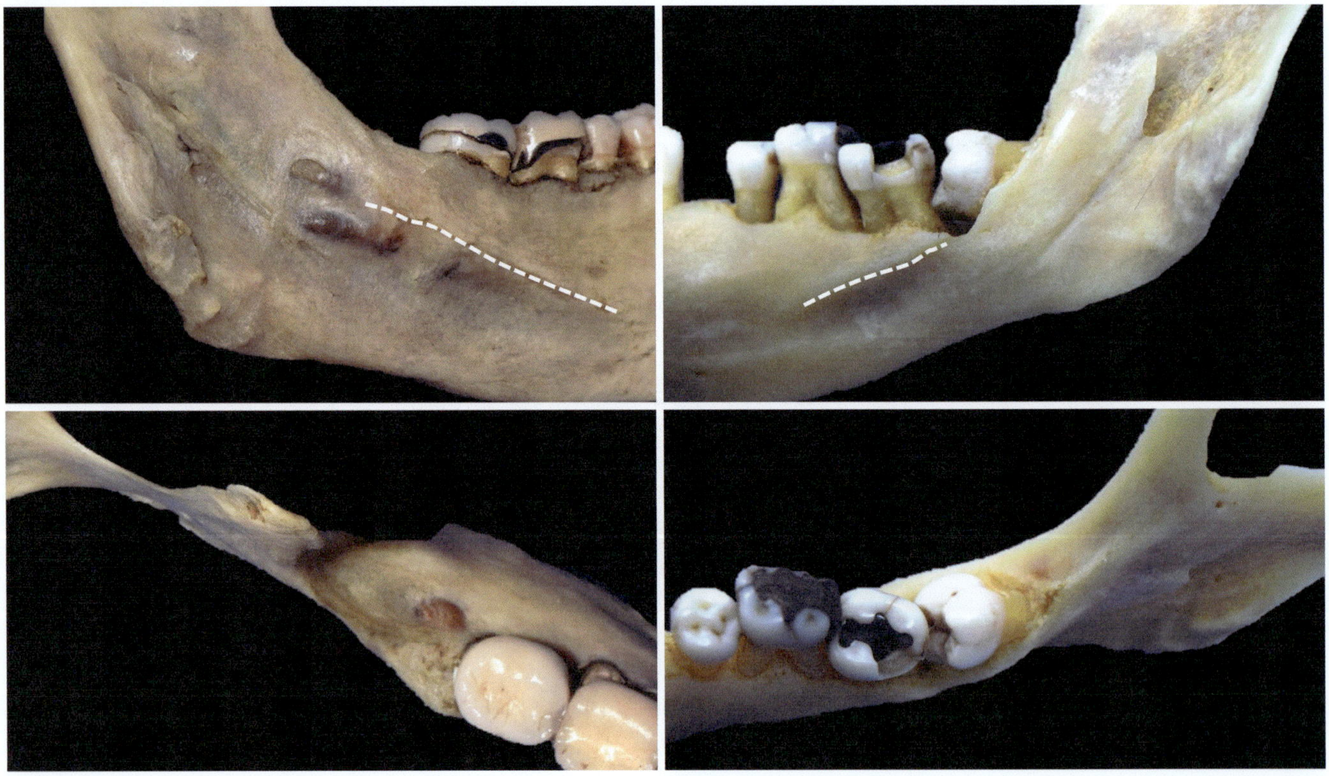

Fig. 3.112 Impacted lower third molar. It is easy to understand why perforation of the lingual cortical plate or displacement of the impacted lower wisdom tooth/fragment to the sublingual and submandibular spaces could lead to lingual nerve paresthesia. The lingual nerve runs just above the mylohyoid muscle. The muscle's origin (mylohyoid line) is shown as the dashed lines

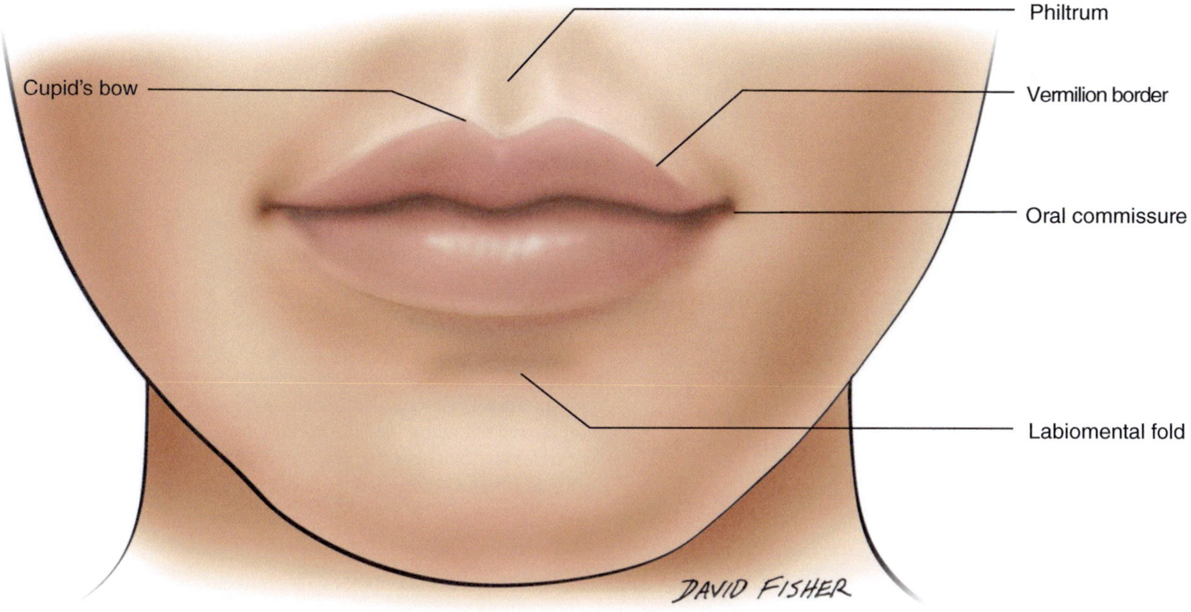

Fig. 3.113 Surface anatomy of the lip. © Fisher/Tubbs 2020. All Rights Reserved

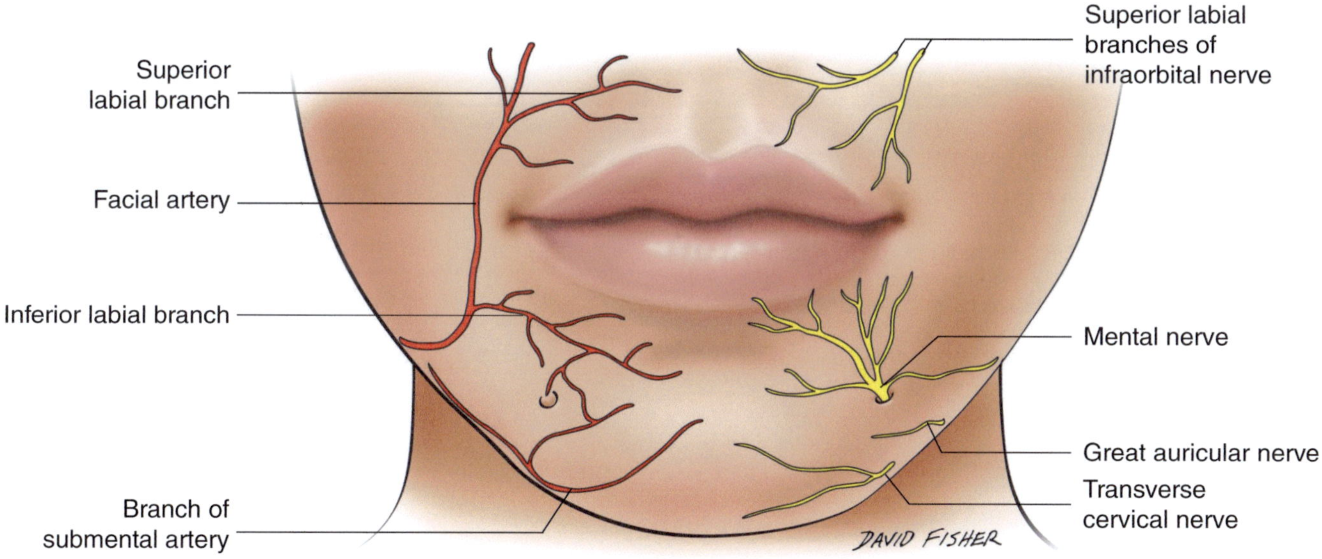

Fig. 3.114 Blood supply and sensory innervation of the lips. © Fisher/Tubbs 2020. All Rights Reserved

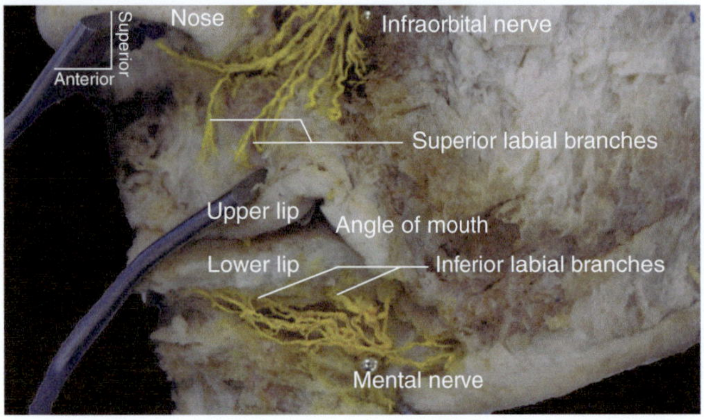

Fig. 3.115 Extraoral dissection showing the superior labial branches of the infraorbital nerve and inferior labial branches of the mental nerve innervating the upper and lower lips, respectively

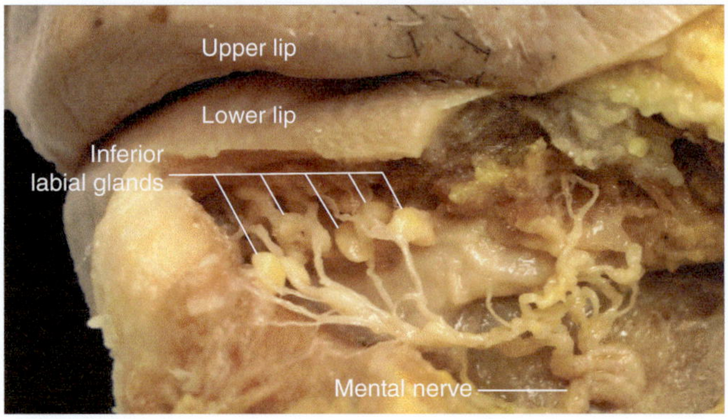

Fig. 3.117 Extraoral dissection (a part of the orbicularis oris is removed) showing the inferior labial glands here innervated by the inferior labial branches of the mental nerve. The postganglionic parasympathetic fibers to these glands might originate from the otic ganglion

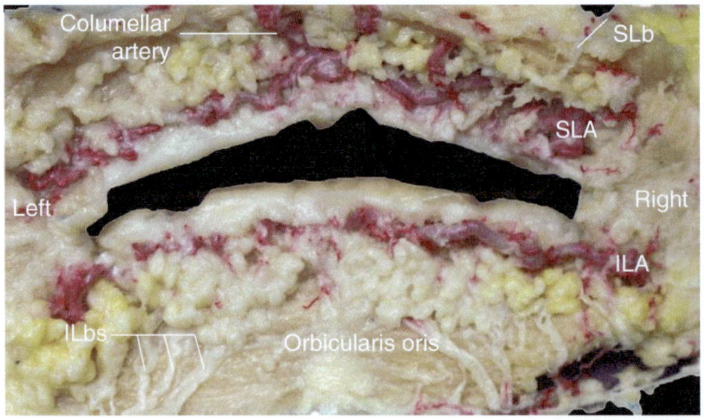

Fig. 3.116 Posterior view of the upper and lower lips. The superior labial (SLA) and inferior labial (ILA) arteries supply the upper and lower lips, respectively. The superior labial branch (SLb) of the infraorbital nerve and inferior labial branch (ILb) of the mental nerve innervate the upper and lower lips, respectively. Note that the superior labial glands are larger in size in the midline, whereas, the inferior labial glands are larger in size around the corner of the mouth

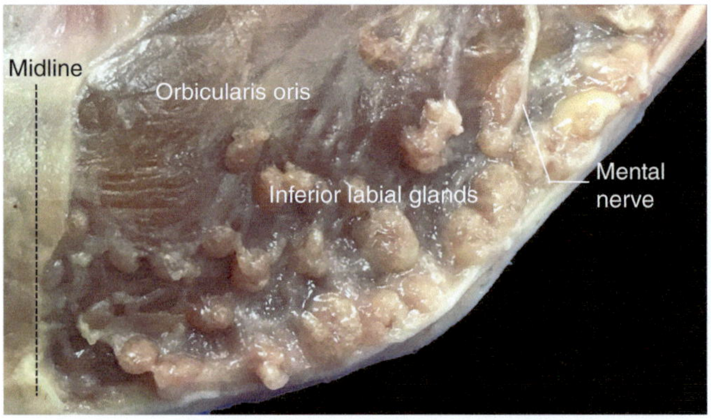

Fig. 3.118 Intraoral dissection (labial mucosa is removed) showing the inferior labial glands with an innervation from the inferior labial branches of the mental nerve. Note that the glands are located on the surface of the orbicularis oris muscle

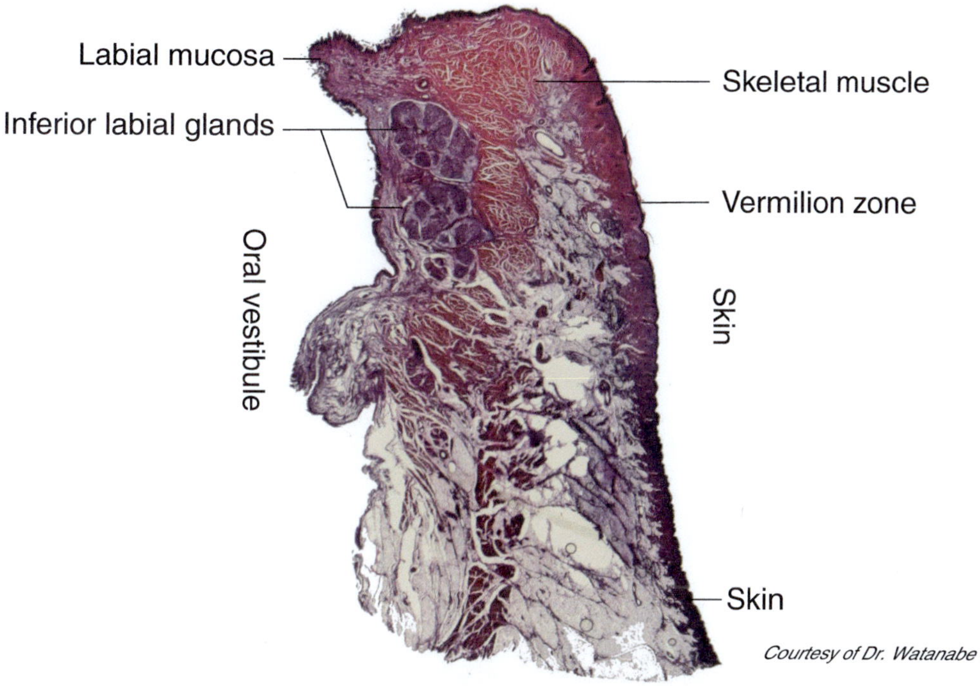

Fig. 3.119 Parasagittal section of the lower lip. Between the skin and mucosa, the vermilion zone is covered with a specialized keratinized stratified squamous epithelium. The epithelium is thin near the skin but gradually thickens as it approaches the mucosa and then becomes thick abruptly when it reaches the mucosa (Standring 2015). Note the inferior labial glands are located just beneath the labial mucosa

3.11 Temporomandibular Joint

Summary

The temporomandibular joint (TMJ) is classified as a synovial joint that allows elevation, rotation, permits gliding, and depression and normally functions in mastication, biting, suckling, yawning, swallowing, and speaking. The mandibular fossa, the articular eminence of the temporal bone, and the mandibular condyle all contribute to the TMJ. The articular surfaces of the TMJ are uniquely lined with fibrocartilage rather than the normal hyaline cartilage. Its joint cavity is divided into superior and inferior joint spaces by an articular disc, and the disc attaches to the capsule. The main muscles that allow for TMJ articulation are the masseter, temporalis, and medial and lateral pterygoid muscles known as the muscles of mastication. From a clinical perspective, understanding the anatomy of the TMJ is significant for TMJ surgery, diagnosis of temporomandibular joint disorders, and related diseases and treatments.

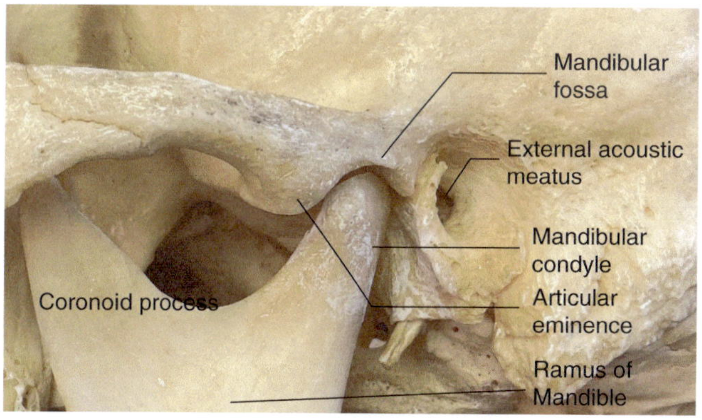

Fig. 3.120 The mandibular fossa, the articular eminence of the temporal bone, and the mandibular condyle form the TMJ. Note the external acoustic meatus is located just behind the TMJ

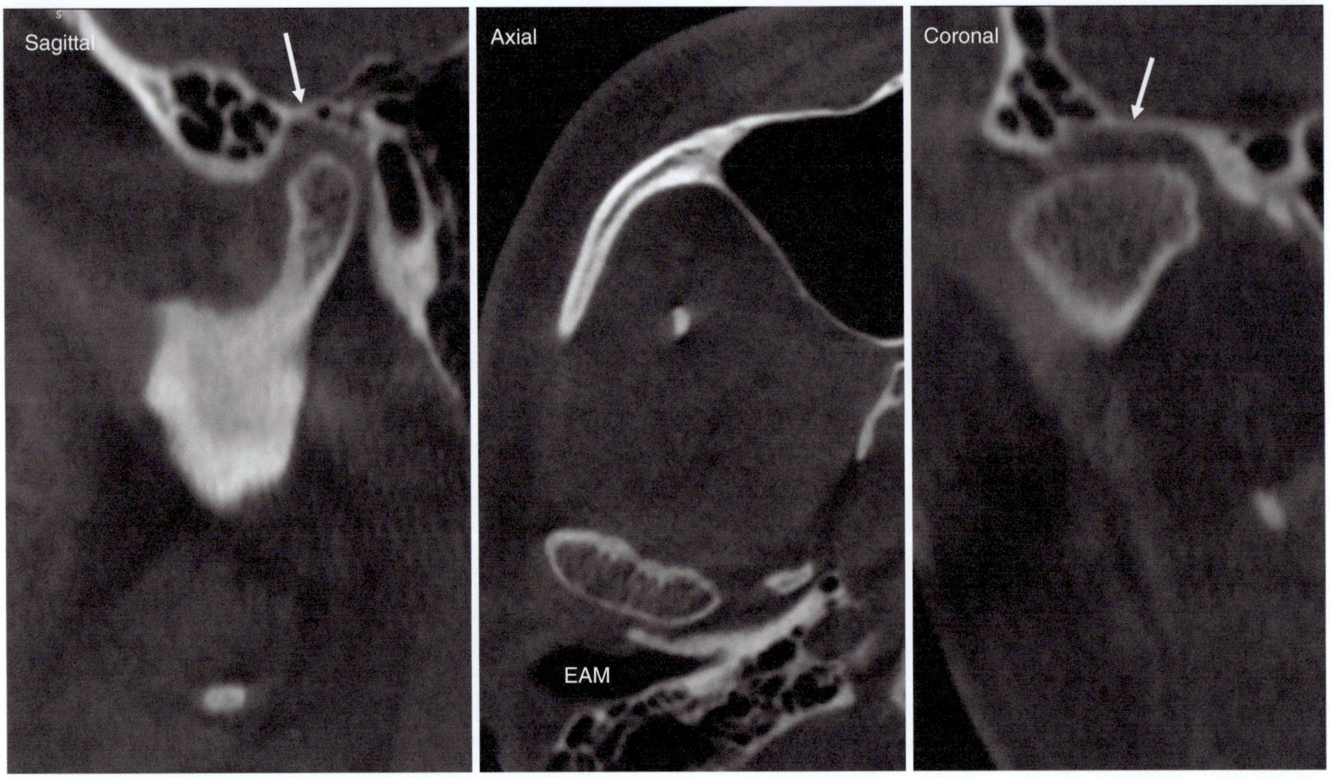

Fig. 3.121 CBCT images of the TMJ. The external acoustic meatus (EAM) is positioned just behind the condyle. The thinnest part of the mandibular fossa (arrows) is 1.0–1.2 mm (Al-Koshab et al. 2015)

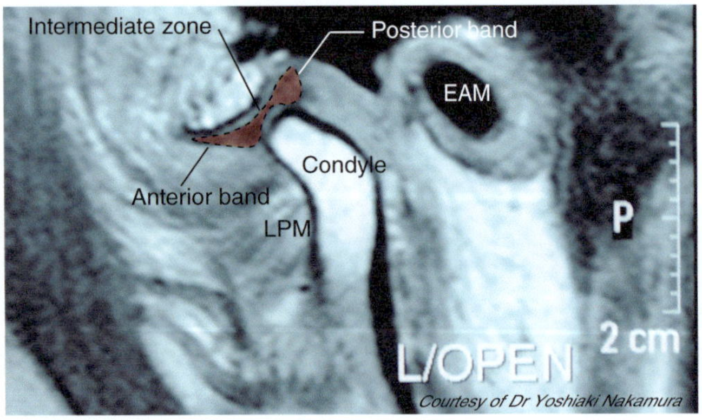

Fig. 3.122 Sagittal MRI image of the right TMJ. The articular disc has three distinct parts: anterior band, thinner intermediate zone, and posterior band. The intermediate zone lacks vascularity and acts as the force-accepting segment. The external acoustic meatus (EAM) is positioned just posterior to the condyle. Note that the disc (red area) appears as a "bow tie." LPM lateral pterygoid muscle

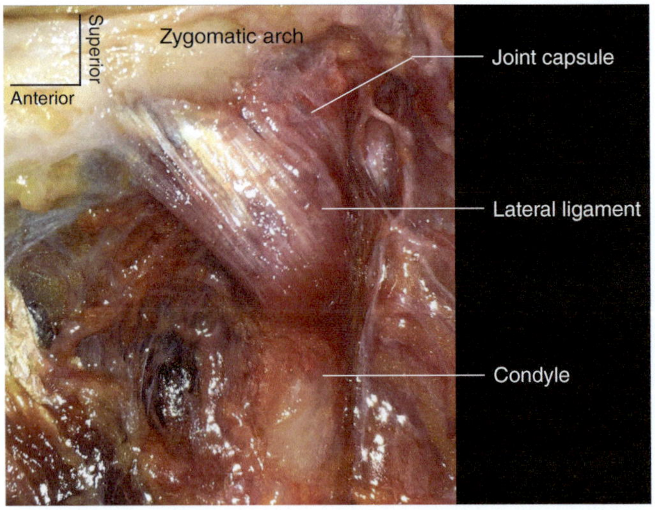

Fig. 3.123 Cadaveric dissection of the left TMJ. Note both the capsule and lateral ligament attach to the condyle and zygomatic arch

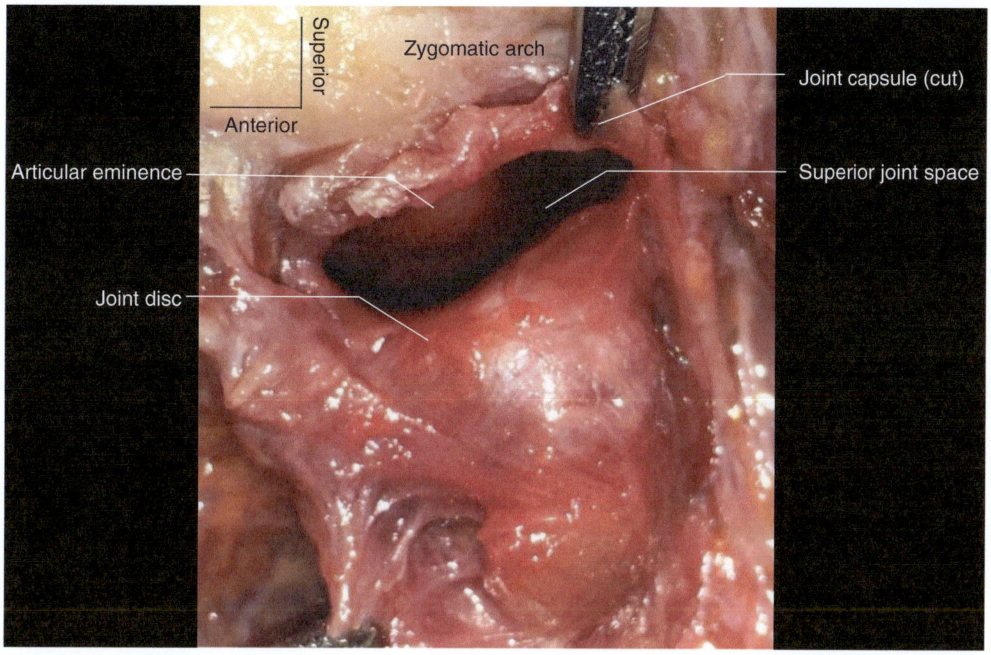

Fig. 3.124 Cadaveric dissection of the left TMJ. Note both the capsule and lateral ligament were incised and the superior joint space is being observed

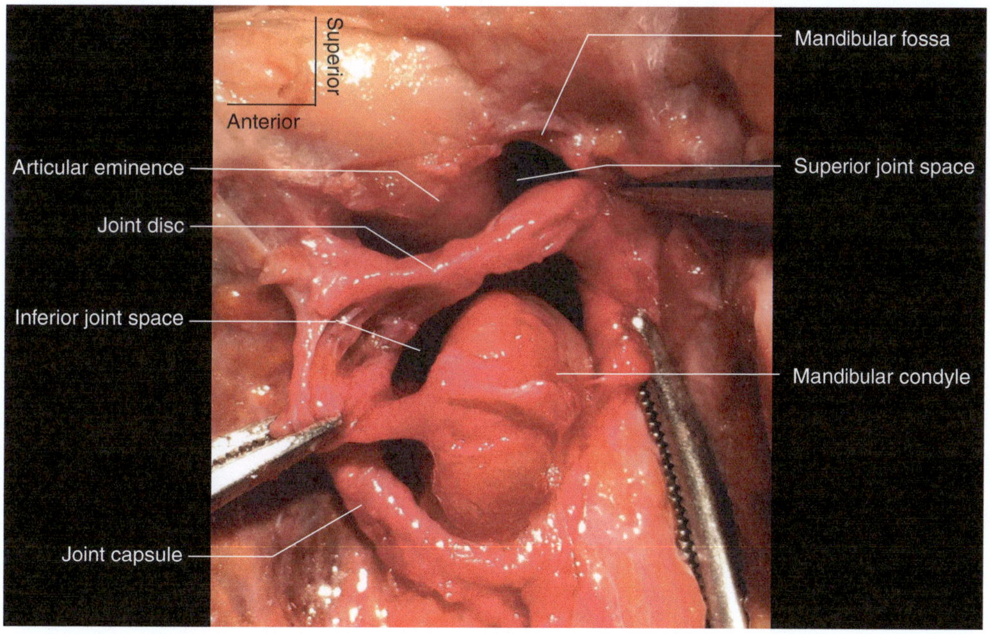

Fig. 3.125 Cadaveric dissection of the left TMJ. The joint disc has been opened. The inferior joint space is now observed between the joint disc and condyle

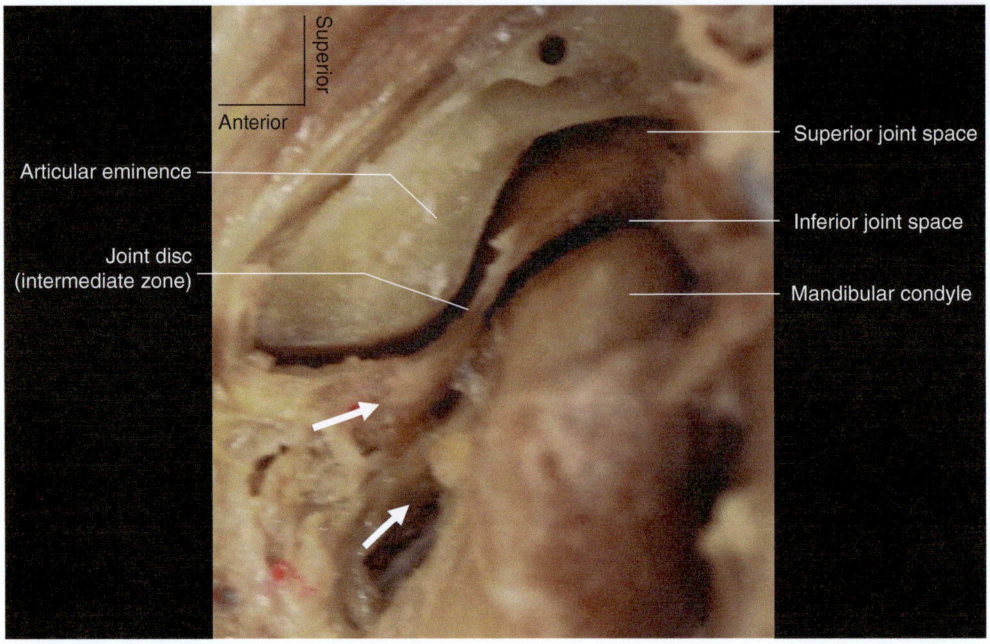

Fig. 3.126 Cadaveric dissection of the left TMJ. Note the lateral pterygoid muscle inserts into both the disc and neck of the condyle (arrows)

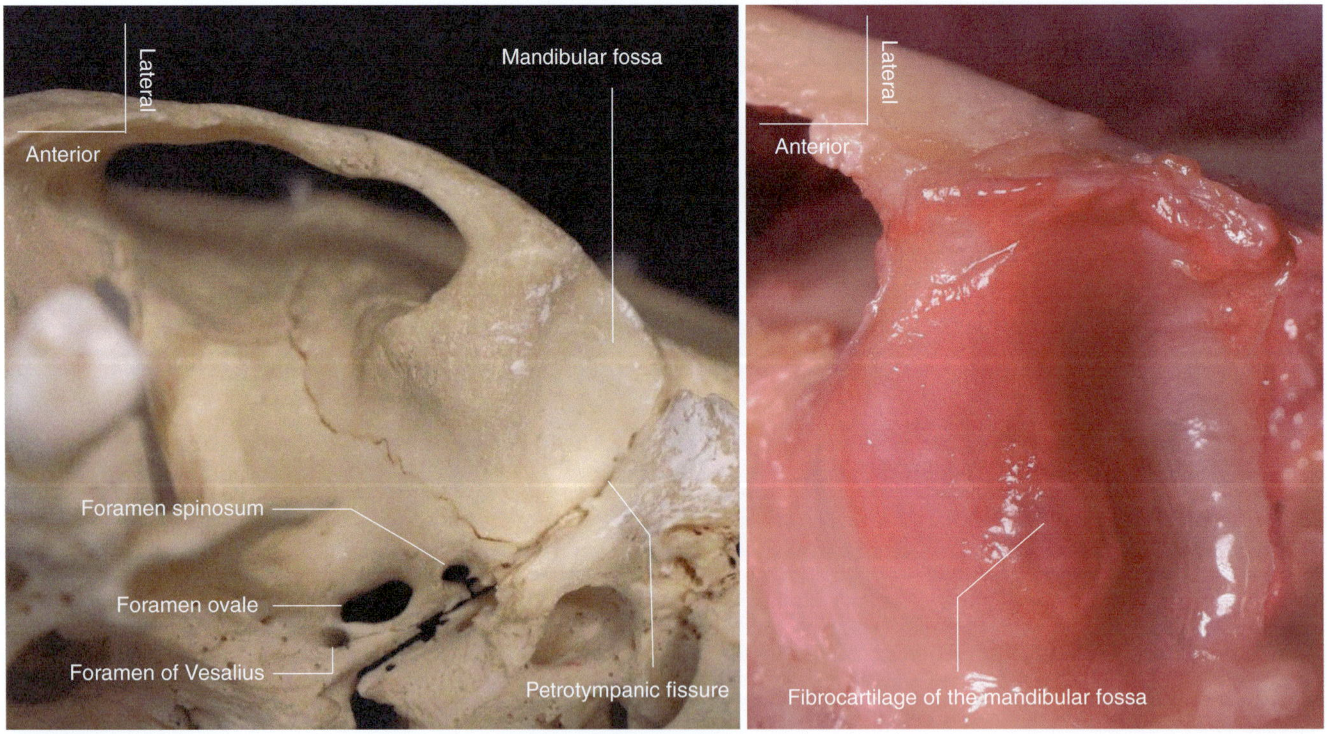

Fig. 3.127 Inferior view of the mandibular fossa. The presence of fibrocartilage rather than hyaline cartilage is important because it has the ability to repair and remodel. The thinnest portion of the mandibular fossa may be lined with synovial membranes

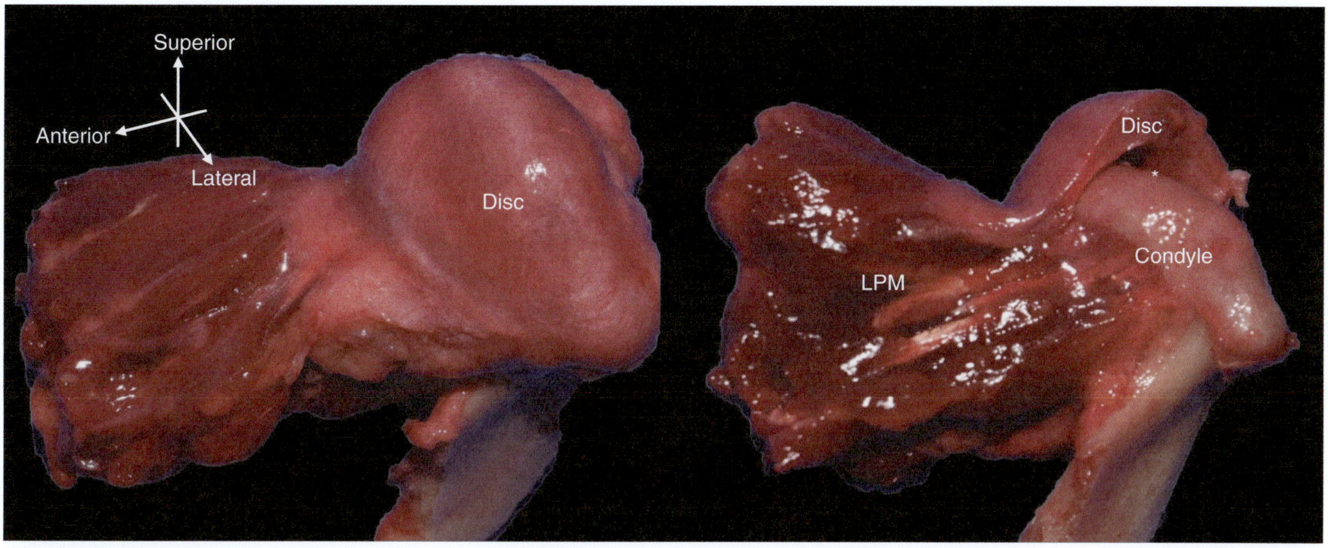

Fig. 3.128 Superolateral view of the joint disc. The disc does not look like a plate/sheet which is often shown in sagittal images but rather as a cap that covers the entire condyle (left figure). The lateral pterygoid muscle (LPM) inserts into the disc and neck of the condyle (right figure). The inferior joint space* is observed between the disc and condyle

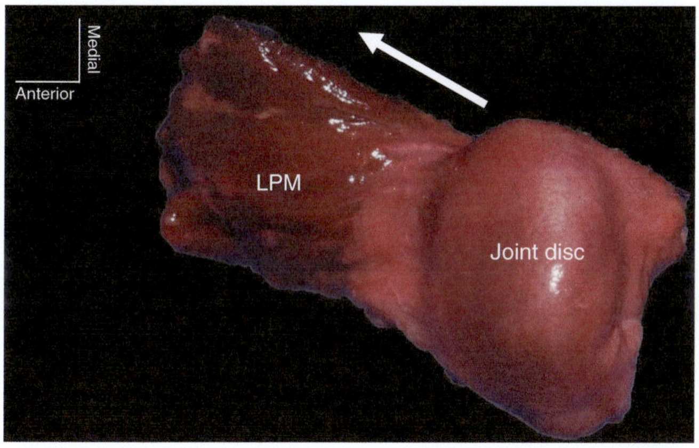

Fig. 3.129 Superior view of the joint disc and lateral pterygoid muscle (LPM). The LPM originates from the lateral plate of the pterygoid process so that the LPM courses anteromedial to posterolateral. As a result, the LPM inserts into only the anterior and medial parts of the disc and neck of the condyle, not the lateral part. This is one of the reasons why the mandible deviates to the contralateral side when the unilateral lateral pterygoid muscle contracts (arrow)

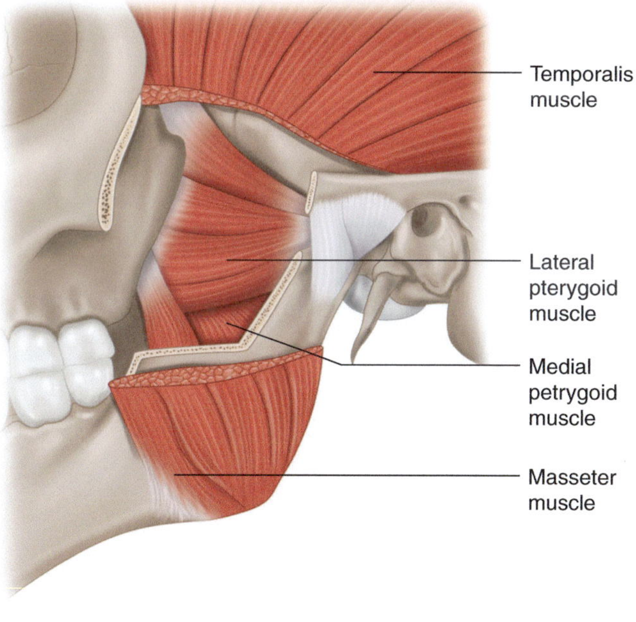

Fig. 3.130 Lateral view of the four muscles of masstication. The zygomatic arch and coronoid process have been resected

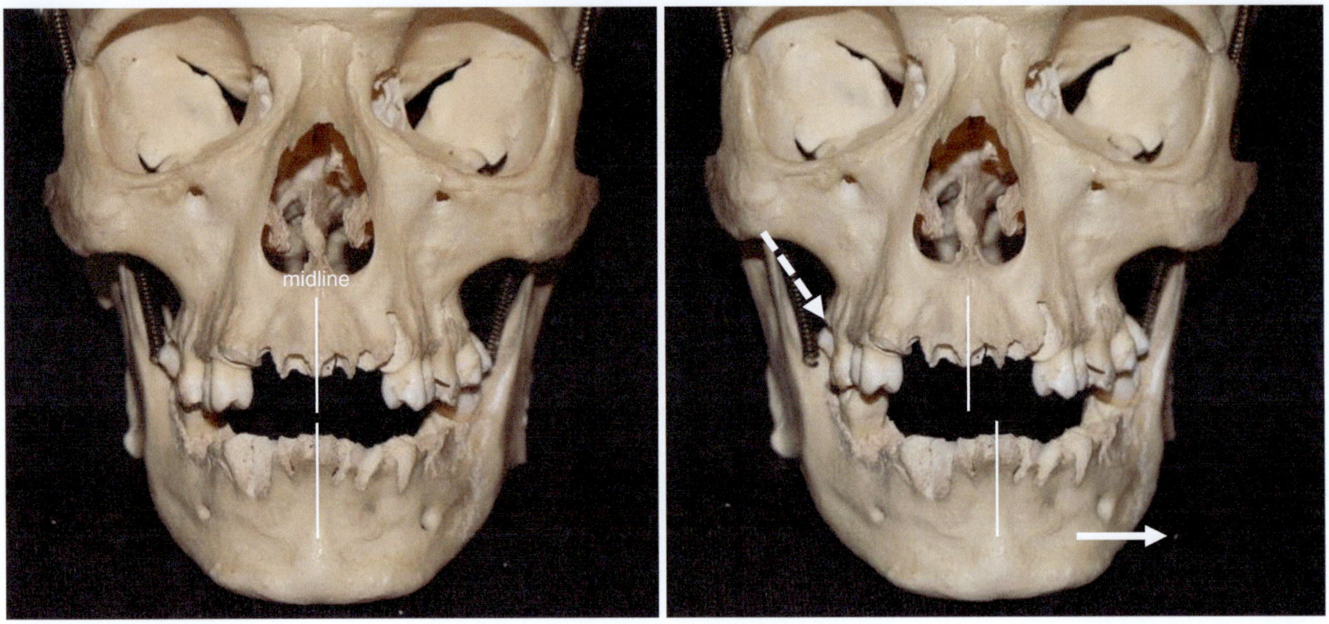

Fig. 3.131 Unilateral lateral pterygoid muscle contraction (dashed arrow) moves the jaw to the contralateral side (arrow)

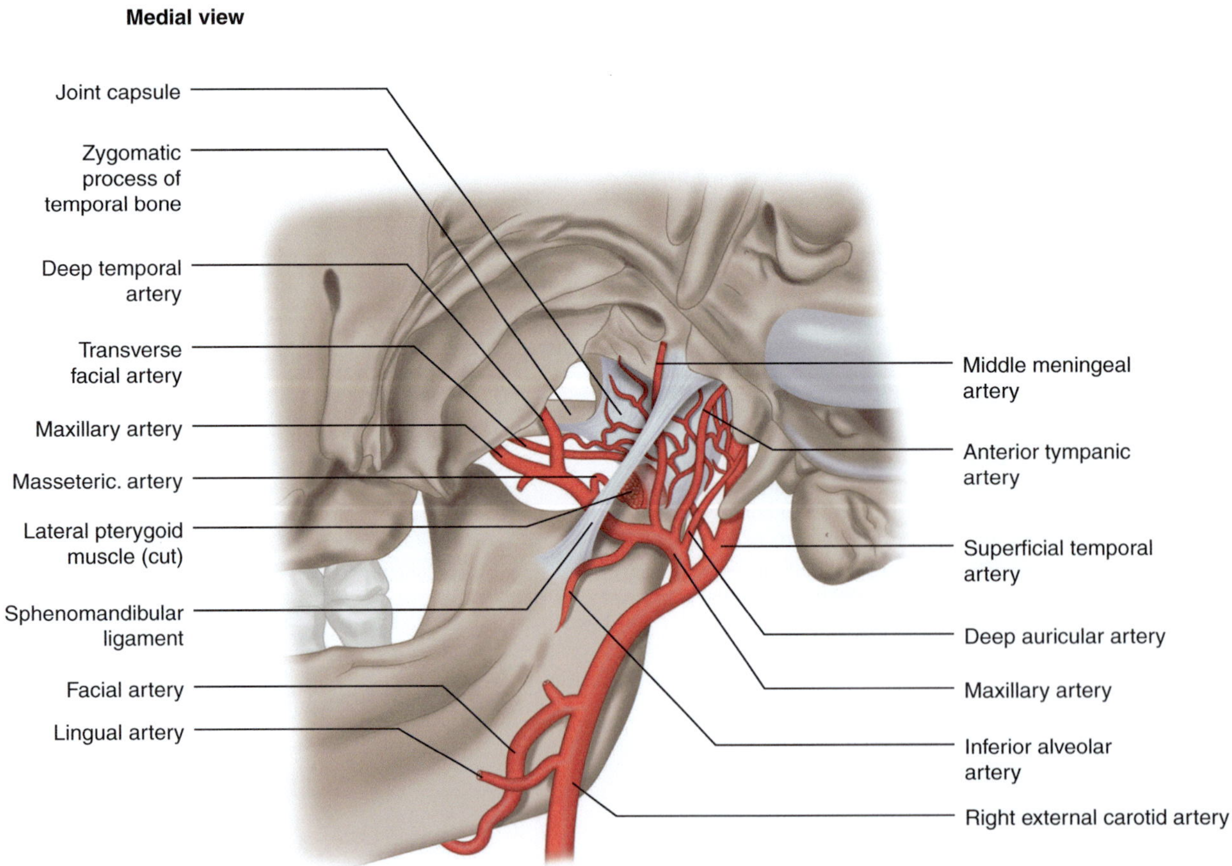

Fig. 3.132 Medial view of the blood supply of the TMJ

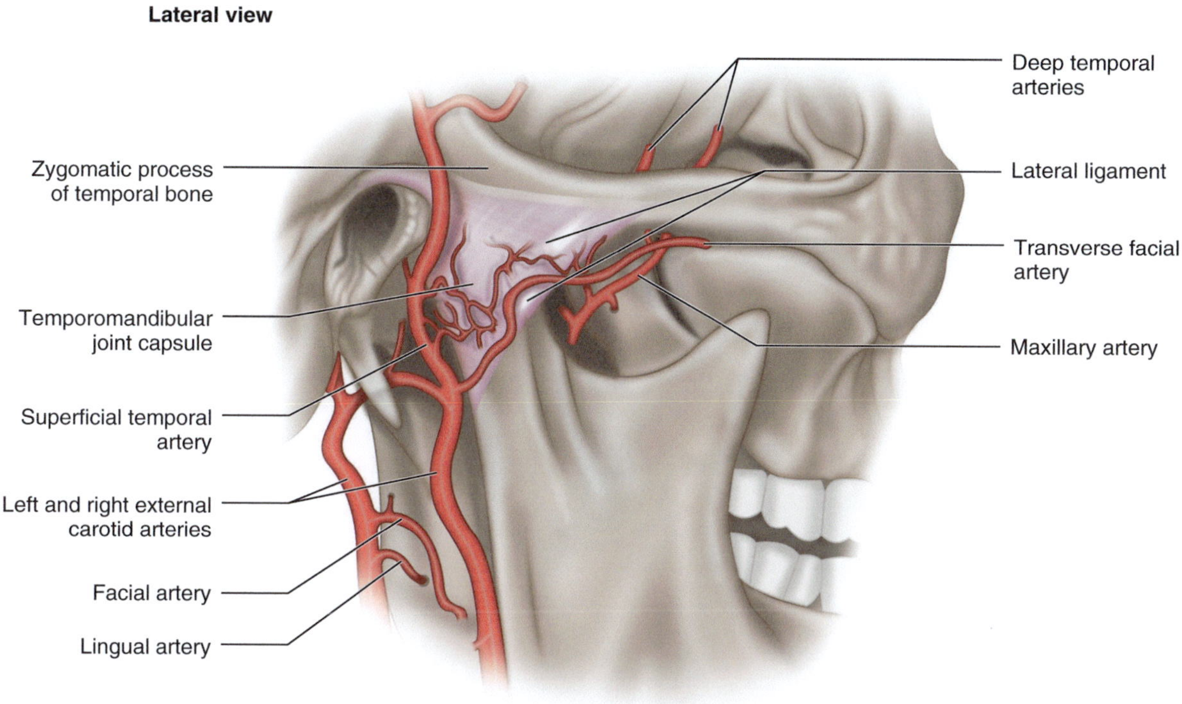

Fig. 3.133 Lateral view of the blood supply of the TMJ

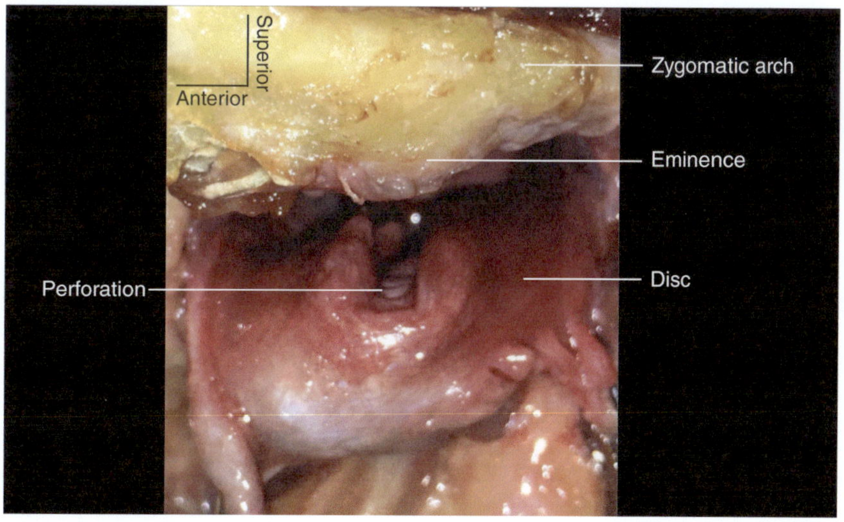

Fig. 3.134 Perforation of the left joint disc (superolateral view)

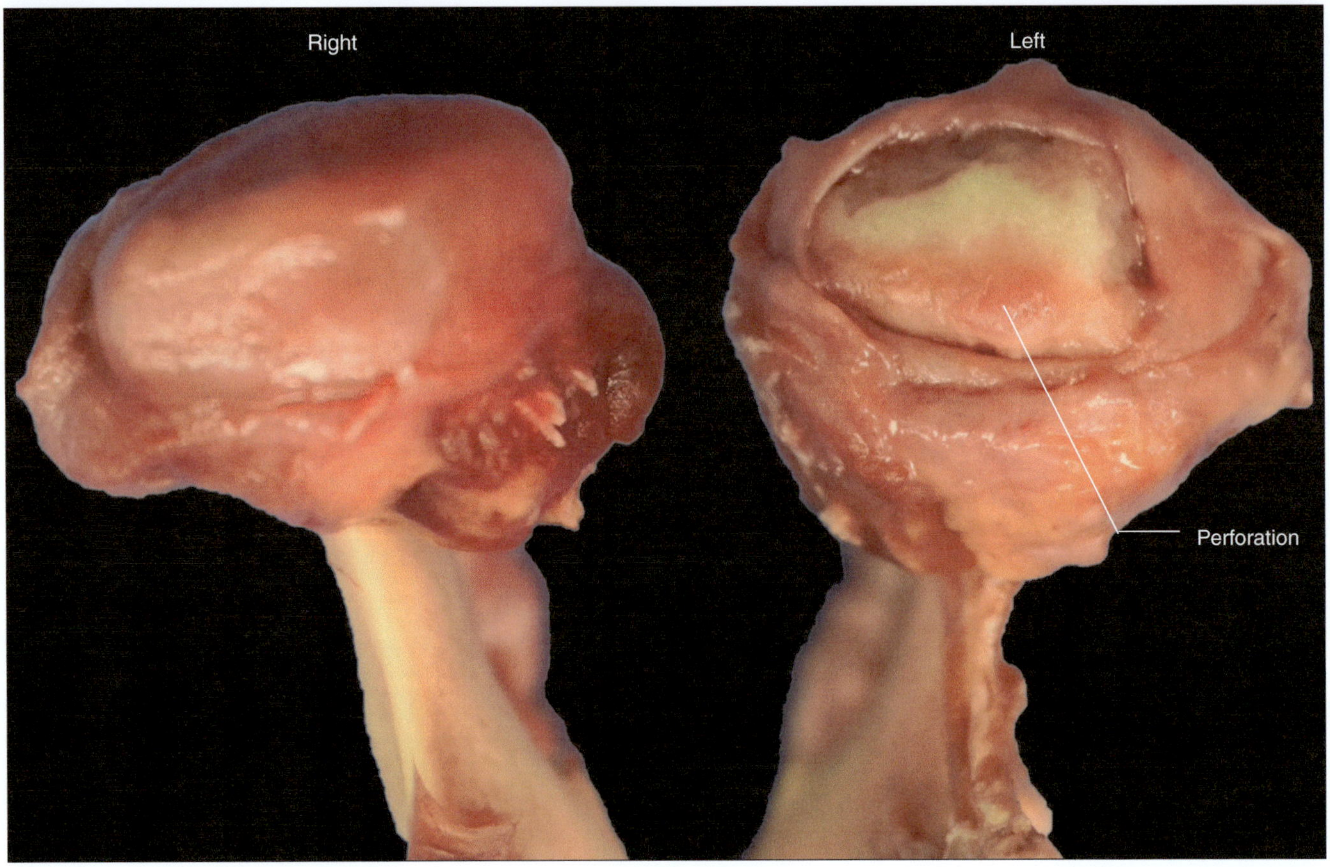

Fig. 3.135 Perforation of the left joint disc (anterosuperior view)

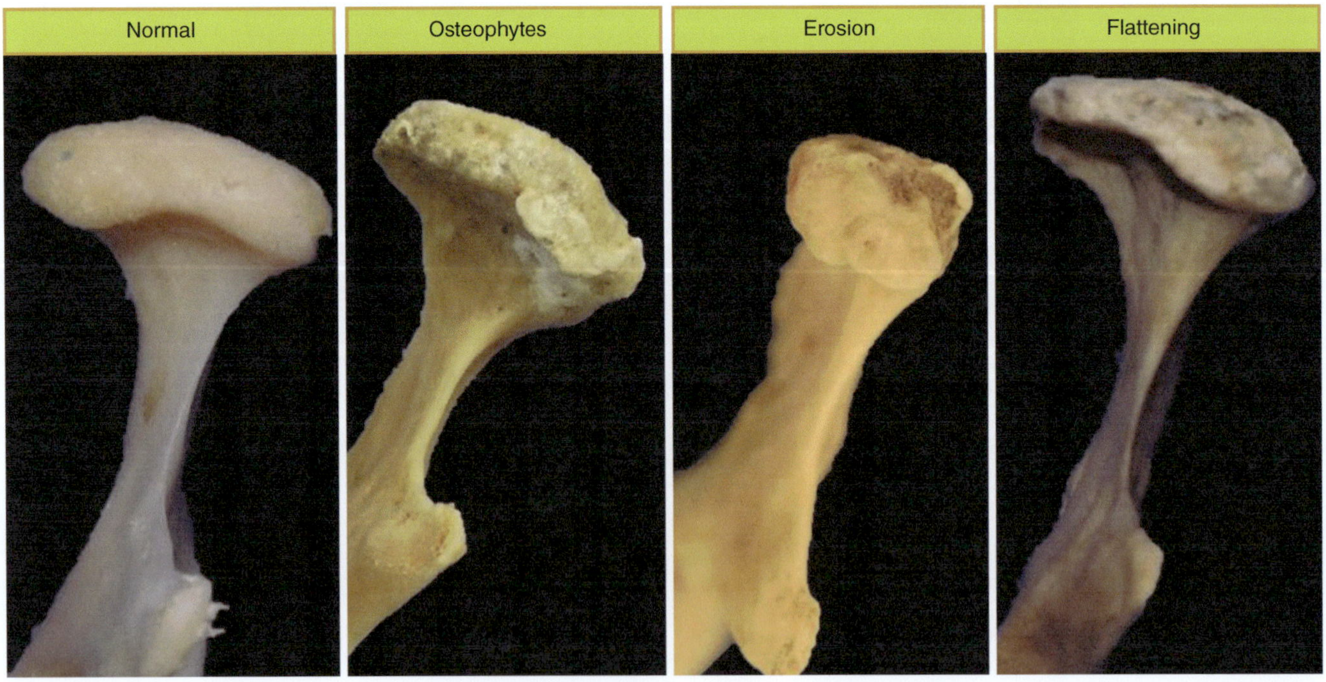

Fig. 3.136 Variations of the structural change of the head of the condyle

References

Al-Koshab M, Nambiar P, John J. Assessment of condyle and glenoid fossa morphology using CBCT in south-east Asians. PLoS One. 2015;10(3):e0121682. https://doi.org/10.1371/journal.pone.0121682.

Carter RB, Keen E. The intramandibular course of the inferior alveolar nerve. J Anat. 1971;108(Pt 3):433.

Chitsazi MT, Shirmohammadi A, Faramarzi M, Esmaieli F, Chitsazi S. Evaluation of the position of the posterior superior alveolar artery in relation to the maxillary sinus using the cone-beam computed tomography scans. J Clin Exp Dent. 2017;9:e394–9.

Danesh-Sani SA, Movahed A, ElChaar ES, Chong Chan K, Amintavakoli N. Radiographic evaluation of maxillary sinus lateral wall and posterior superior alveolar artery anatomy: a cone beam computed tomographic study. Clin Implant Dent Relat Res. 2017;19:151–60.

Gosau M, Rink D, Driemel O, Draenert FG. Maxillary sinus anatomy: a cadaveric study with clinical implications. Anat Rec (Hoboken). 2009;292:352–4.

Hafeez NS, Ganapathy S, Sondekoppam R, Johnson M, Merrifield P, Galil KS. Anatomical variations of the greater palatine nerve in the greater palatine canal. J Can Dent Assoc. 2015;81:f14.

Iwanaga J, Tubbs RS. Buccal nerve dissection via an intraoral approach: correcting an error regarding buccal nerve blockade. J Oral Maxillofac Surg. 2019;77(6):1154–e1.

Iwanaga J, Saga T, Tabira Y, Nakamura M, Kitashima S, Watanabe K, Yamaki KI. The clinical anatomy of accessory mental nerves and foramina. Clin Anat. 2015;28(7):848–56.

Iwanaga J, Watanabe K, Saga T, Tabira Y, Kitashima S, Kusukawa J, Yamaki K. Accessory mental foramina and nerves: application to periodontal, periapical, and implant surgery. Clin Anat. 2016;29(4):493–501. https://doi.org/10.1002/ca.22635.

Iwanaga J, Kamura Y, Tanaka T, Watanabe K, Kusukawa J, Oskouian RJ, Tubbs RS. A new space of the face: the bucco-mandibular space. Clin Anat. 2017;30(7):958–962. https://doi.org/10.1002/ca.22964.

Iwanaga J, Nakamura K, Alonso F, Kirkpatrick C, Oskouian RJ, Watanabe K, Tubbs RS. Anatomical study of the so-called "retromolar gland": distinguishing normal anatomy from oral cavity pathology. Clin Anat. 2018;31(4):462–5. https://doi.org/10.1002/ca.23047.

Iwanaga J, Kikuta S, Tanaka T, Kamura Y, Tubbs RS. Review of risk assessment of major anatomical variations in clinical dentistry: accessory foramina of the mandible. Clin Anat. 2019a;32(5):672–7.

Iwanaga J, Wong TL, Kikuta S, Tubbs RS. Stafne bone cavity: a rare cadaveric case report. Anat Cell Biol. 2019b;52(3):354–6.

Iwanaga J, Katafuchi M, Matsushita Y, Kato T, Horner K, Tubbs RS. Anatomy of the mandibular canal and surrounding structures: part I: morphology of the superior wall of the mandibular canal. Ann Anat. 2020a;232:151580. https://doi.org/10.1016/j.aanat.2020b.151580.

Iwanaga J, Anand MK, Jain MN, Nagata M, Matsushita Y, Ibaragi S, Kusukawa J, Tubbs RS. Microsurgical anatomy of the superior wall of the mandibular canal and surrounding structures: suggestion for new classifications for dental implantology. Clin Anat. 2020b;33(2):223–31. https://doi.org/10.1002/ca.23456.

Kikuta S, Iwanaga J, Nakamura K, Hino K, Nakamura M, Kusukawa J. The retromolar canals and foramina: radiographic observation and application to oral surgery. Surg Radiol Anat. 2018 Jun;40(6):647–52. https://doi.org/10.1007/s00276-018-2005-5.

Kikuta S, Iwanaga J, Kusukawa J, Tubbs RS. The mental artery: anatomical study and literature review. J Anat. 2020;236(3):564–9. https://doi.org/10.1111/joa.13113.

Kilic C, Kamburoğlu K, Ozen T, Balcioglu HA, Kurt B, Kutoglu T, Ozan H. The position of the mandibular canal and histologic feature of the inferior alveolar nerve. Clin Anat. 2010;23(1):34–42. https://doi.org/10.1002/ca.20889. PMID: 19918867.

Klosek SK, Rungruang T. Anatomical study of the greater palatine artery and related structures of the palatal vault: considerations for palate as the subepithelial connective tissue graft donor site. Surg Radiol Anat. 2009;31:245–50.

Lekholm U, Zarb GA. Patient selection and preparation. In: Branemark PI, Zarb GA, Albrektsson T, editors. Tissue-integrated prostheses: osseointegration in clinical dentistry. Chicago: Quintessence Publ Co; 1985. p. 199–209.

Lovasova K, Kachlik D, Rozpravkova M, Matusevska M, Ferkova J, Kluchova D. Three-dimensional CAD/CAM imaging of the maxillary sinus in ageing process. Ann Anat. 2018;218:69–82.

Matani JD, Kheur MG, Kheur SM, Jambhekar SS. The anatomic inter relationship of the neurovascular structures within the inferior Alveolar Canal: a cadaveric and histological study. J Maxillofac Oral Surg. 2014;13(4):499–502. https://doi.org/10.1007/s12663-013-0563-y.

Misch CE. Bone character: second vital implant criterion. Dent Today. 1988;7:39–40.

Misch CE. Density of bone: effect on treatment plans, surgical approach, healing, and progressive bone loading. Int J Oral Implantol. 1990;6:23–31.

Misch CE. Contemporary implant dentistry. 2nd ed. St. Louis, MO: Mosby; 1999.

Motamedi MH, Gharedaghi J, Mehralizadeh S, Navi F, Badkoobeh A, Valaei N, Azizi T. Anthropomorphic assessment of the retromolar foramen and retromolar nerve: anomaly or variation of normal anatomy? Int J Oral Maxillofac Surg. 2016;45(2):241–4. https://doi.org/10.1016/j.ijom.2015.10.017.

Naitoh M, Hiraiwa Y, Aimiya H, Gotoh K, Ariji E. Accessory mental foramen assessment using cone-beam computed tomography. Oral Surg Oral Med Oral Pathol Oral Radiol Endodontol. 2009a;107(2):289–94.

Naitoh M, Hiraiwa Y, Aimiya H, Ariji E. Observation of bifid mandibular canal using cone-beam computerized tomography. Int J Oral Maxillofac Implants. 2009b;24(1):155–9.

Neiva RF, Gapsli R, Wang HL. Morphometric analysis of implant-related anatomy in Caucasian skulls. J Periodontol. 2004;75(8):1061–7.

Nortjé CJ, Farman AG, Grotepass FW. Variations in the normal anatomy of the inferior dental (mandibular) canal: a retrospective study of panoramic radiographs from 3612 routine dental patients. Br J Oral Surg. 1977;15(1):55–63.

Pandharbale AA, Gadgil RM, Bhoosreddy AR, Kunte VR, Ahire BS, Shinde MR, Joshi SS. Evaluation of the posterior superior alveolar artery using cone beam computed tomography. Pol J Radiol. 2016;81:606–10.

Standring S, editor. Gray's anatomy: the anatomical basis of clinical practice. London: Elsevier Health Sciences; 2015.

Takezawa K, Ghabriel M, Townsend G. The course and distribution of the buccal nerve: clinical relevance in dentistry. Aust Dent J. 2018;63(1):66–71. https://doi.org/10.1111/adj.12543. Epub 2017 Sep 8. PMID: 28646596.

Tehranchi M, Taleghani F, Shahab S, Nouri A. Prevalence and location of the posterior superior alveolar artery using cone-beam computed tomography. Imag Sci Dent. 2017;47:39–44.

Yu SK, Lee MH, Jeon YH, Chung YY, Kim HJ. Anatomical configuration of the inferior alveolar neurovascular bundle: a histomorphometric analysis. Surg Radiol Anat. 2016;38(2):195–201. https://doi.org/10.1007/s00276-015-1540-6.

4 Maxillofacial Anatomy and Anatomical Spaces

4.1 Overview of Anatomical Spaces

Summary
The anatomical spaces of the face are defined as loose connective tissues bordered by the mucosa, bone, muscles, and fasciae and which contain vessels, nerves, salivary glands and ducts, and muscles. Infections and tumors can spread via these spaces to reach the mediastinum, for example. Also, pathology in these spaces can cause dysfunction of adjacent nerves.

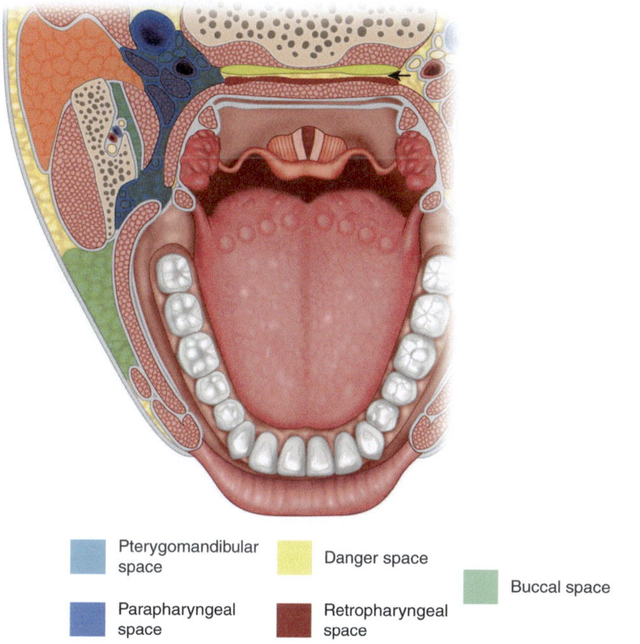

Fig. 4.1 Axial view of the spaces. Note the alar fascia (arrow) dividing the space located posterior to the posterior pharyngeal wall into the retropharyngeal and "danger" spaces

J. Iwanaga, R. S. Tubbs, *Atlas of Oral and Maxillofacial Anatomy*, https://doi.org/10.1007/978-3-030-78327-3_4

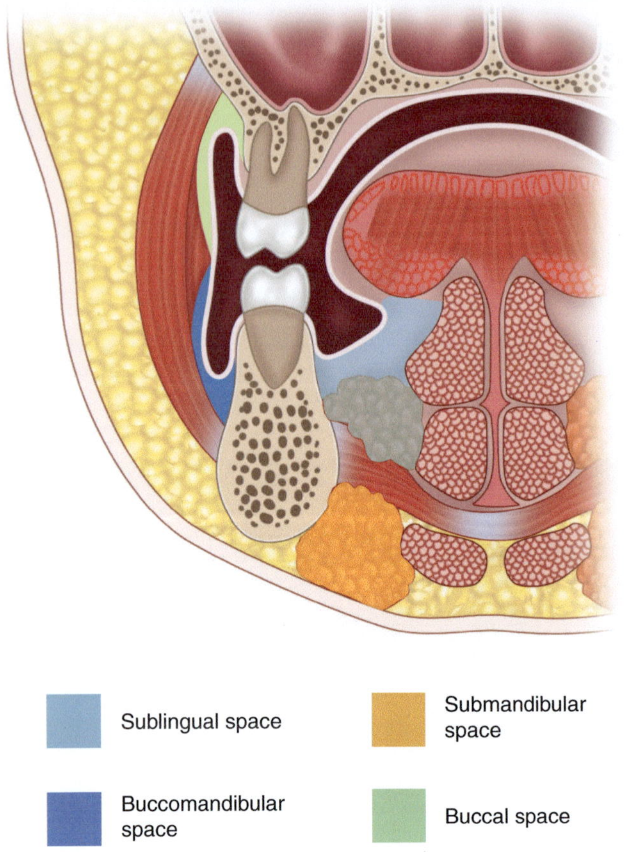

Fig. 4.2 Coronal view of the spaces. The buccomandibular space is a separate space from the buccal space and was first reported in 2017 (Iwanaga et al. 2017)

4.2 Nose, Nasal Cavity, and Paranasal Sinuses

Summary

The nose and nasal cavity consist of the frontal, nasal, maxillary, ethmoid, lacrimal, inferior nasal concha, palatine, and sphenoid bones and major alar, minor alar, septal nasal, vomeronasal, and accessory nasal cartilages. In general, there are three pairs of nasal conchae, the superior and middle conchae are parts of the ethmoid bone, and the inferior nasal concha is a separate bone. Below each concha exists a nasal meatus (superior, middle, and inferior) which is a pathway for air and accommodates the openings of the paranasal sinuses (maxillary sinus, frontal sinus, sphenoidal sinus, and ethmoidal cells) and nasolacrimal duct. The main blood supply is from the sphenopalatine branch of the maxillary artery and anterior and posterior ethmoidal branches of the ophthalmic artery (a small area of the nostril is supplied by the collumellar branch of the facial artery). The innervation is via the nasopalatine nerve (V2), anterior ethmoidal nerve (V1), and internal nasal branch of the infraorbital nerve (V2).

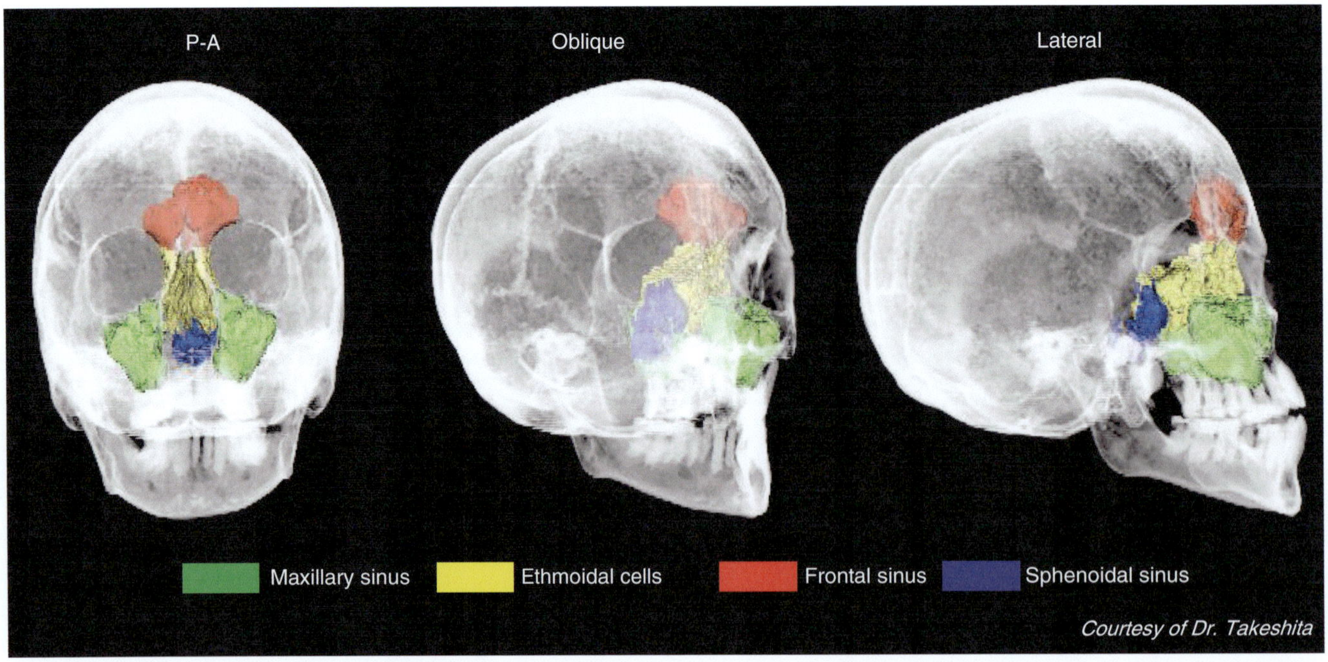

Fig. 4.3 Paranasal sinuses in a patient with a dentulous mandible

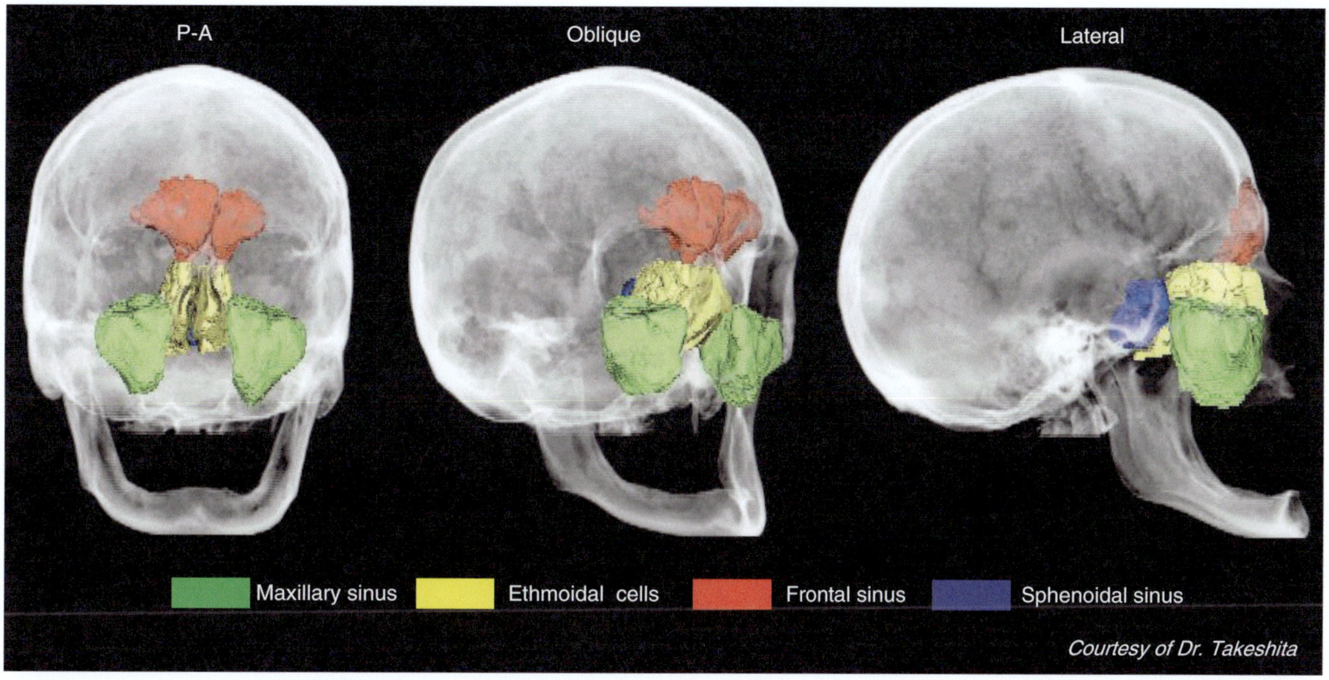

Fig. 4.4 Paranasal sinuses in a patient with an edentulous mandible. The volume of the maxillary sinus increases after upper tooth loss

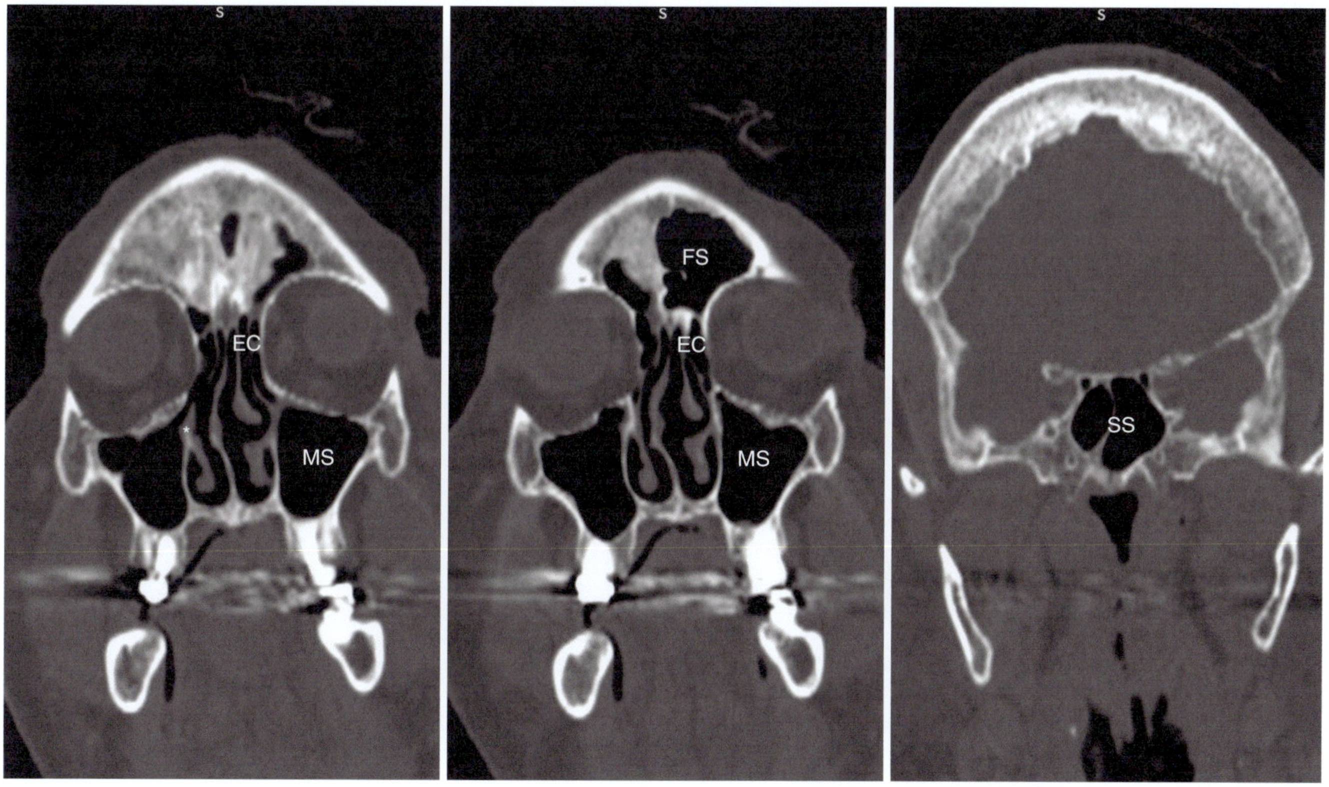

Fig. 4.5 The paranasal sinuses on coronal CT images. Note the opening of the maxillary sinus into the middle nasal meatus which is observed above the uncinate process (*) on the far left image. *EC* ethmoid cells; *MS* maxillary sinus; *FS* frontal sinus; *SS* sphenoid sinus

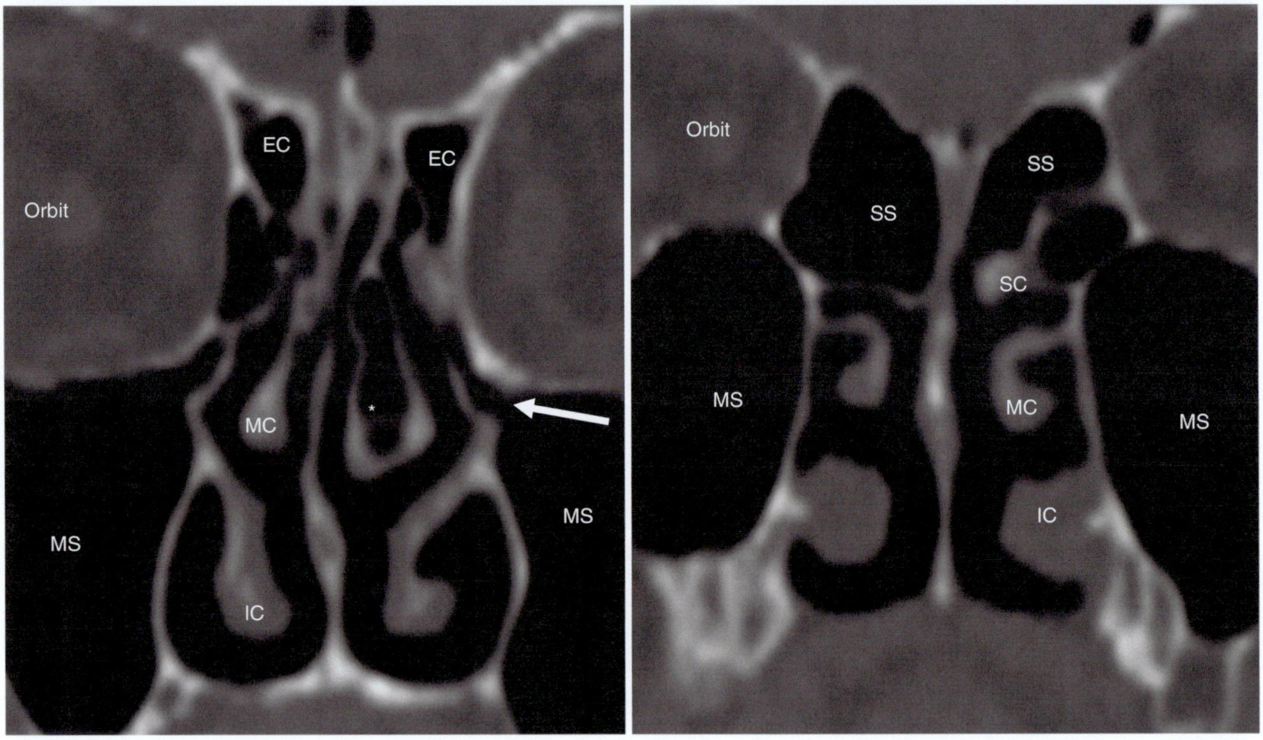

Fig. 4.6 The nasal cavity on coronal CT images. Note the ethmoidal bulla (*) is observed medial to the opening of the maxillary sinus into the middle meatus on the left image (arrow). *EC* ethmoid cells; *MS* maxillary sinus; *FS* frontal sinus; *SS* sphenoid sinus; *IC* inferior concha; *MC* middle concha; and *SC* superior concha

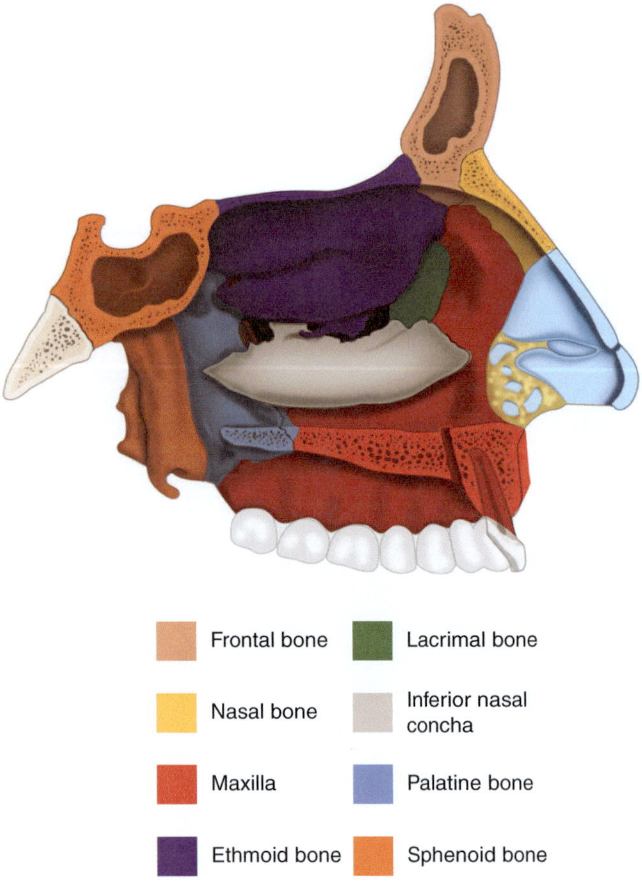

Fig. 4.7 Medial view of the bony structures in of the nasal cavity

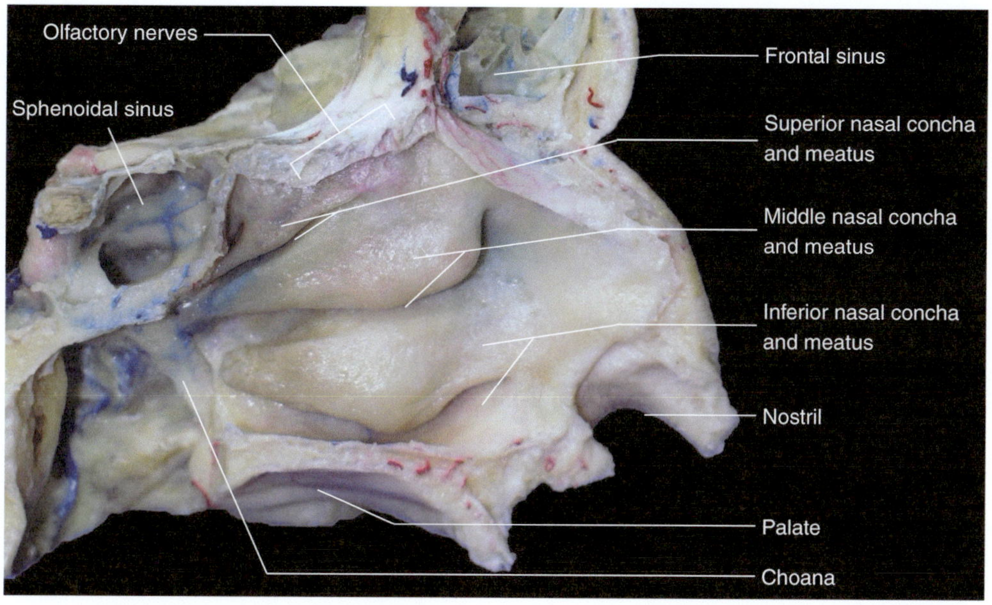

Fig. 4.8 Medial view of the nasal cavity

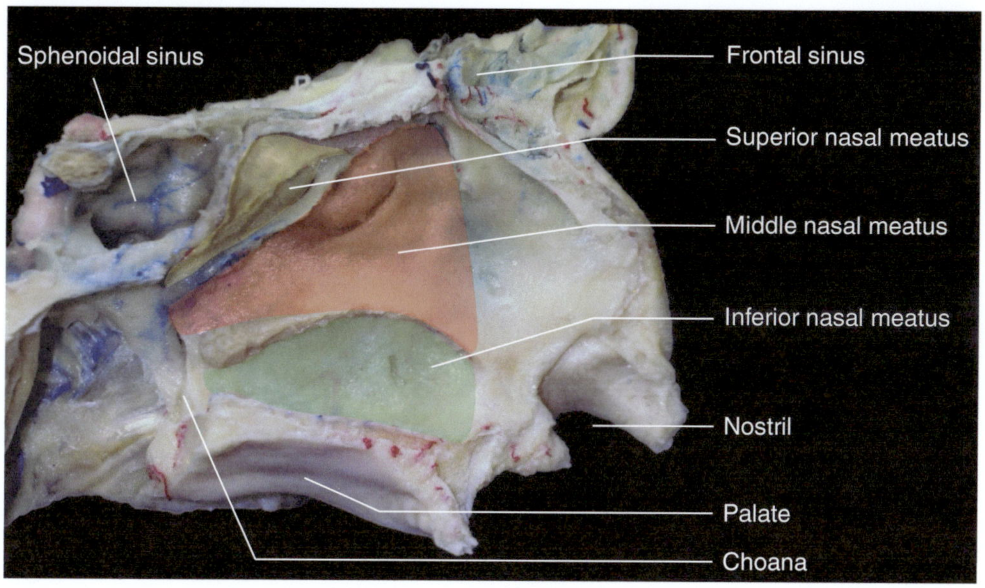

Fig. 4.9 Medial view of the nasal cavity. Note the superior, middle, and inferior nasal conchae are removed

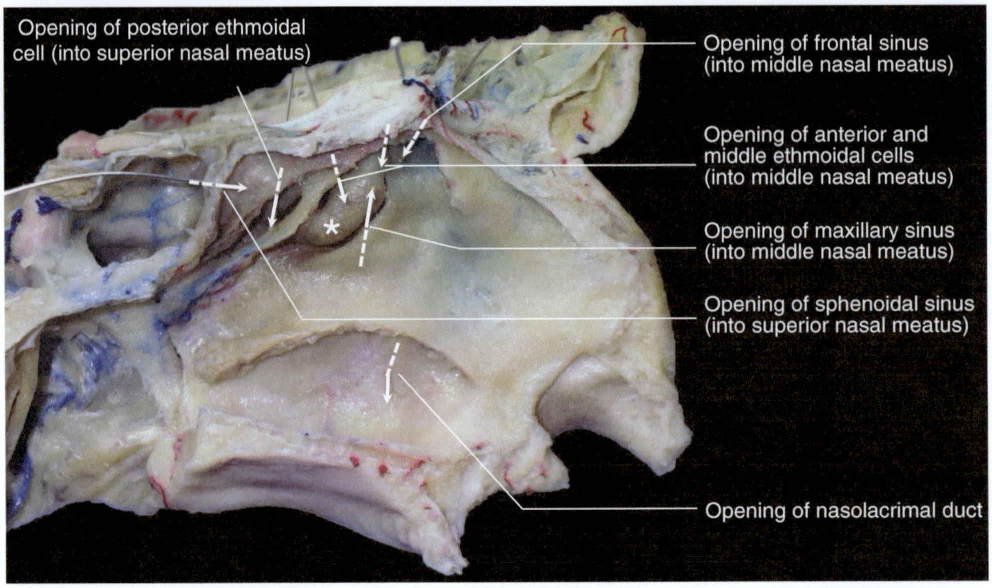

Fig. 4.10 Medial view of the nasal cavity showing the openings of the paranasal sinuses and nasolacrimal duct
*Ethmoidal bulla

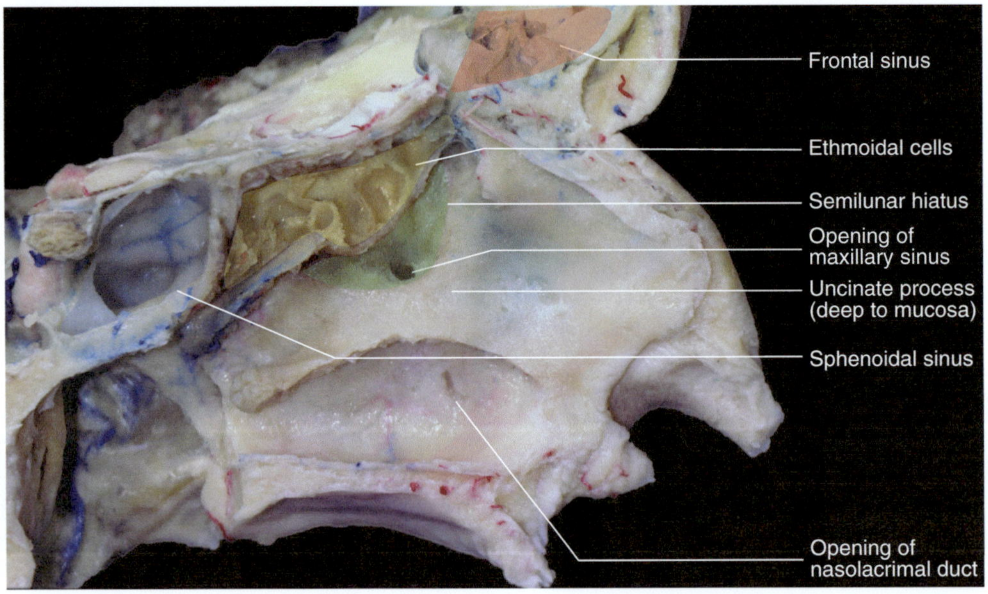

Fig. 4.11 Medial view of the nasal cavity. The medial wall of the ethmoidal cells and ethmoidal bulla are removed

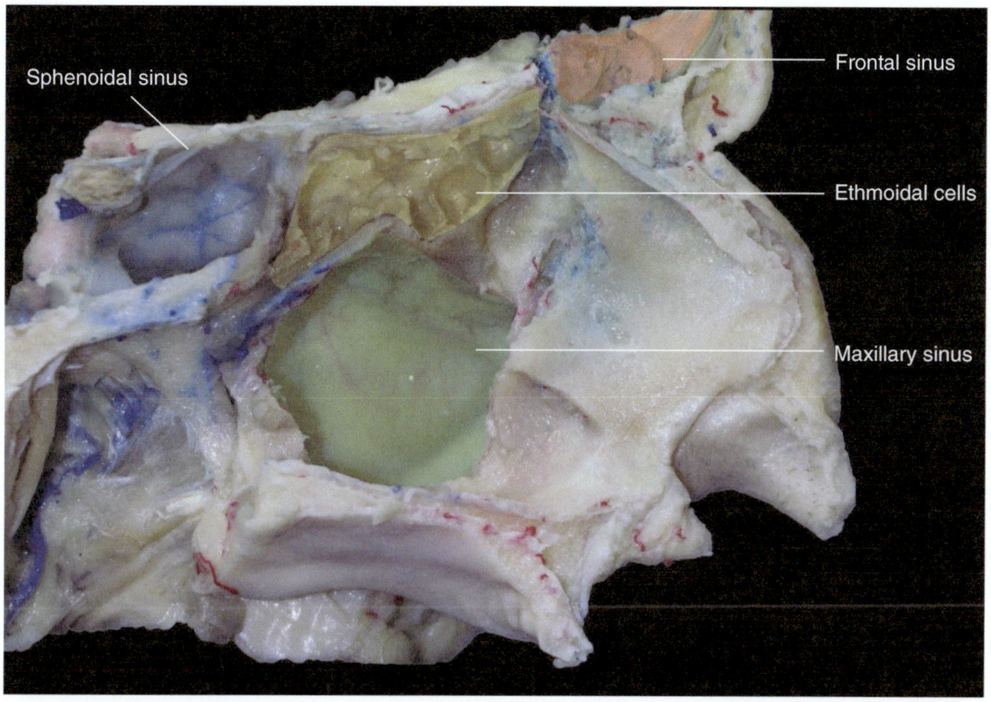

Fig. 4.12 Medial view of the nasal cavity. Note that the four paranasal sinuses are shown

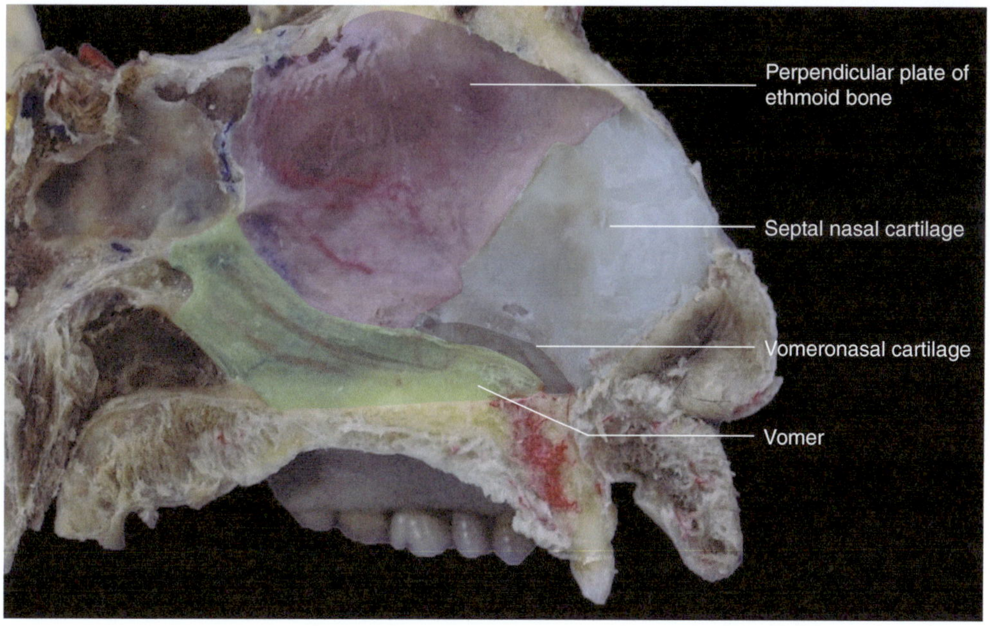

Fig. 4.13 Medial view of the nasal septum

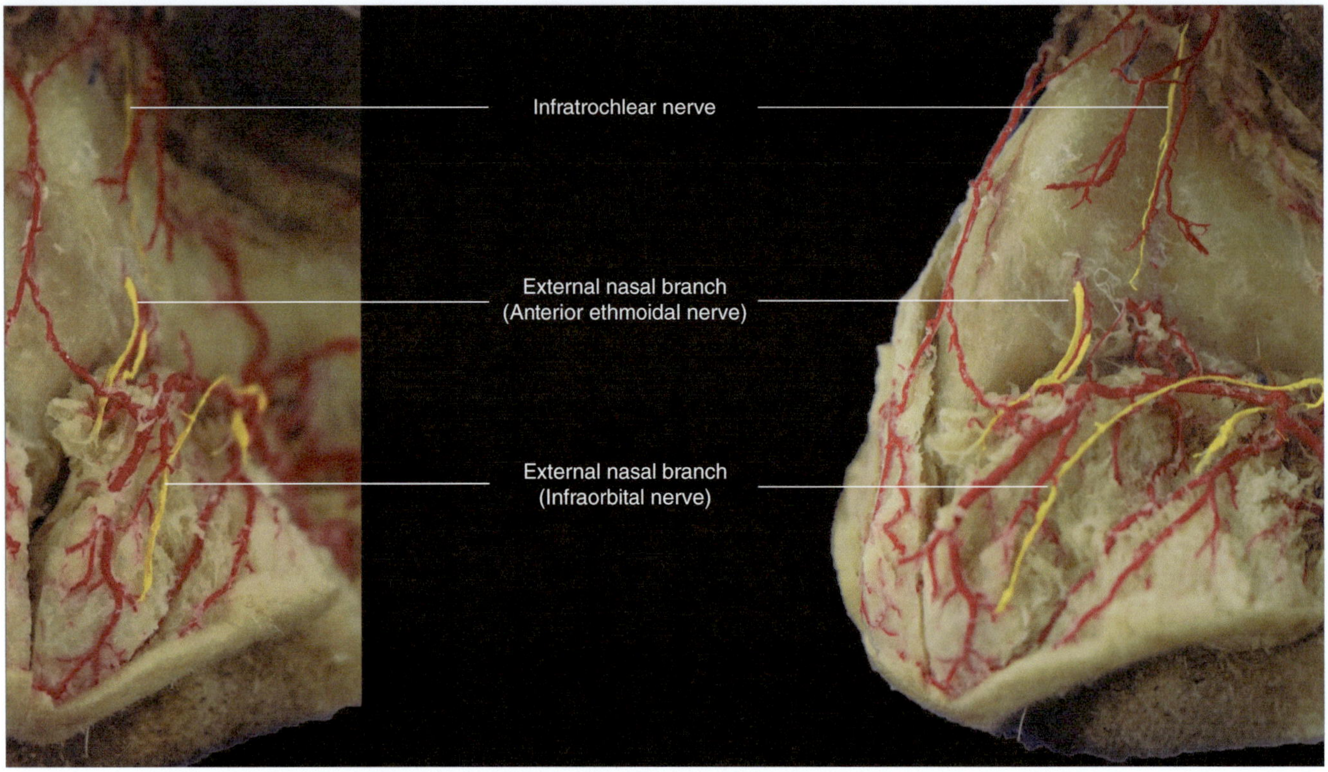

Fig. 4.14 Innervation of the external nose

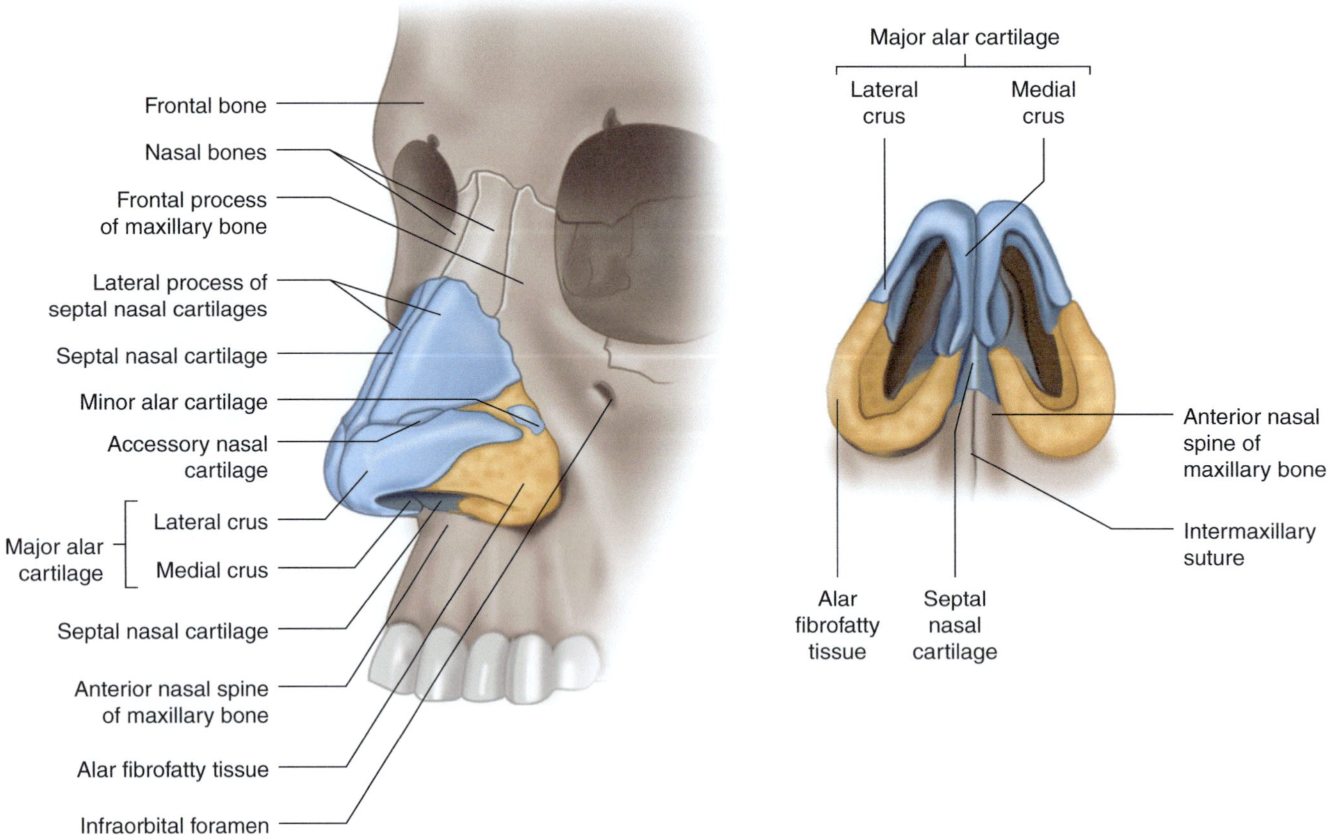

Fig. 4.15 Schematic drawing of the nasal cartilages

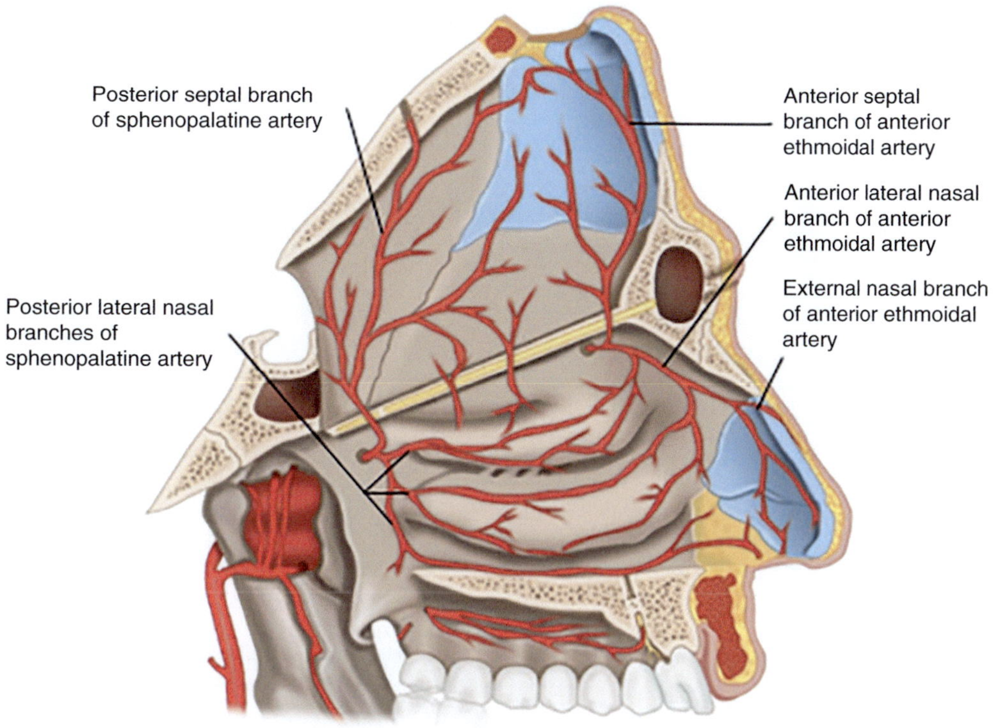

Fig. 4.16 Blood supply of the nasal cavity

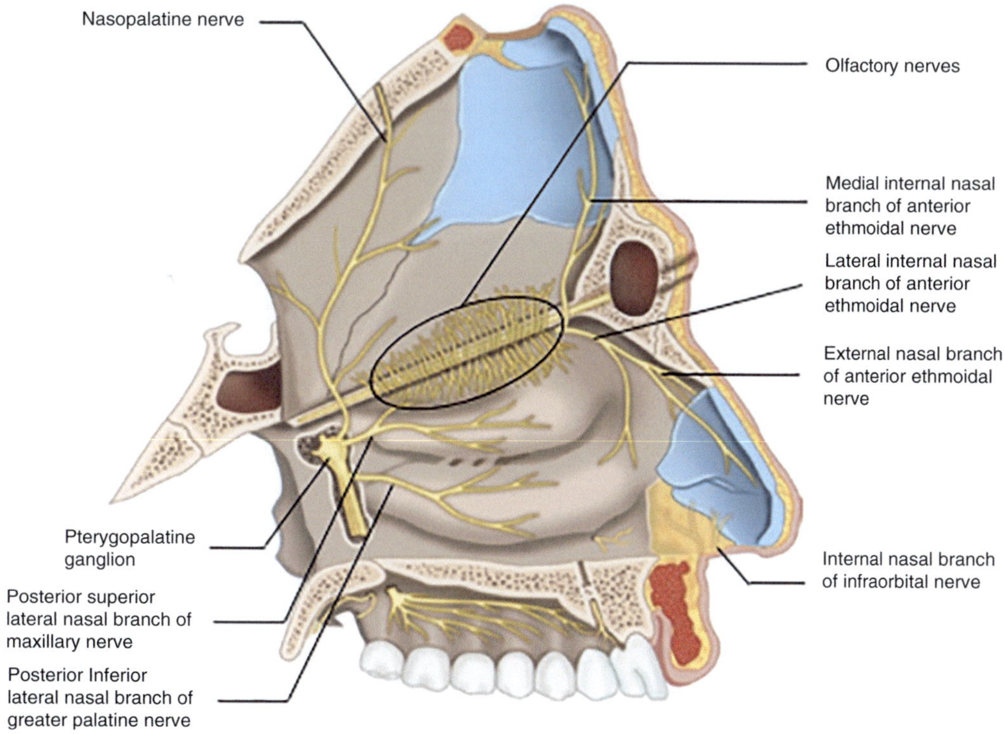

Fig. 4.17 Innervation of the nasal cavity and nasal septum

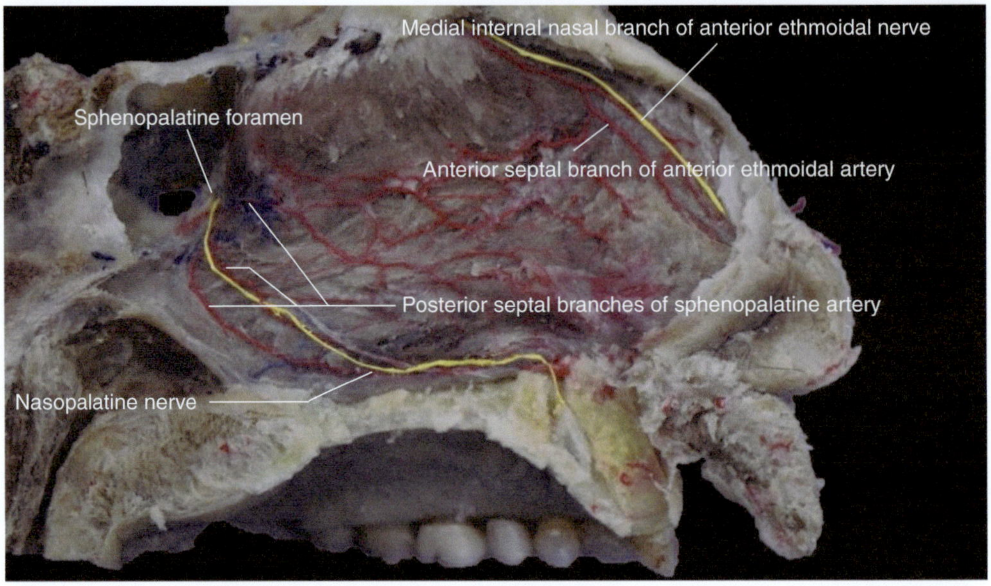

Fig. 4.18 Blood supply and innervation of the nasal cavity

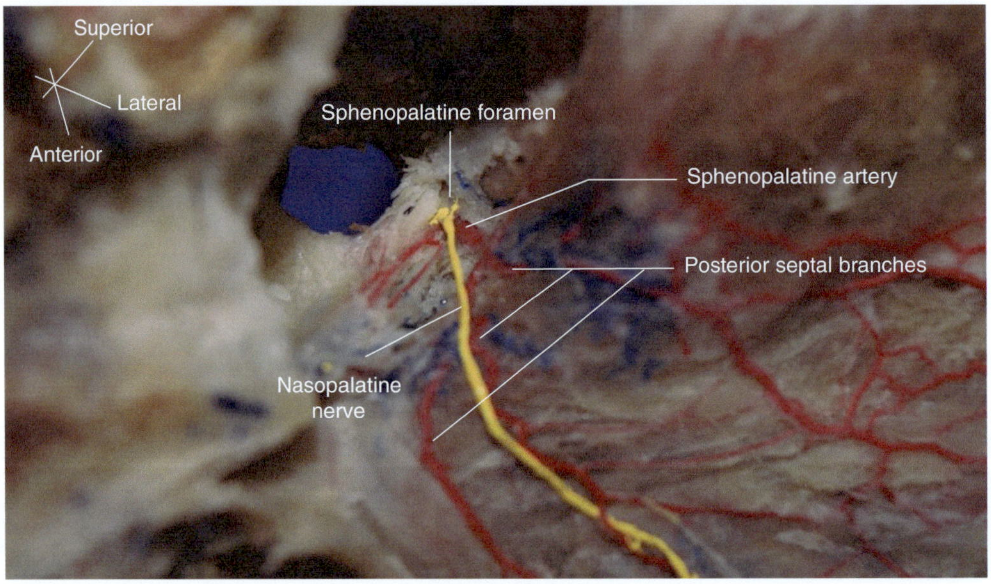

Fig. 4.19 Origin of the sphenopalatine artery and nasopalatine nerve via the sphenopalatine foramen

4.3 Orbit

Summary

Vision is carried out by the optic nerve. To move the eyeball, cranial nerves III, IV, and VI enter the orbit via superior orbital fissure. Tears are produced in the lacrimal gland and function to prevent dryness of the cornea. The excessive fluid is collected by the medially located nasolacrimal duct to drain into the inferior nasal meatus. The orbit receives arterial branches from the ophthalmic, facial, and transverse facial arteries. Importantly, the superior and inferior ophthalmic veins drain into the cavernous sinus so that infections in the orbit can affect the cavernous sinus. In this section, the anatomy of the orbit will be shown.

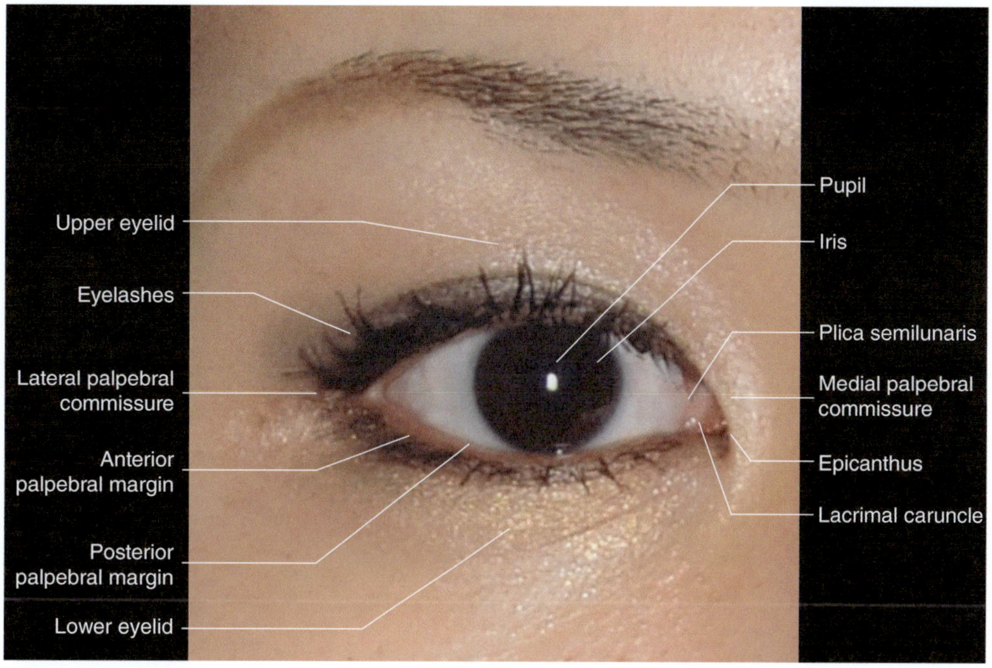

Fig. 4.20 Anterior view of the right eye. The epicanthus (or epicanthal fold) is seen in one-third of healthy young North American Caucasians (Farkas and Cheung 1979) and around 50-90% of Koreans and Japanese (Lai et al. 2012)

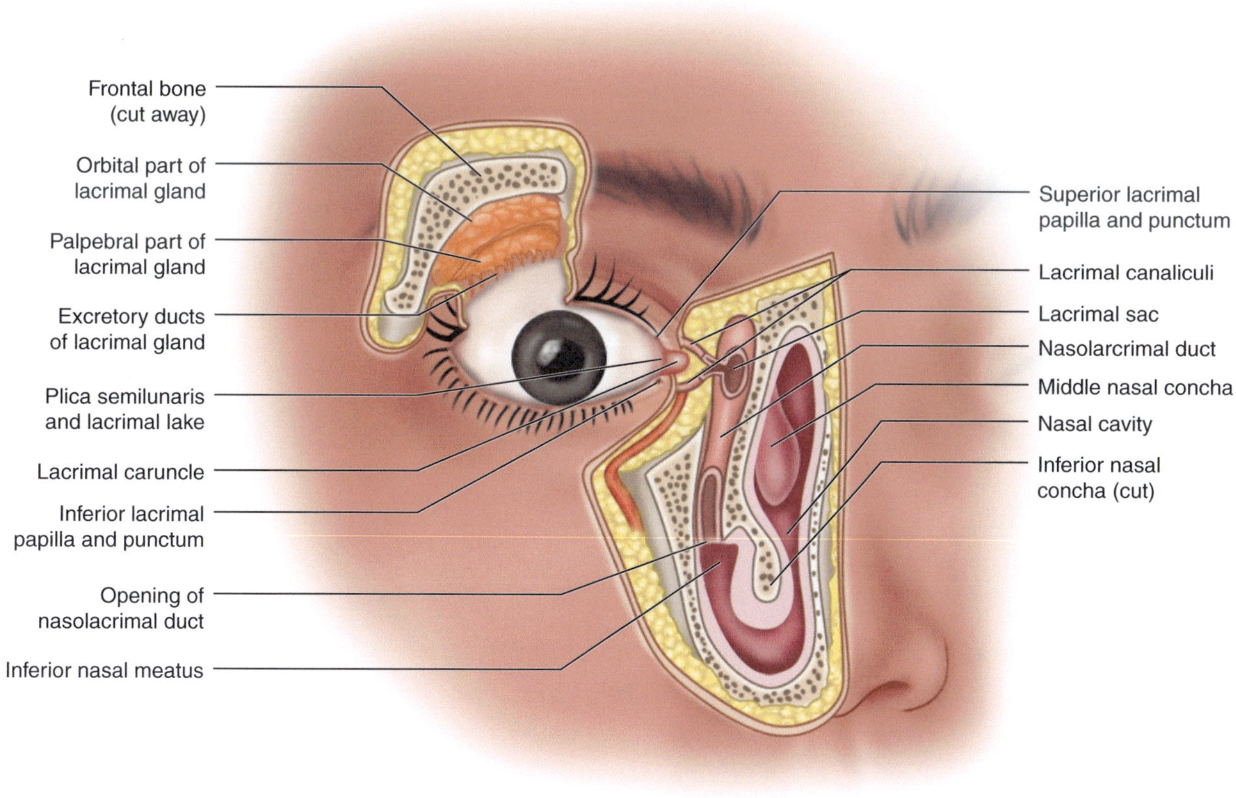

Fig. 4.21 Pathway of the tears which are produced in the lacrimal gland which is innervated by the lacrimal nerve, a branch of V1. The autonomic fibers that travel along the lacrimal nerve to the gland are derived from the facial nerve

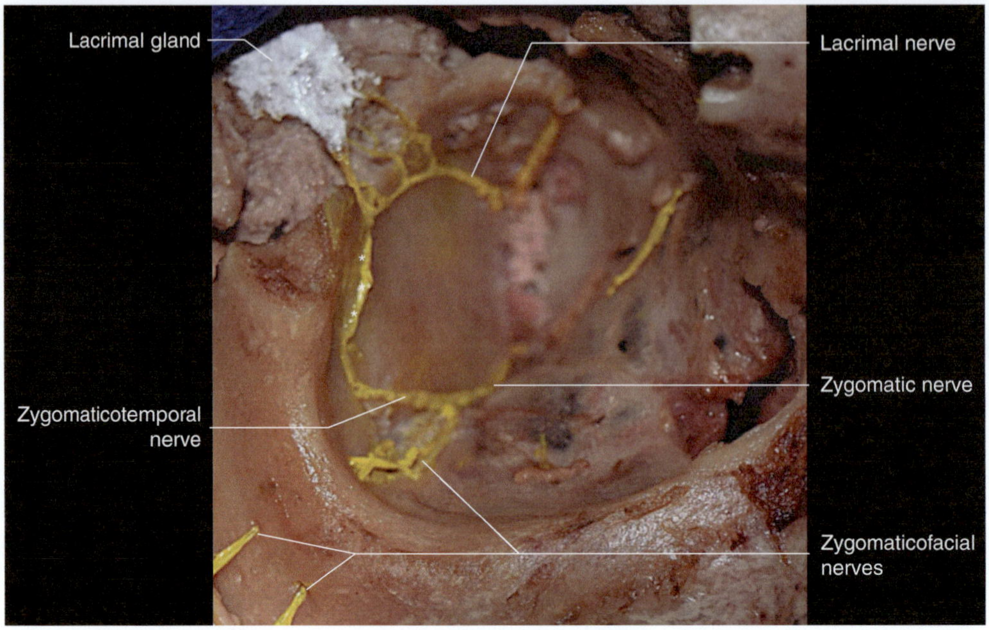

Fig. 4.22 Anterior view of the right orbit. The postganglionic parasympathetic fibers for the lacrimal gland originate from the pterygopalatine ganglion via the zygomaticotemporal nerve which sends a communicating branch (*) to the lacrimal nerve to supply the parasympathetic fibers

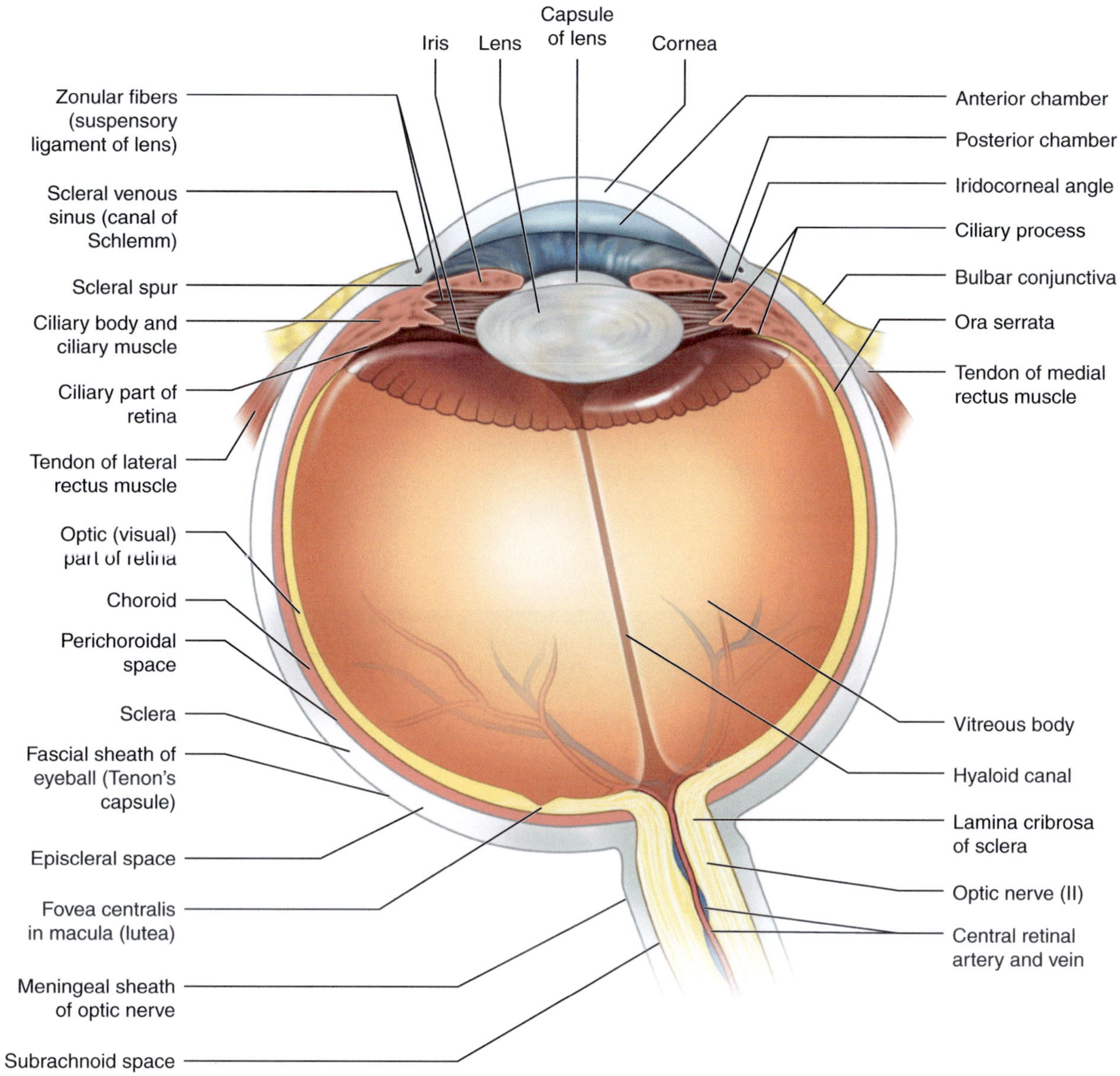

Fig. 4.23 Axial section of the left eyeball

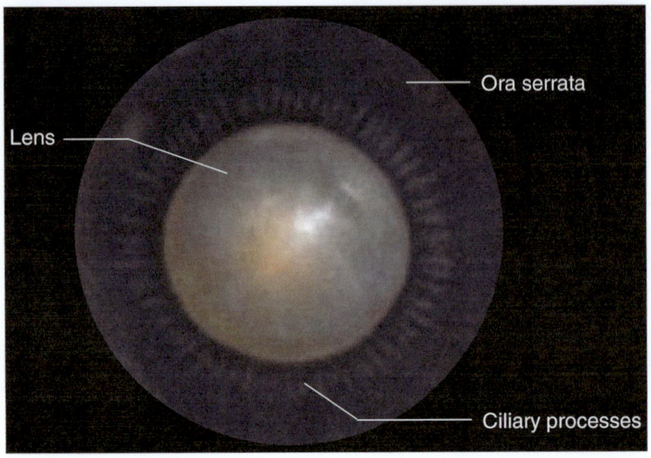

Fig. 4.24 Coronal section of the eyeball. Anterior segment viewed from behind

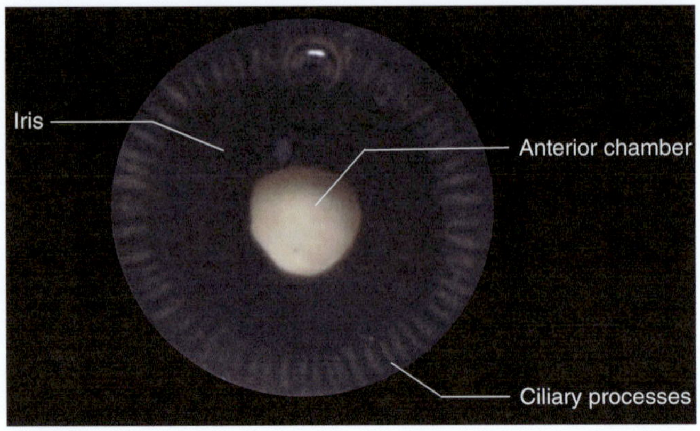

Fig. 4.25 Coronal section of the eyeball. Anterior segment viewed from behind. Lens is removed

Fig. 4.26 Coronal section of the eyeball. Right optic nerve and retinal arterioles are shown

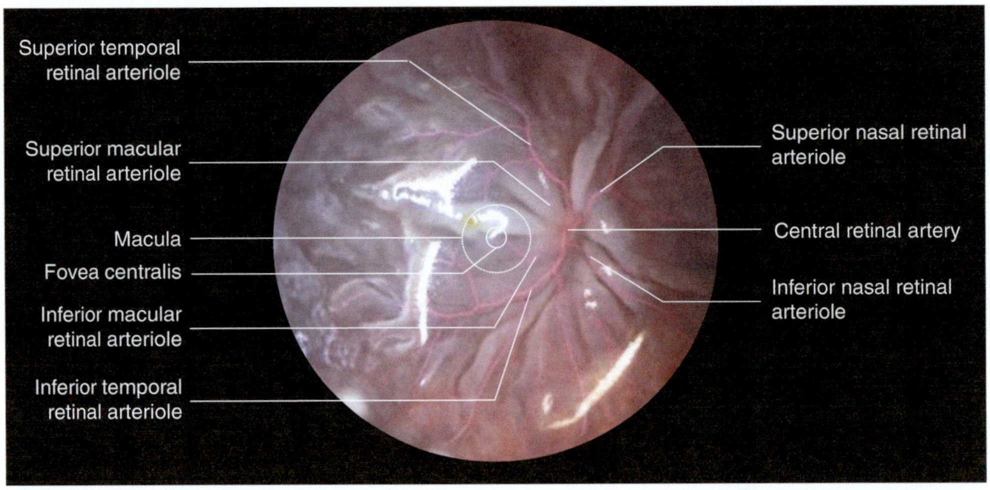

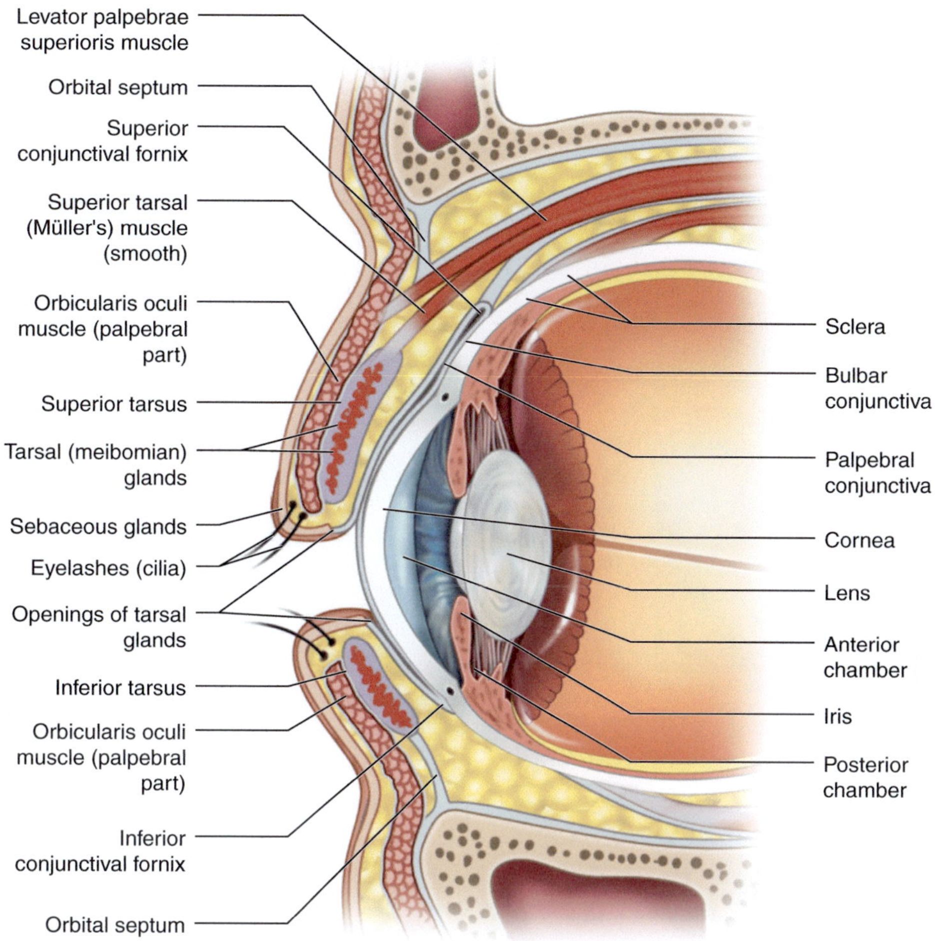

Fig. 4.27 Sagittal image of the orbit

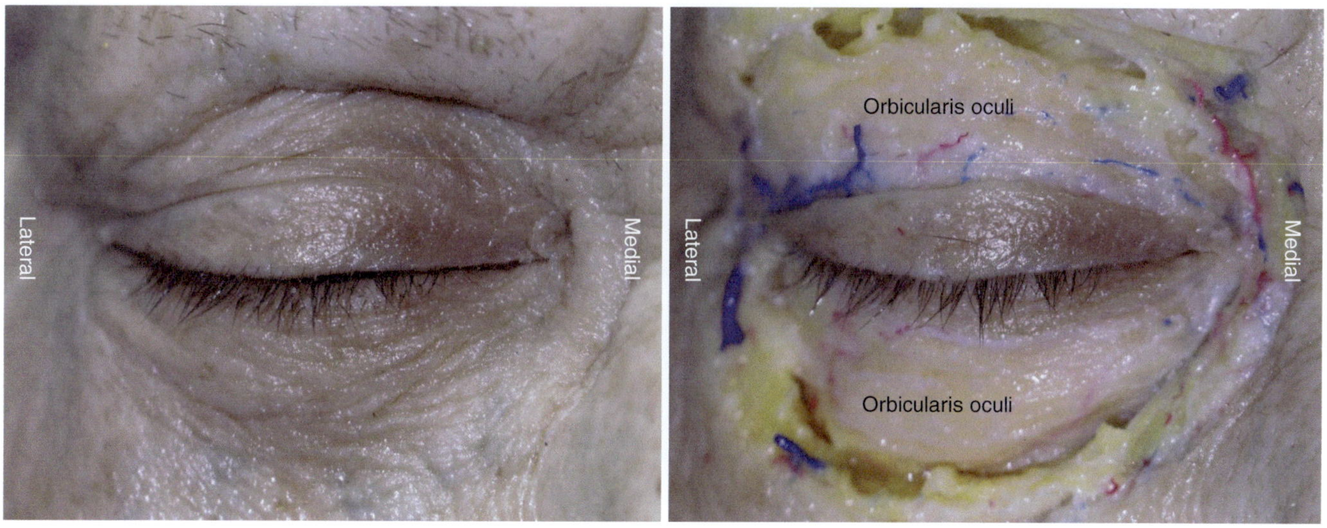

Fig. 4.28 Anterior view of the right eyelids

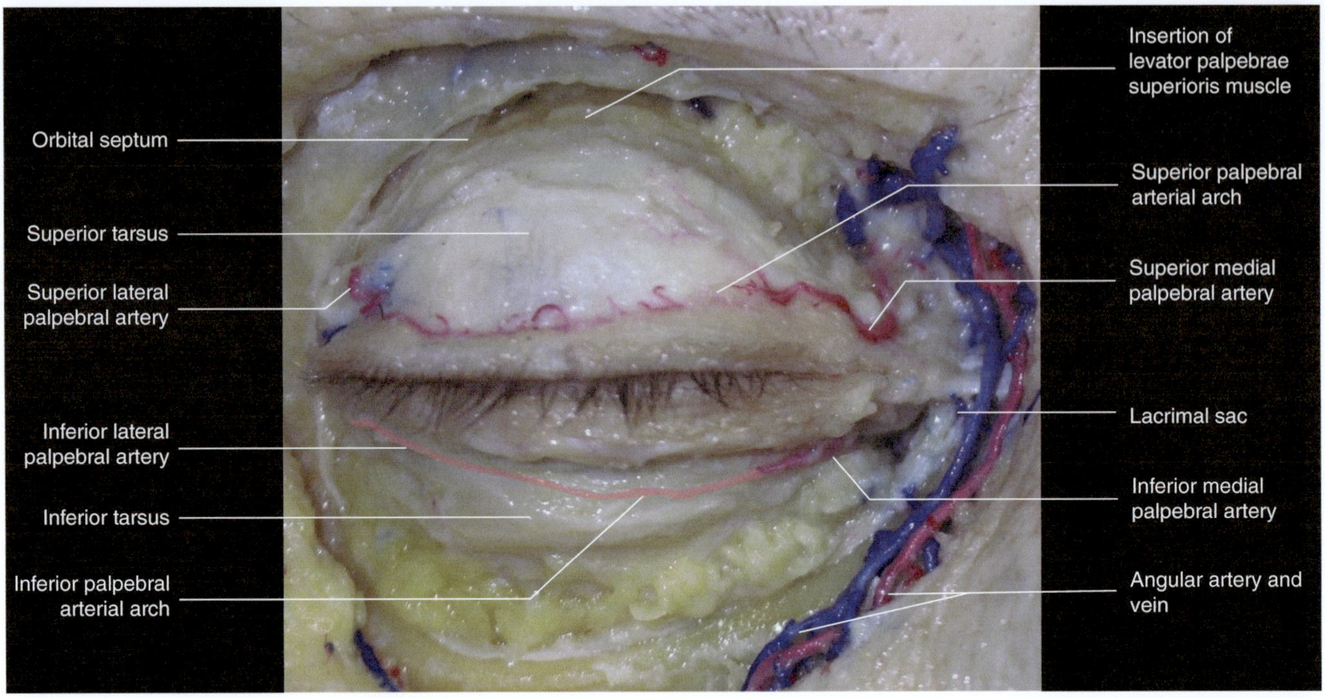

Fig. 4.29 Anterior view of the right eye after removal of the orbicularis oculi

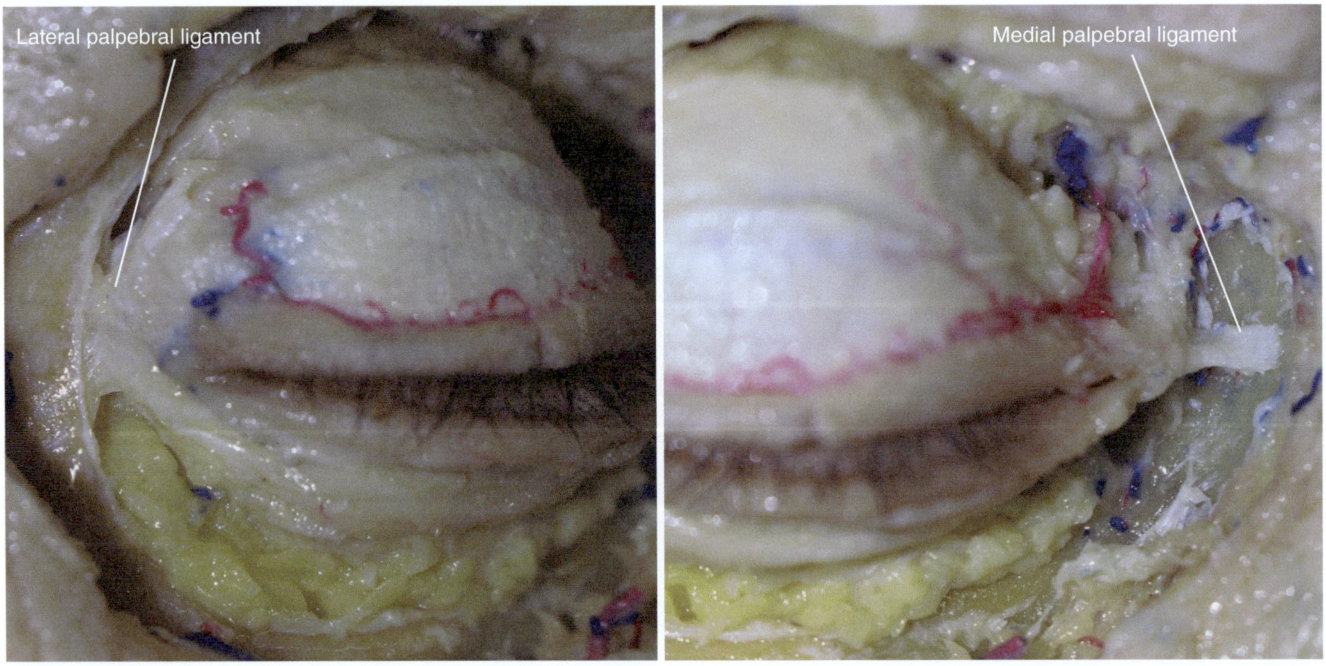

Fig. 4.30 Medial and lateral palpebral ligaments

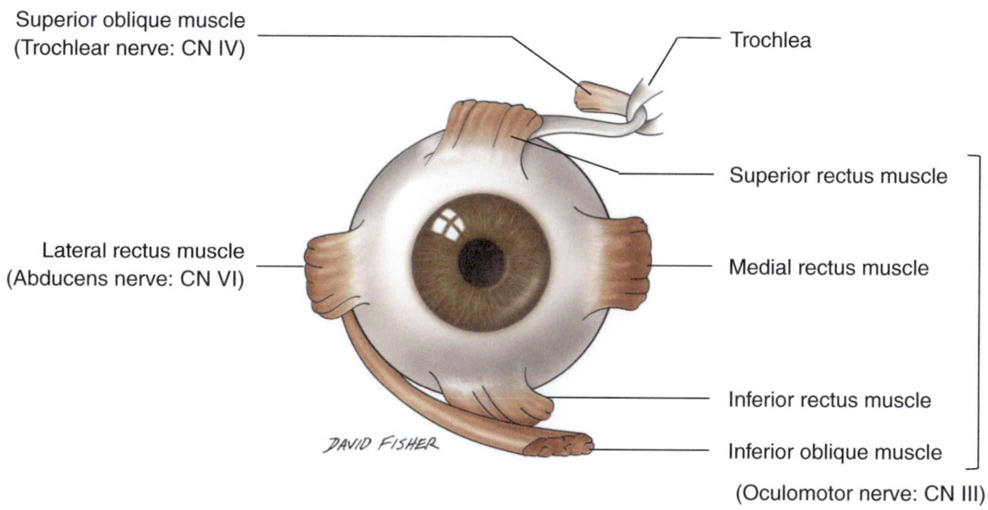

Fig. 4.31 Anterior view of the right extraocular muscles.

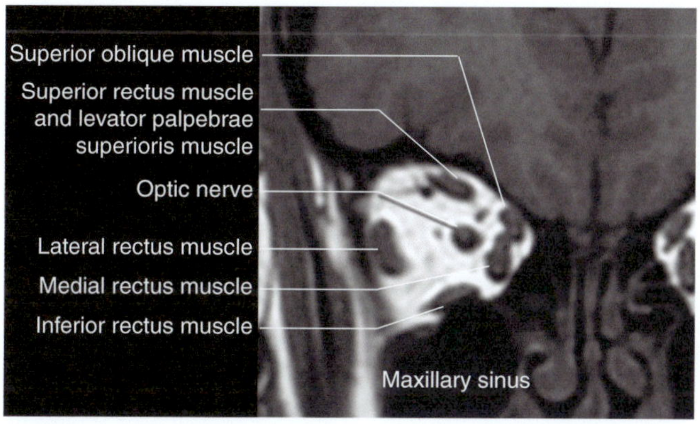

Fig. 4.32 Coronal MRI of the right orbit (posterior to the eyeball)

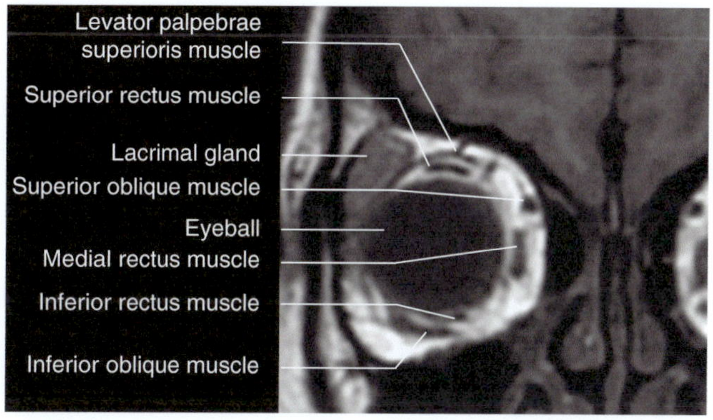

Fig. 4.33 Coronal MRI of the right orbit (middle of the eyeball)

Fig. 4.34 Superior view of the floor of the left anterior cranial fossa

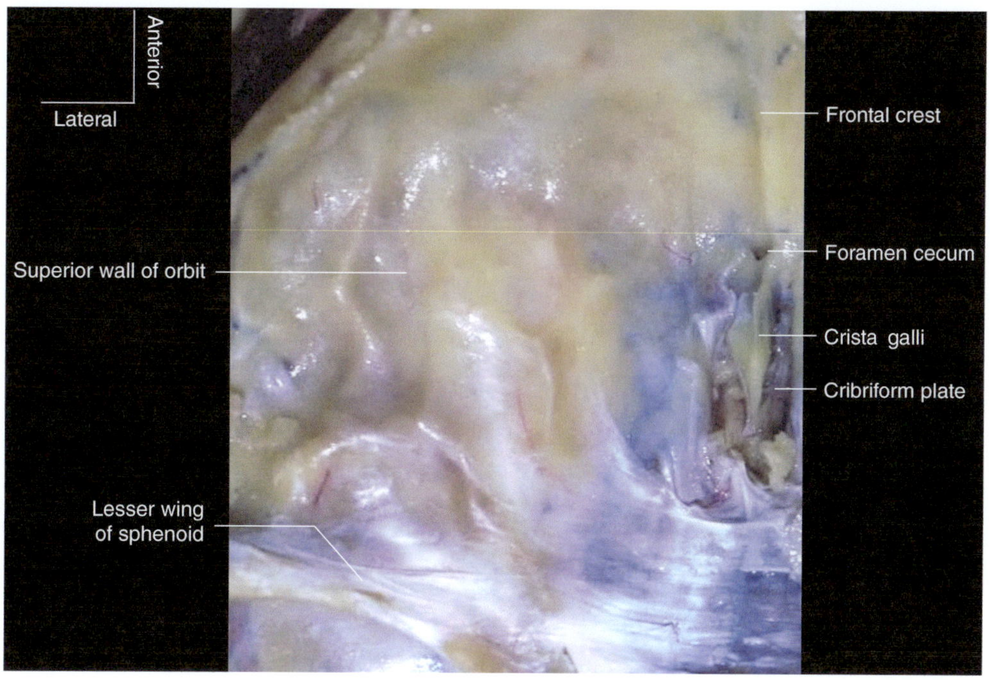

Fig. 4.35 Superior view of the left orbit. The superior walls of the orbit, frontal sinus, ethmoidal cells, and sphenoidal sinus are removed

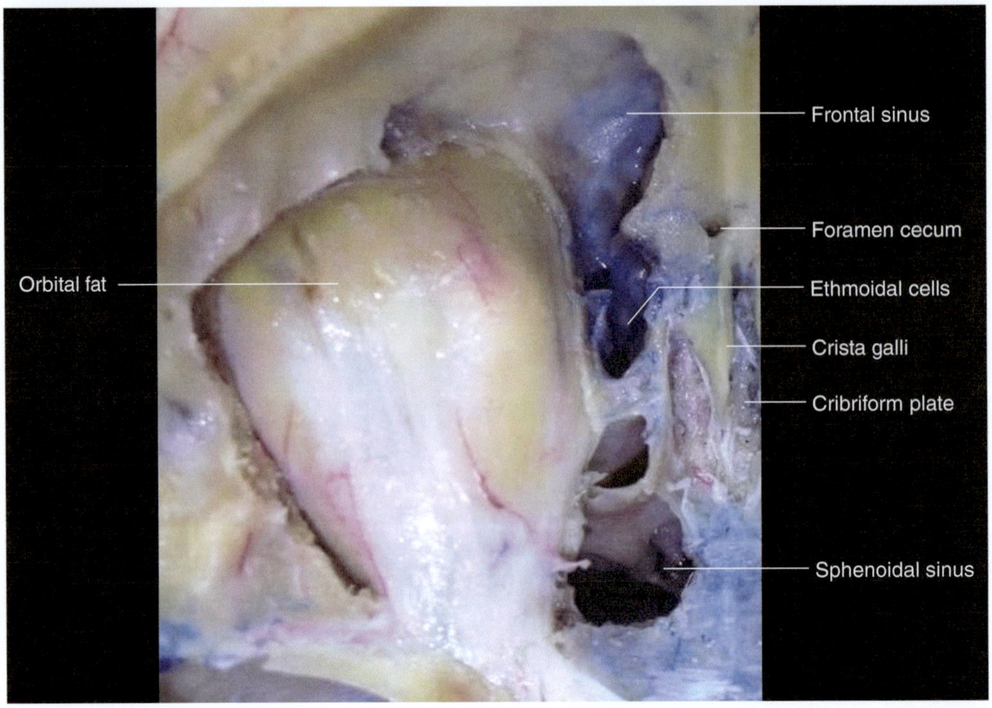

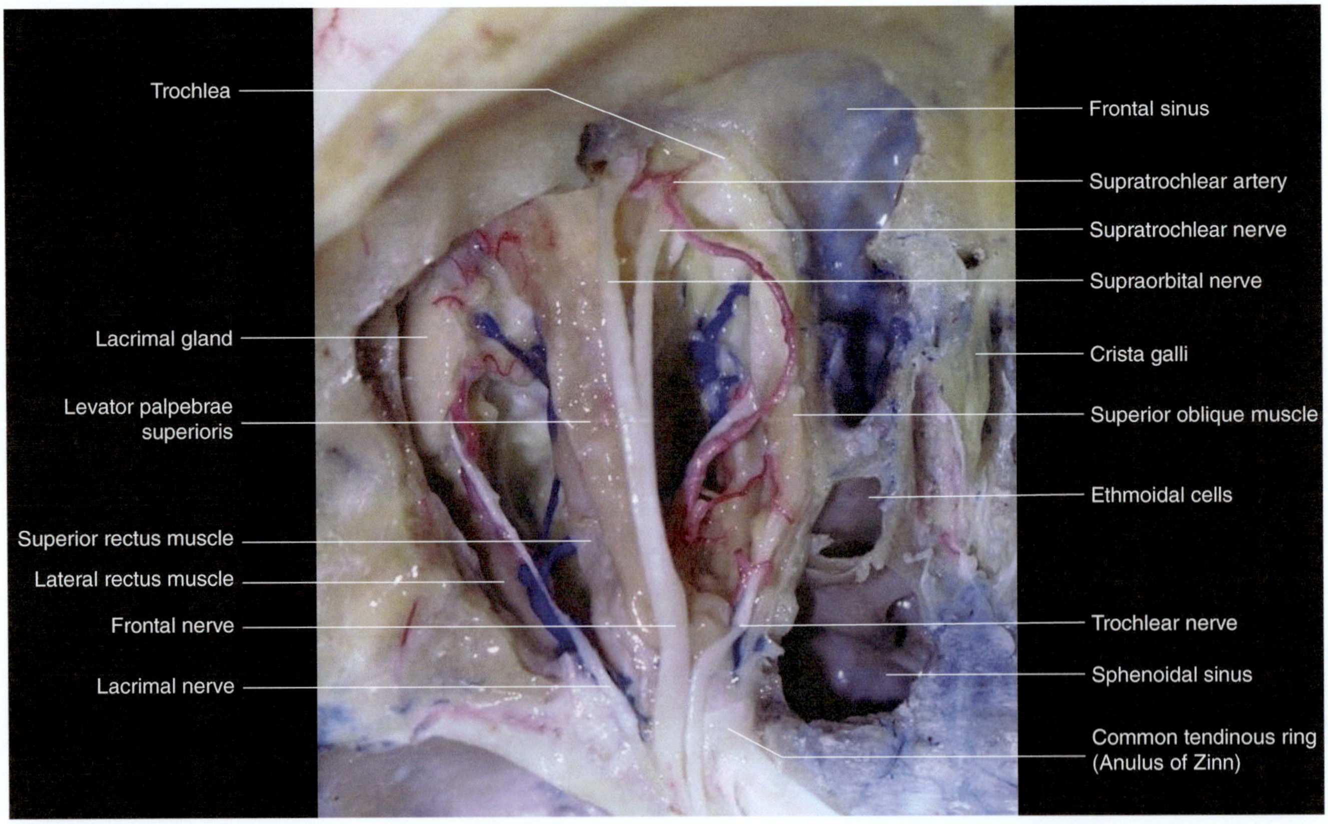

Fig. 4.36 Superior view of the left orbit following removal of the orbital fat

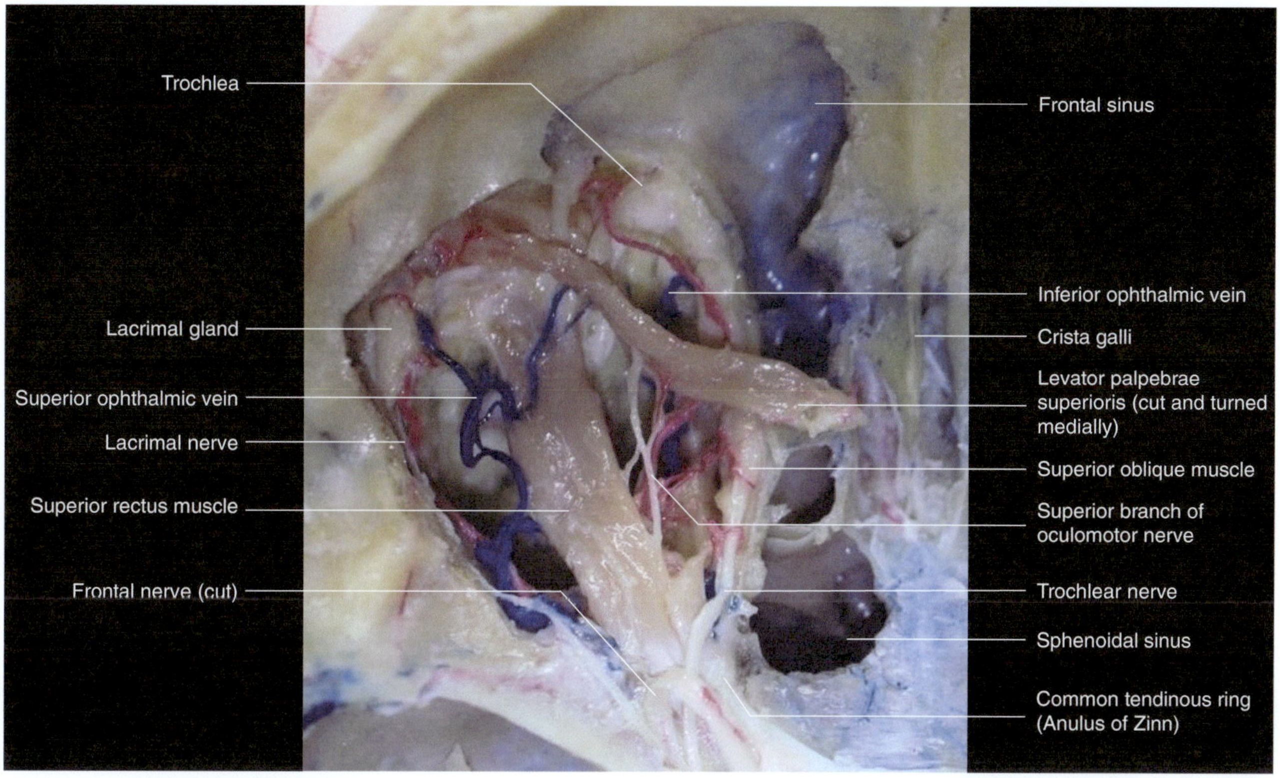

Fig. 4.37 Superior view of the left orbit. The supraorbital and supratrochlear nerves have been resected. The levator palpebrae superioris muscle is cut proximally and turned medially

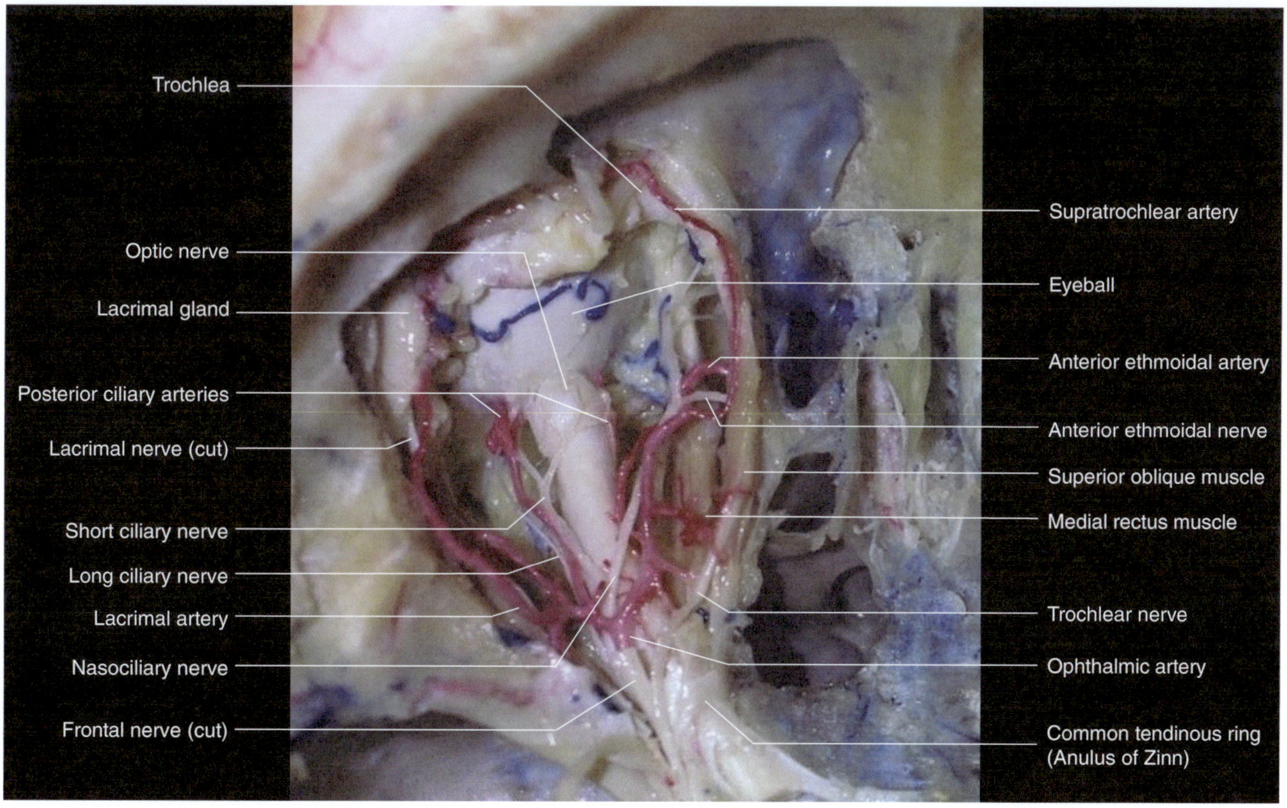

Fig. 4.38 Superior view of the left orbit. The levator palpebrae superioris and superior rectus muscles are removed. Note that the branches of the ophthalmic artery and that the optic nerve is within its meningeal sheath

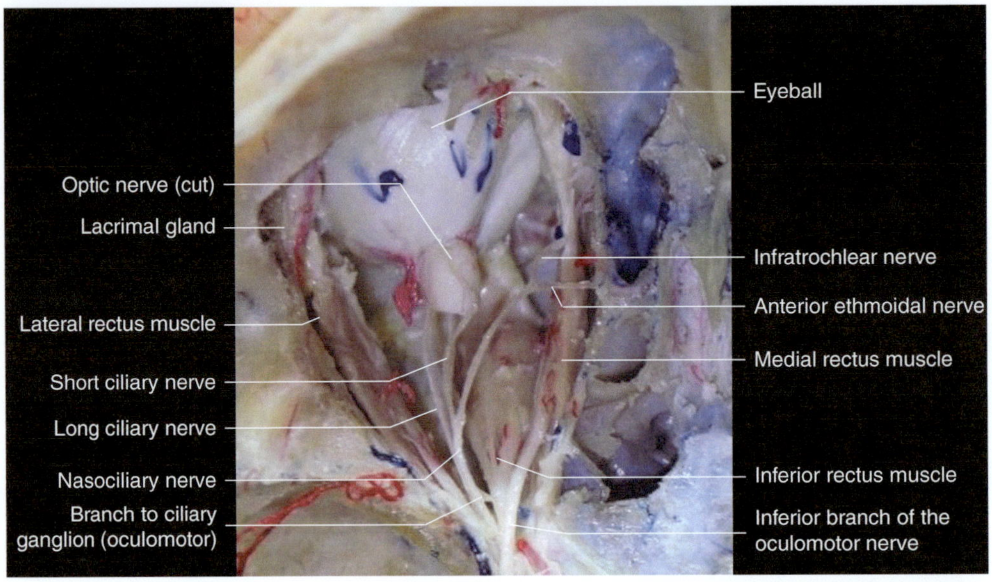

Fig. 4.39 Superior view of the left orbit. Distal two-thirds of the optic nerve is removed and the inferior rectus muscle is shown deep to it. Note the superior branch of the oculomotor nerve is removed

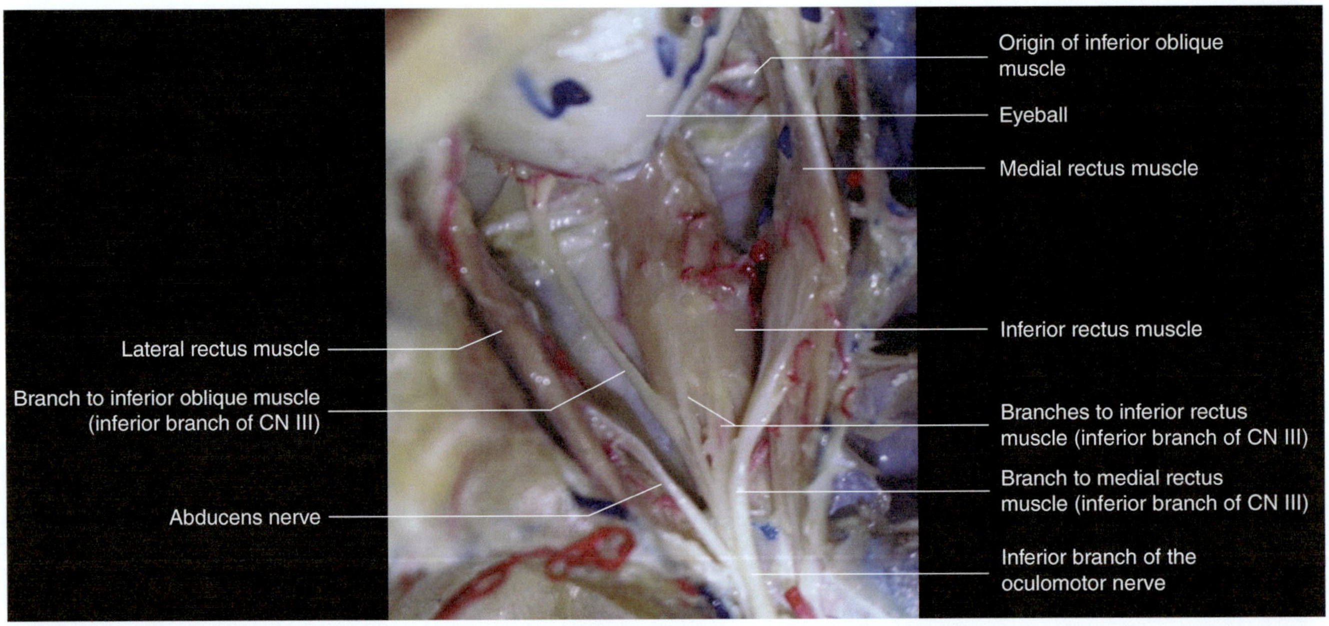

Fig. 4.40 Superior view of the left orbit. The optic and nasociliary nerves have been removed. The distribution of the abducens and the inferior branch of the oculomotor nerves are shown

4.4 Ear

Summary
The ear consists of external, middle, and internal parts. The major function of the ear is hearing and balance. The external ear channels sound to the tympanic membrane. The middle ear, also known as the tympanic cavity contains the three ear ossicles, i.e., malleus, incus, and stapes. The ossicles transmit sound to the inner ear. The eustachian tube, originating from the tympanic cavity, connects to the nasopharynx and helps the ear drain fluid and equalizes air pressure. The internal ear, the deepest part of the ear, has two different structures and functions. The vestibule contributes to balance and the cochlea is the organ of hearing.

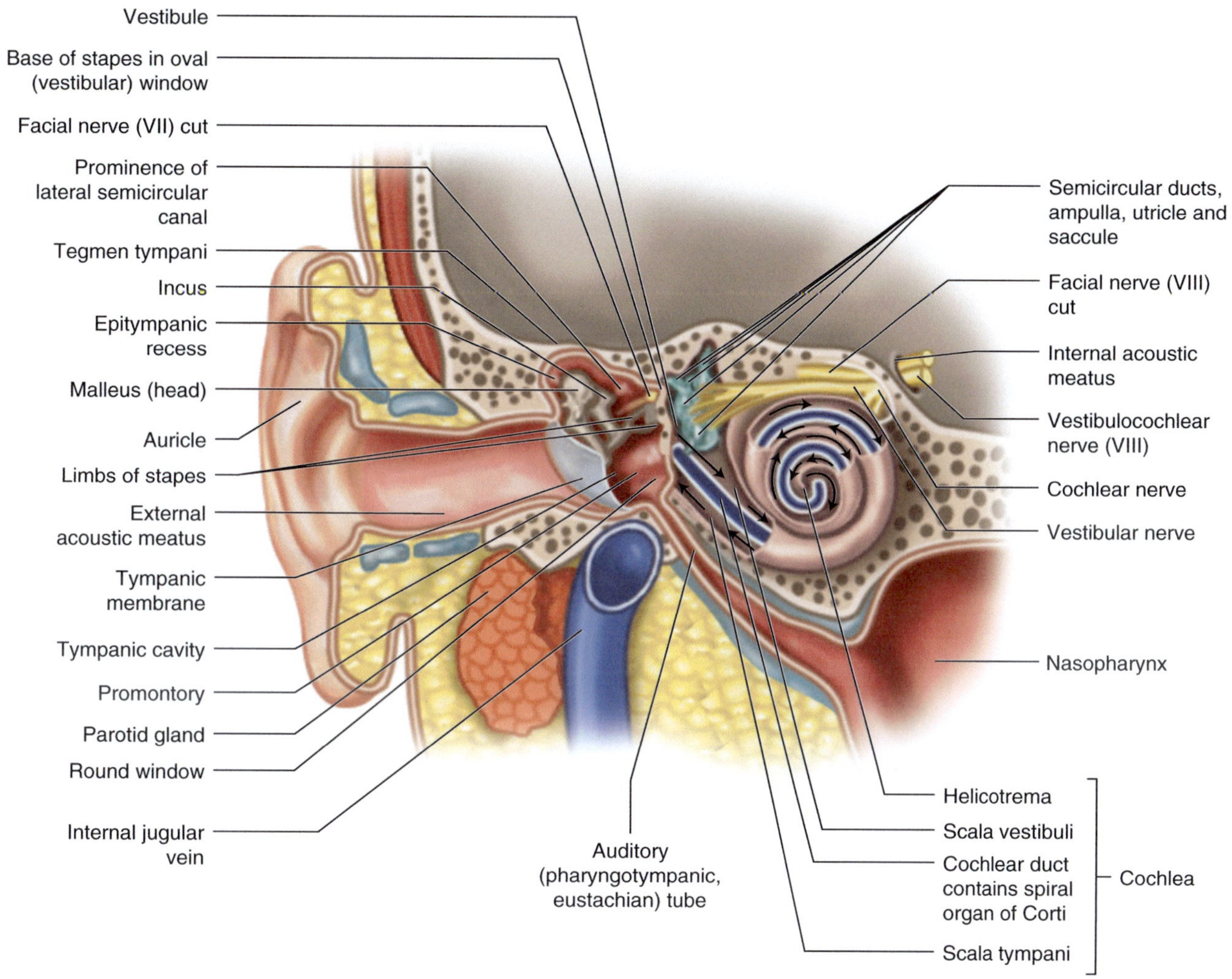

Fig. 4.41 Anterior view of the external, middle, and internal parts of the ear

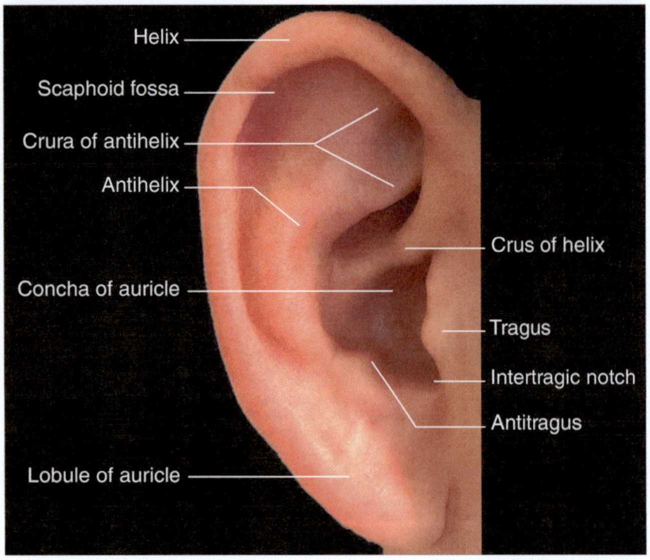

Fig. 4.42 Superficial anatomy of the right auricle

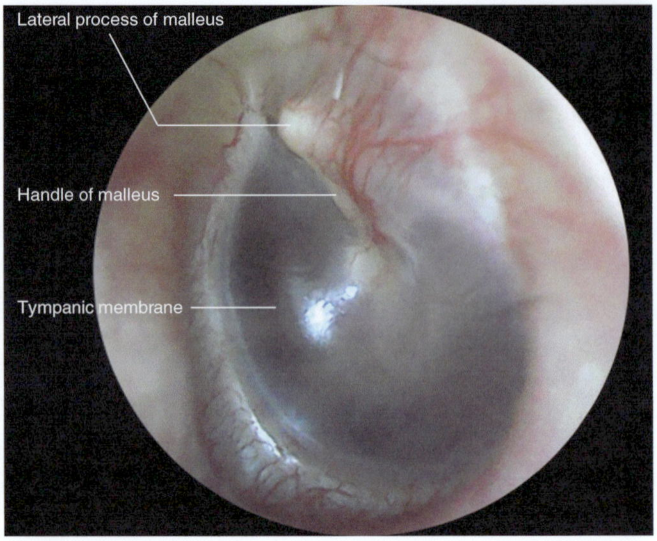

Fig. 4.43 Endoscopic view of the left tympanic membrane

Fig. 4.44 Endoscopic view of the left middle ear (tympanic membrane is removed)

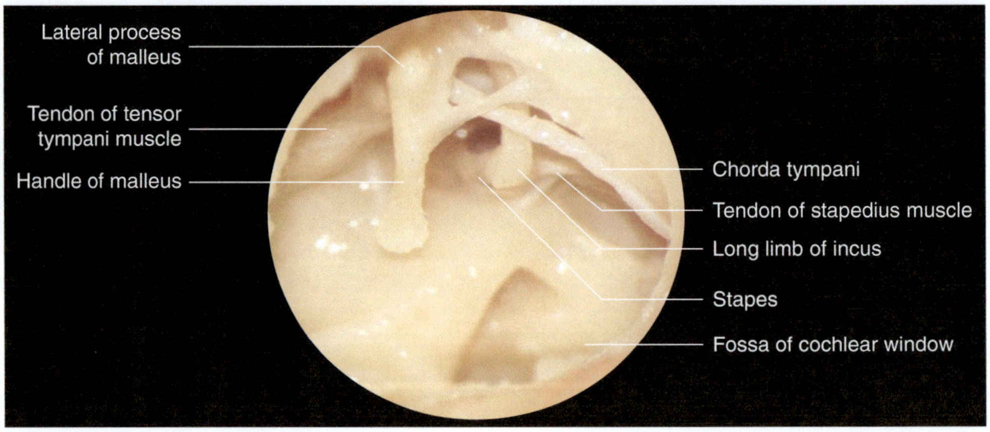

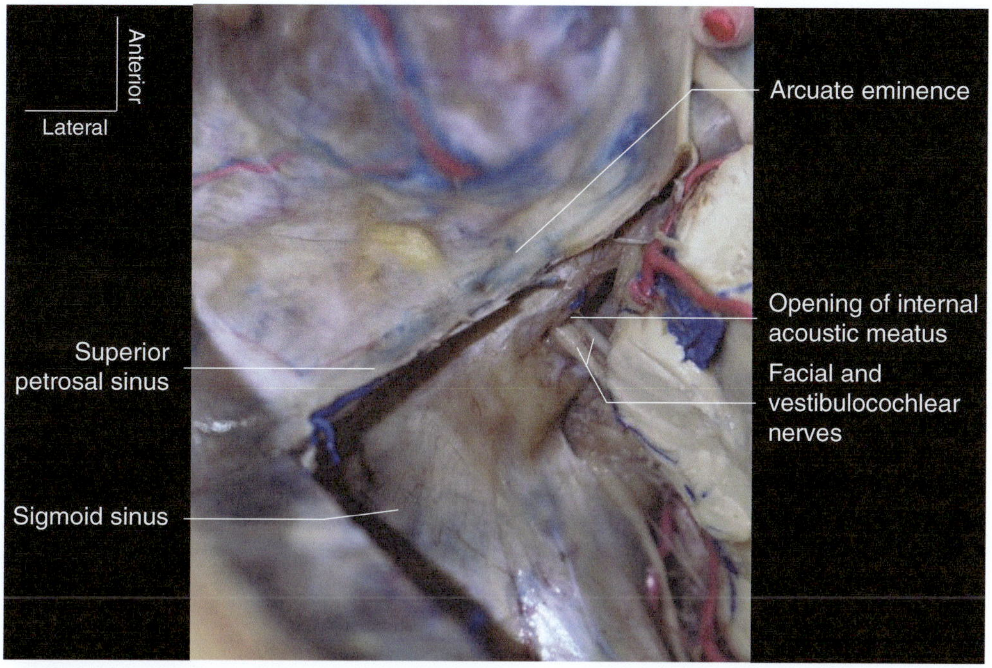

Fig. 4.45 Superior view of the left petrous part of the temporal bone

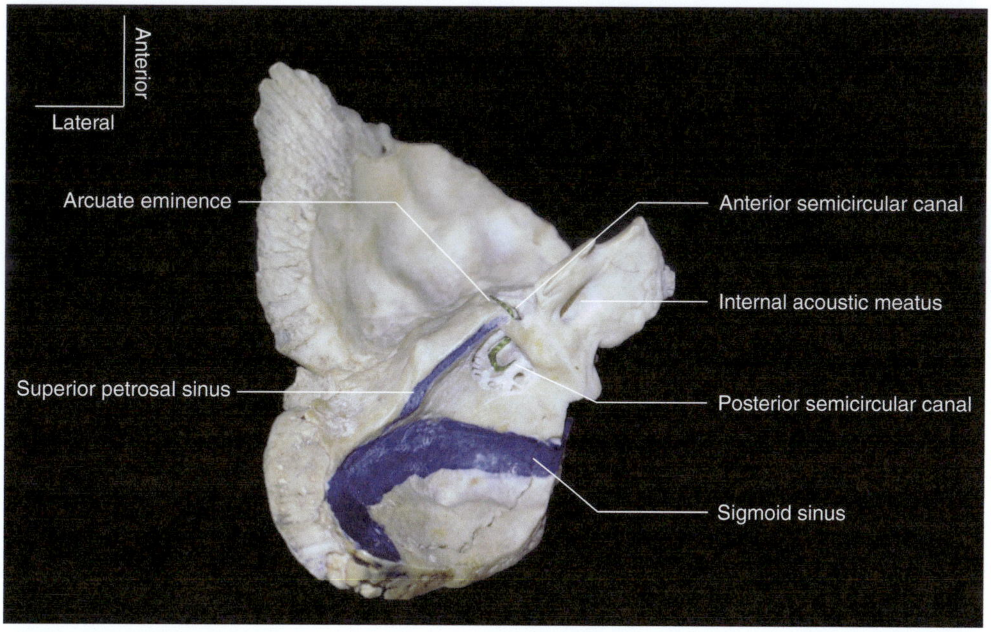

Fig. 4.46 Superior view of the left temporal bone

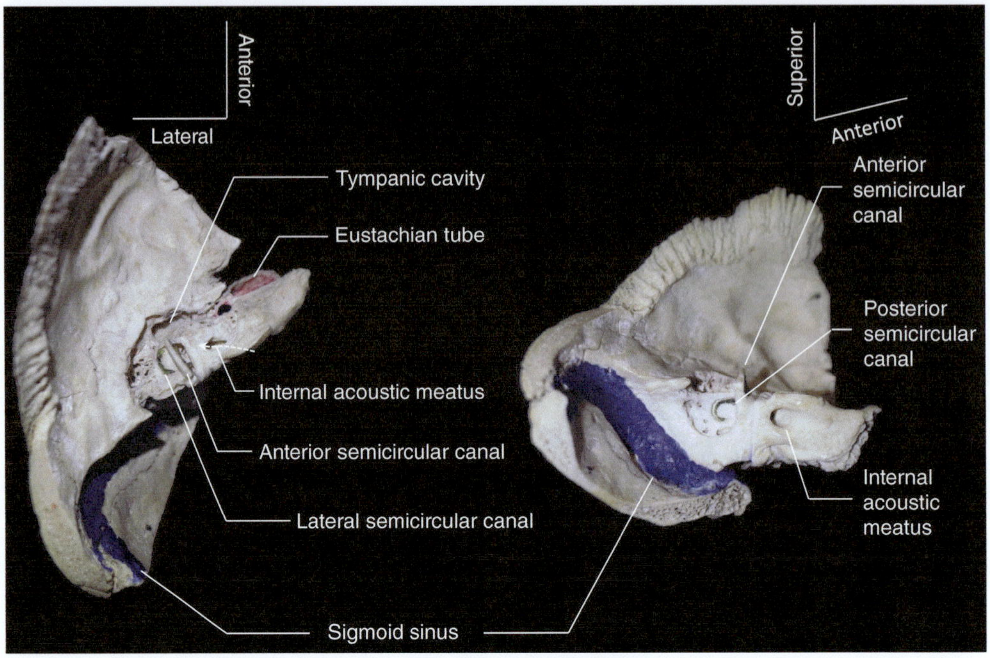

Fig. 4.47 Superior and medial views of the left temporal bone

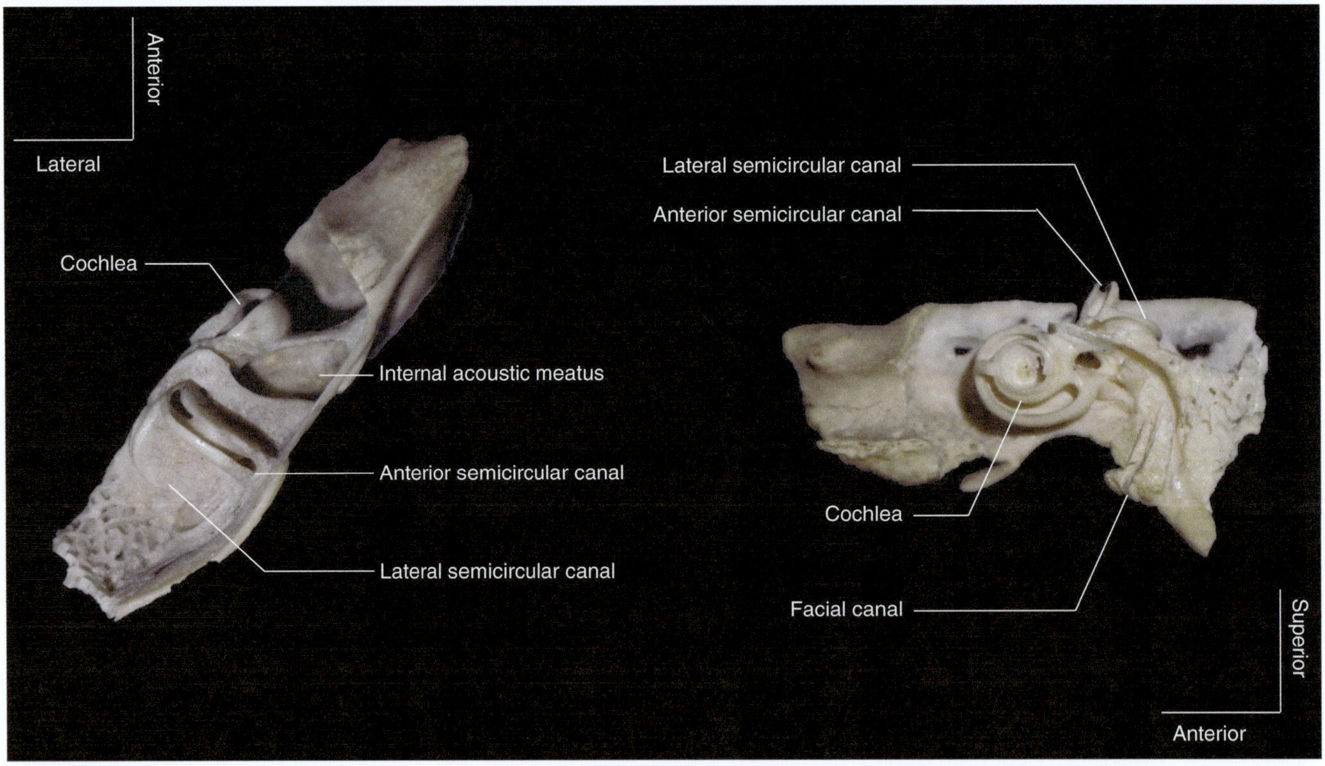

Fig. 4.48 Superior view of the left petrous part of the temporal bone

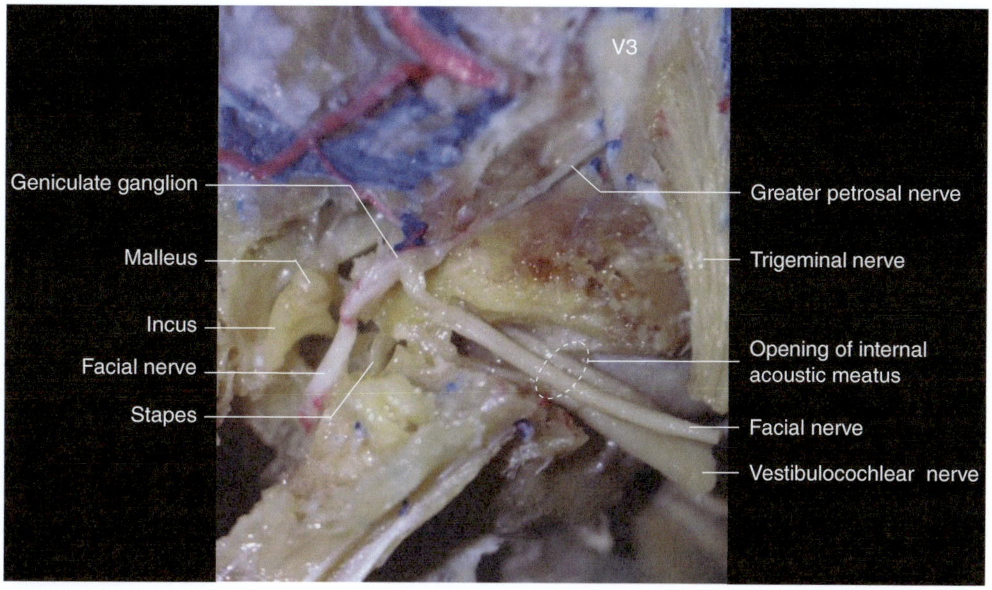

Fig. 4.49 Superior view of the left petrous part of the temporal bone

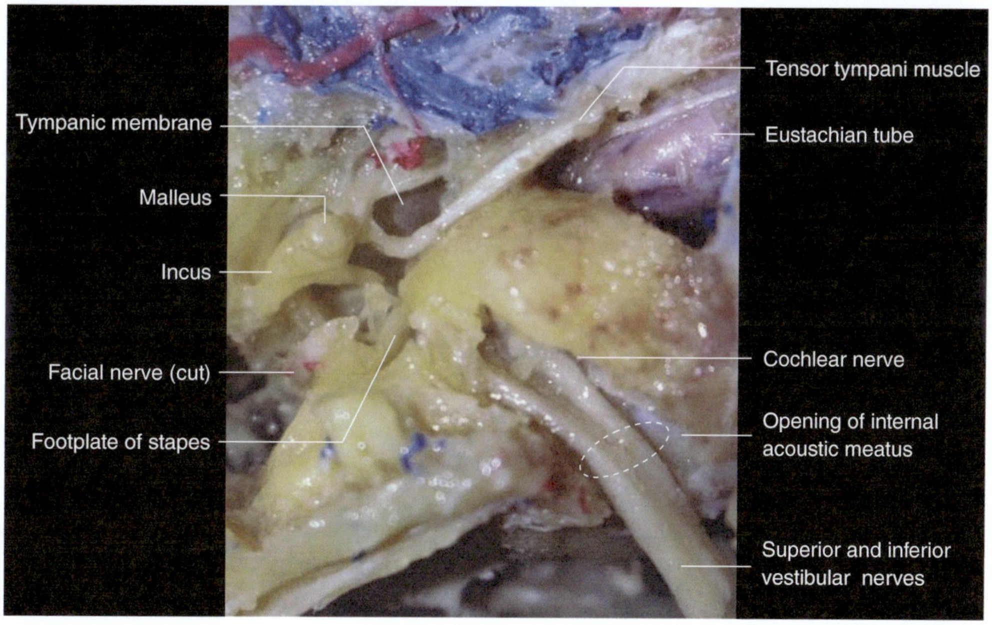

Fig. 4.50 Superior view of the left petrous part. Facial nerve, geniculate ganglion, and greater petrosal nerve are resected

4.5 Pharynx and Parapharyngeal Spaces

Summary

The pharynx is a part of both the upper respiratory system and is divided into three parts: nasopharynx, oropharynx, and laryngopharynx. The function of the pharynx as a part of the respiratory system is for warming, humidifying, and filtering inspired air. As a part of the digestive system, its three pharyngeal constrictor muscles help propel food into the esophagus. The pharynx contains a ring of lymphatic tissue called Waldeyer's ring and this is formed by the lingual, (tubal), palatine, and pharyngeal tonsils. The majority of the blood supply to the pharynx is via the ascending pharyngeal artery and branches of the facial, lingual, and maxillary arteries. The pharynx is innervated by branches of CNs V, IX, and X. The parapharyngeal space is a pathway for the major vessels, cranial nerves, and other anatomical structures. The auditory tubes (eustachian tubes) connect the nasopharynx to the middle ear so that the air pressure in the middle ear can be equalized.

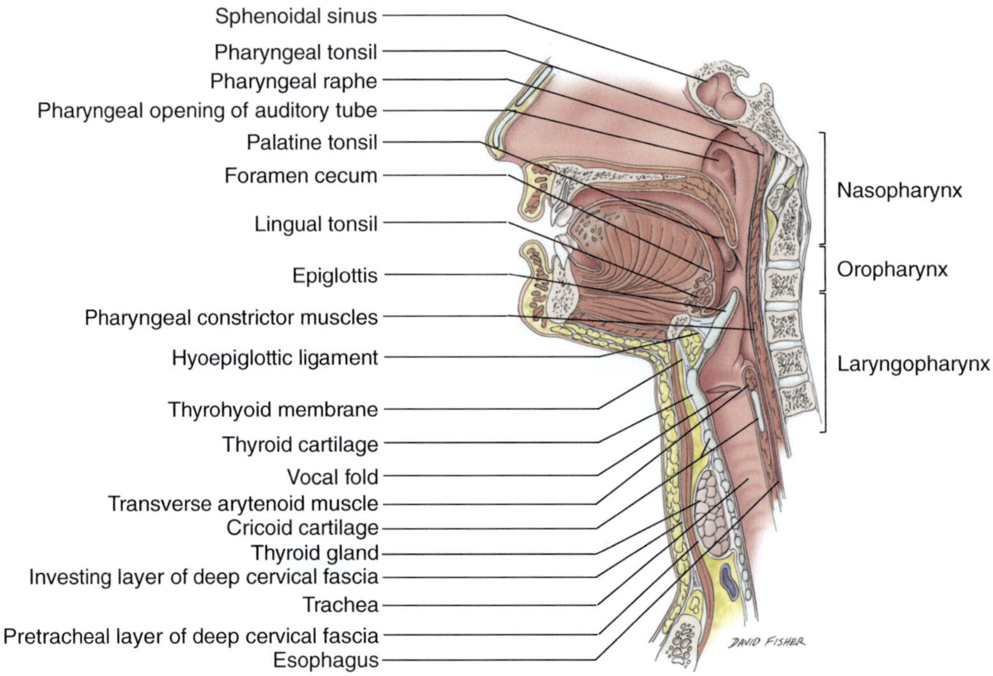

Fig. 4.51 Medial view of the pharynx. The pharynx is divided into three parts: nasopharynx, oropharynx, and laryngopharynx. The nasopharynx borders the skull base superiorly and the inferior edge of the uvula inferiorly; the oropharynx is bordered by the superior edge of the epiglottis inferiorly; the laryngopharynx is bordered by the inferior border of the cricoid cartilage inferioly. Waldeyer's ring is formed by the lingual tonsil, palatine tonsil, and pharyngeal tonsil.

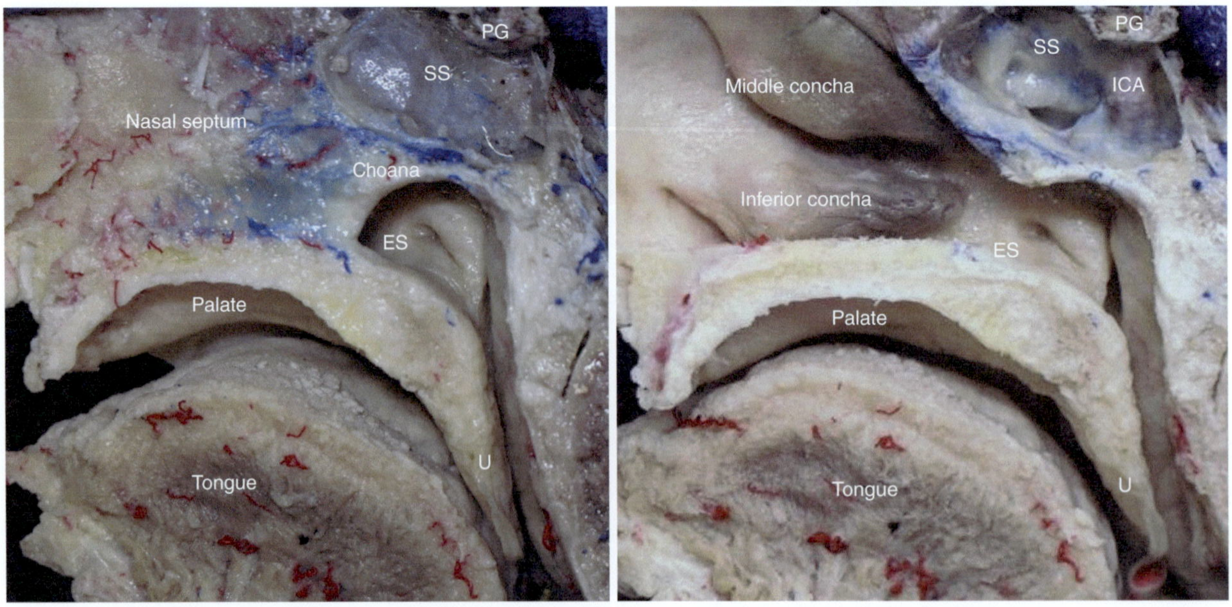

Fig. 4.52 Medial view of the nasopharynx and surrounding structures. Before (left) and after (right) removal of the nasal septum. *ES* eustachian tube, *PG* pituitary gland, *SS* sphenoidal sinus, *U* uvula

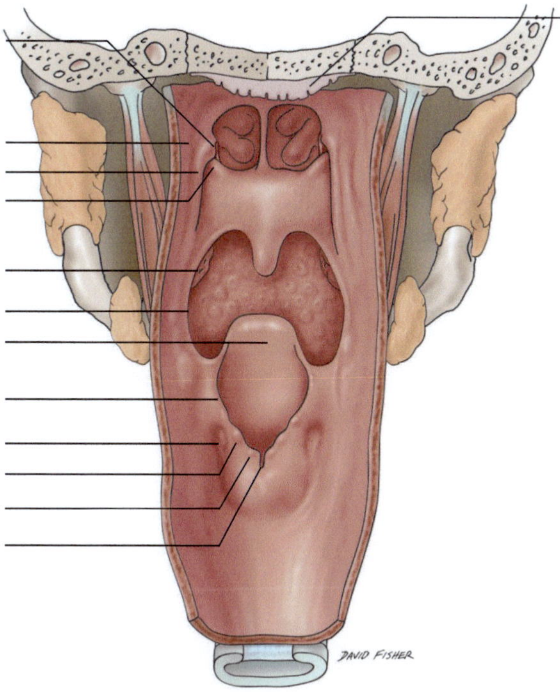

Fig. 4.53 Posterior view of the pharynx. © Fisher/Tubbs 2020. All Rights Reserved

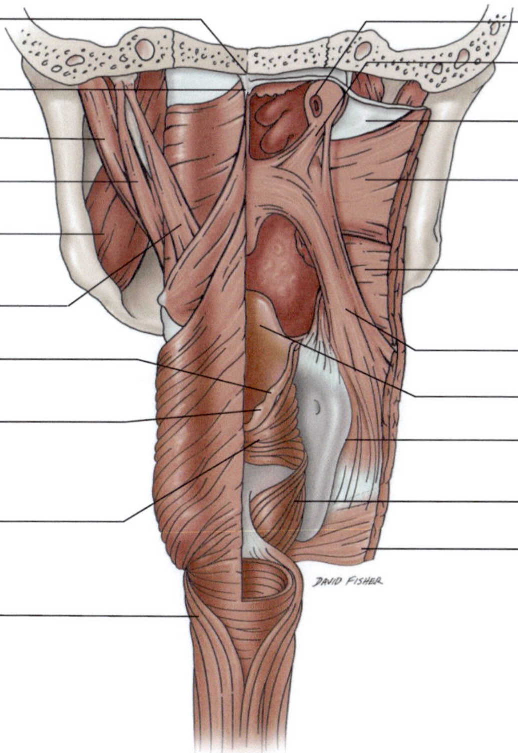

Fig. 4.54 Posterior view of the pharynx. The pharyngeal constrictor muscles are all innervated by the vagus nerve via the pharyngeal plexus. Although it is controversial, the cricopharyngeal part of the inferior pharyngeal constrictor muscle can be supplied by the external branch of the superior laryngeal nerve and recurrent laryngeal nerve (Sakamoto 2013; Standring 2020). © Fisher/Tubbs 2020. All Rights Reserved

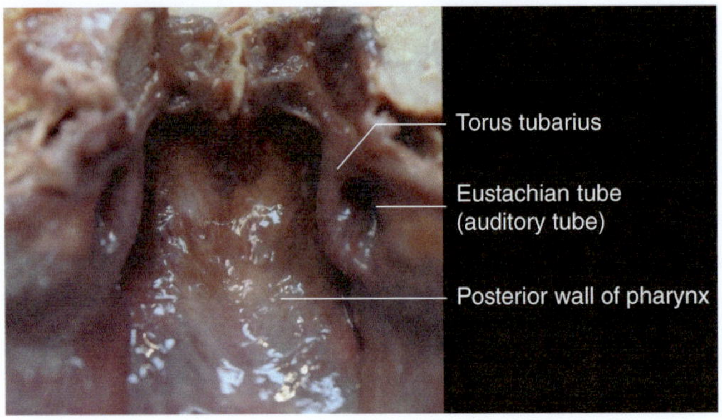

Fig. 4.55 Anterior view of the posterior wall of the pharynx

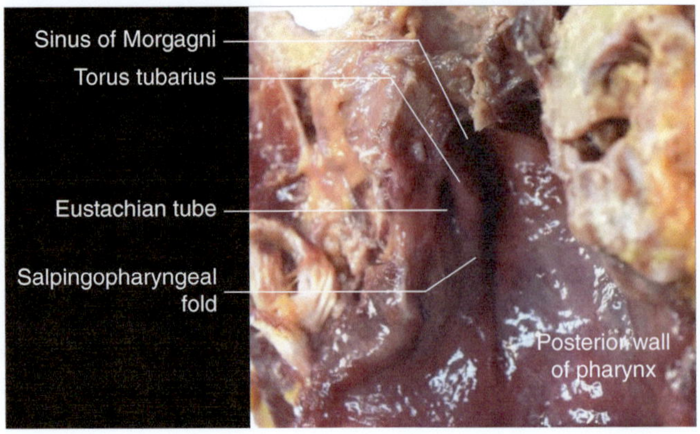

Fig. 4.56 Anteromedial view of the posterior and lateral walls of the pharynx

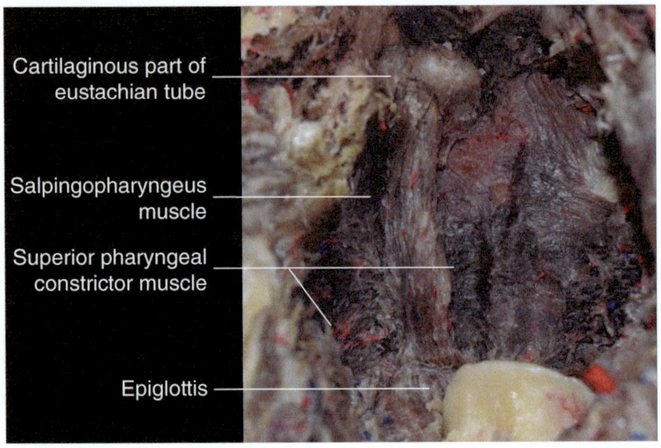

Fig. 4.57 Anteromedial view of the posterior and lateral walls of the pharynx. Note the overlying mucosa has been removed

Fig. 4.58 Anteromedial view of the posterior and lateral walls of the pharynx. Before (left) and after (right) removal of the overlying mucosa

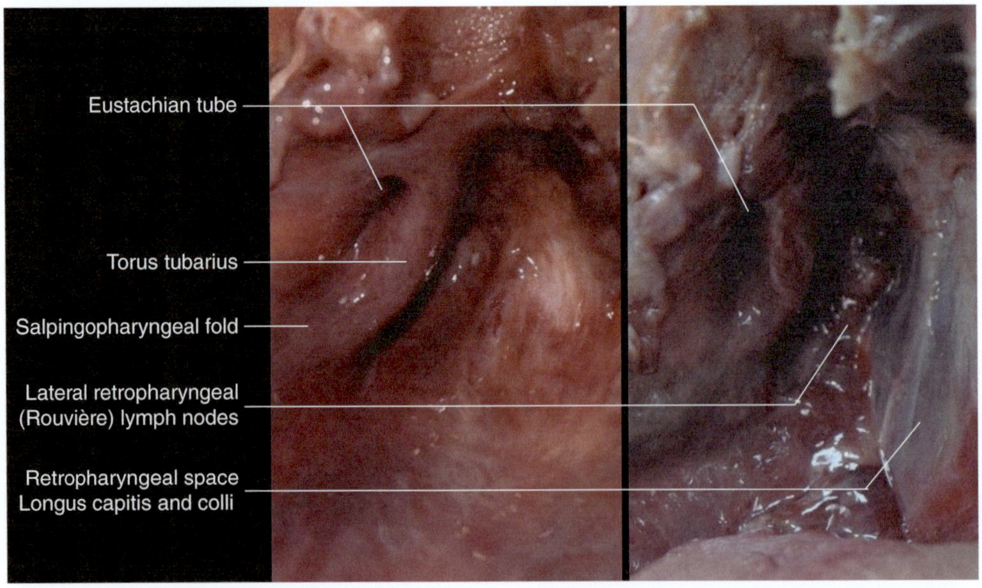

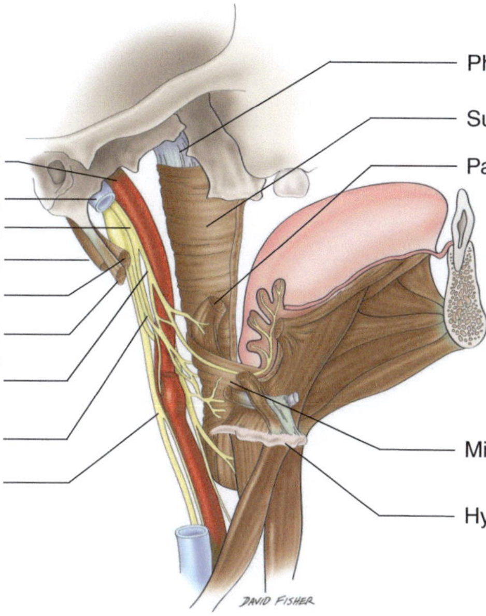

Fig. 4.59 Lateral view of the pharyngeal plexus. © Fisher/Tubbs 2020. All Rights Reserved

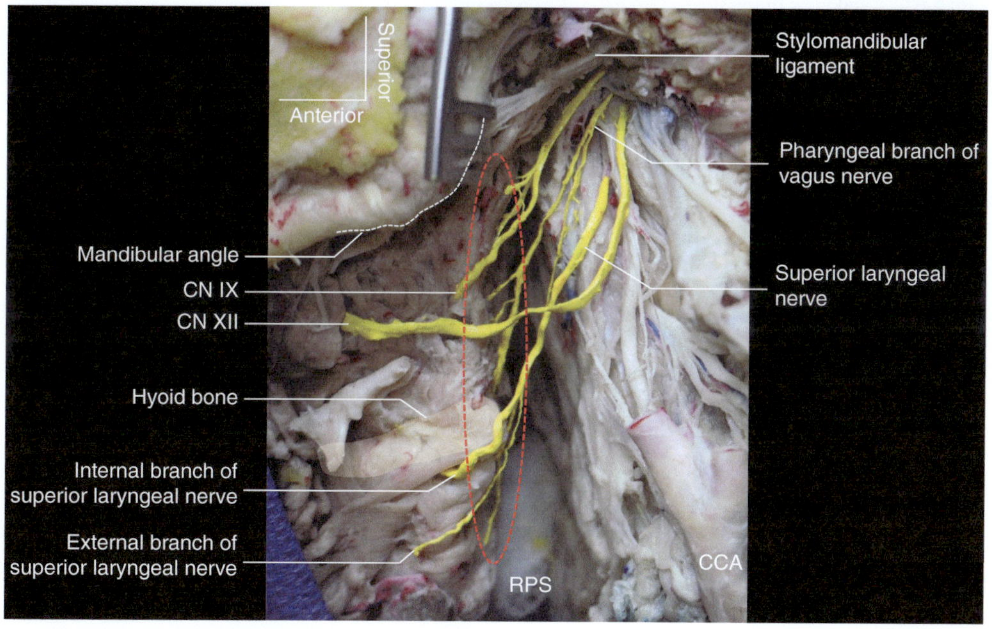

Fig. 4.60 Lateral view of the pharynx. Pharyngeal branches of the vagus and glossopharyngeal nerves form the pharyngeal plexus (red dashed circle). CCA common carotid artery, RPS retropharyngeal space

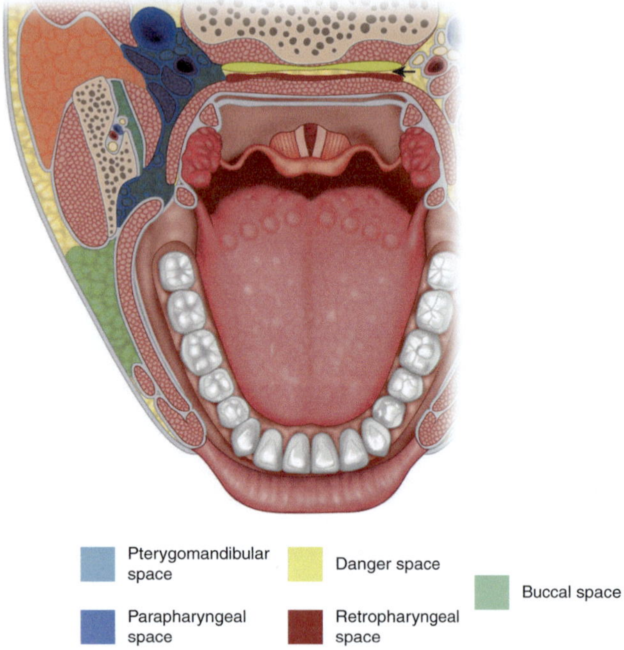

Fig. 4.61 Axial view of the spaces. Note the alar fascia (arrow) divides the space located posterior to the posterior pharyngeal wall into the retropharyngeal and "danger" spaces. The parapharyngeal space is further divided into pre- and poststyloid spaces based on the relationship between the styloid muscles, i.e., stylohyoid, styloglossus, and stylopharyngeus muscles

Fig. 4.62 Axial image of the parapharyngeal space (blue area) and related structures on contrasted computed tomography

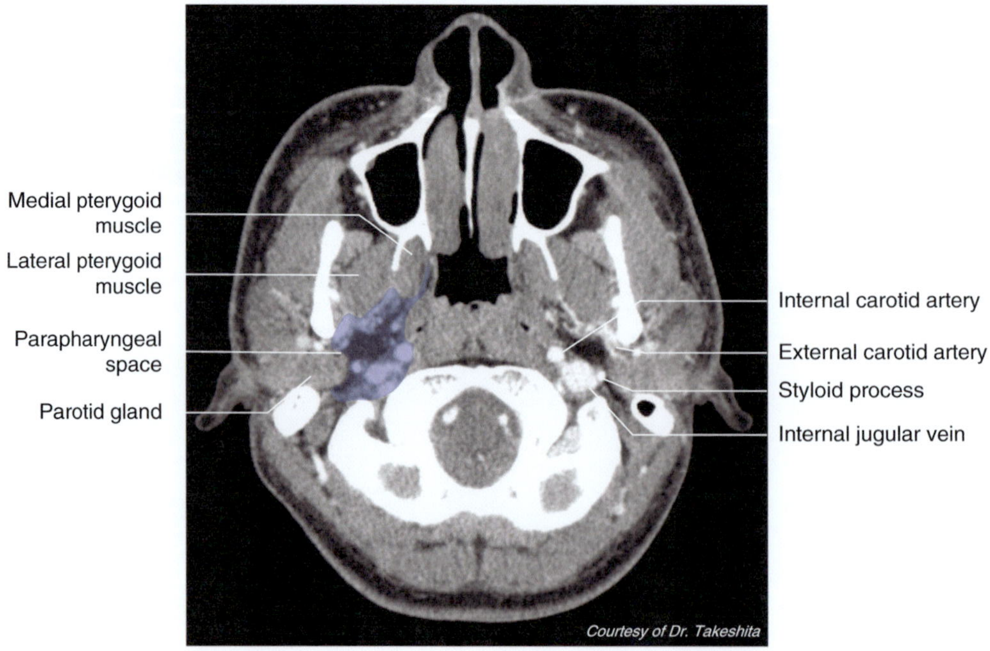

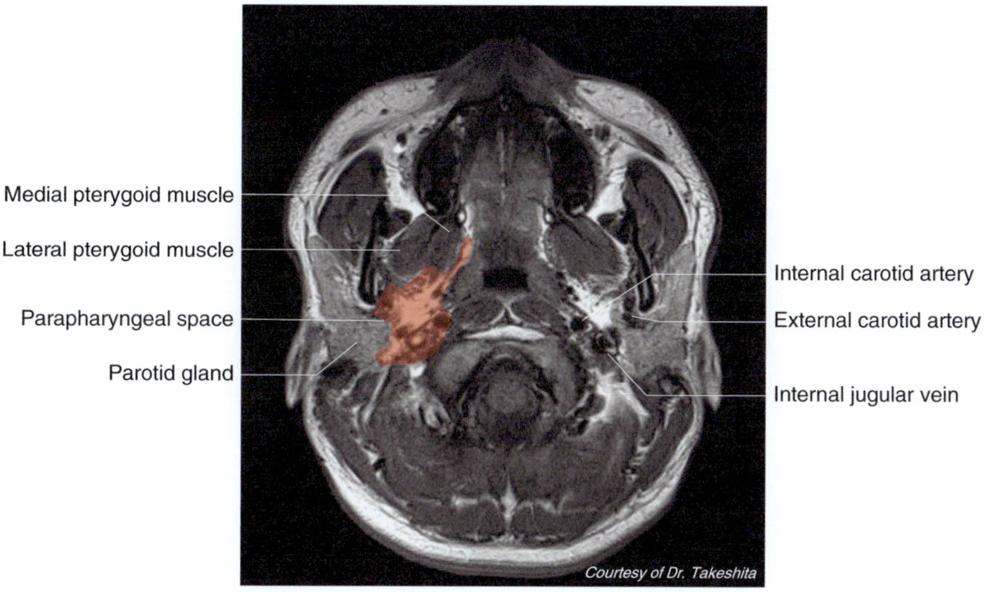

Fig. 4.63 Axial section of the parapharyngeal space (red area) and related structures on magnetic resonance image (T1W1). Note that the adipose tissue in the parapharyngeal space enhances

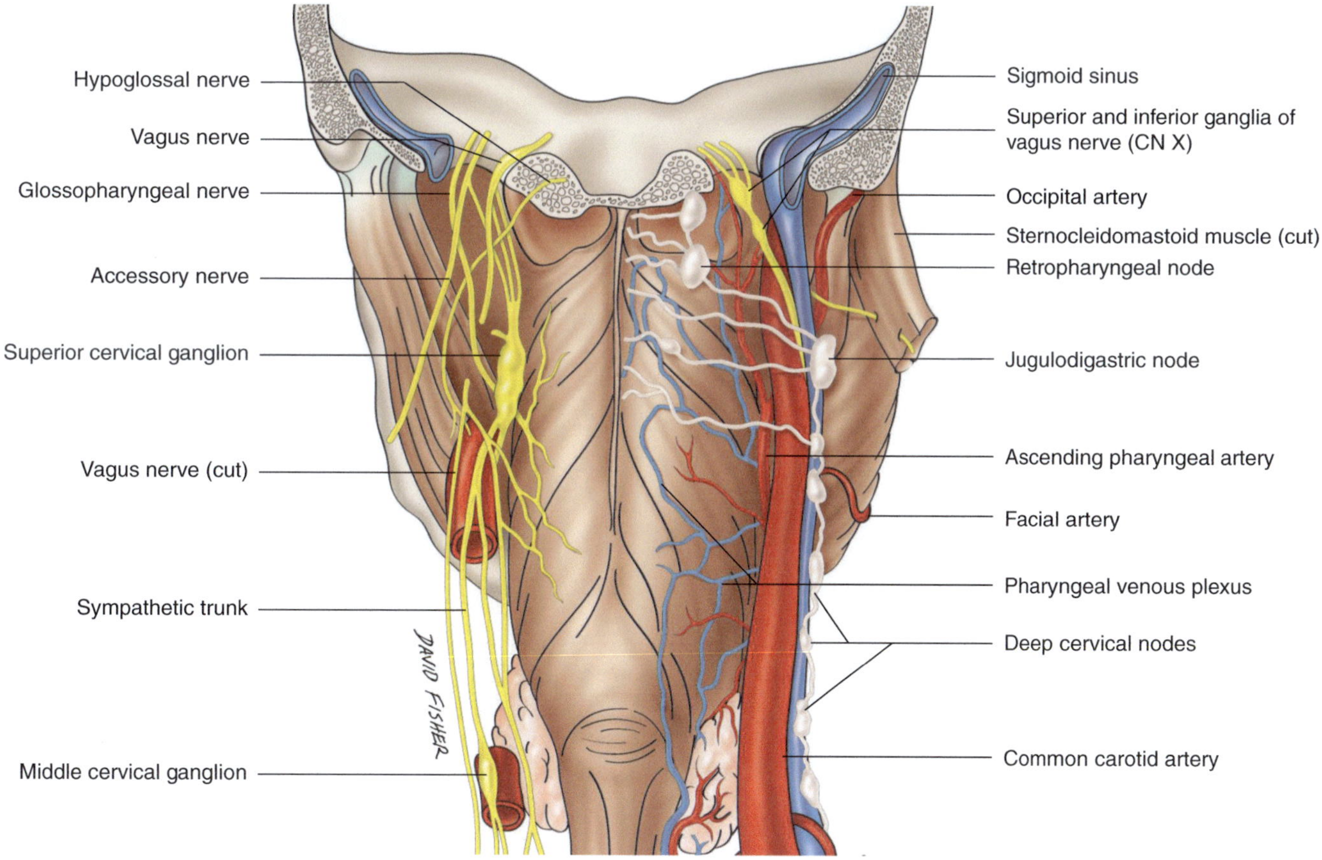

Fig. 4.64 Posterior view of the pharynx and para/retropharyngeal spaces

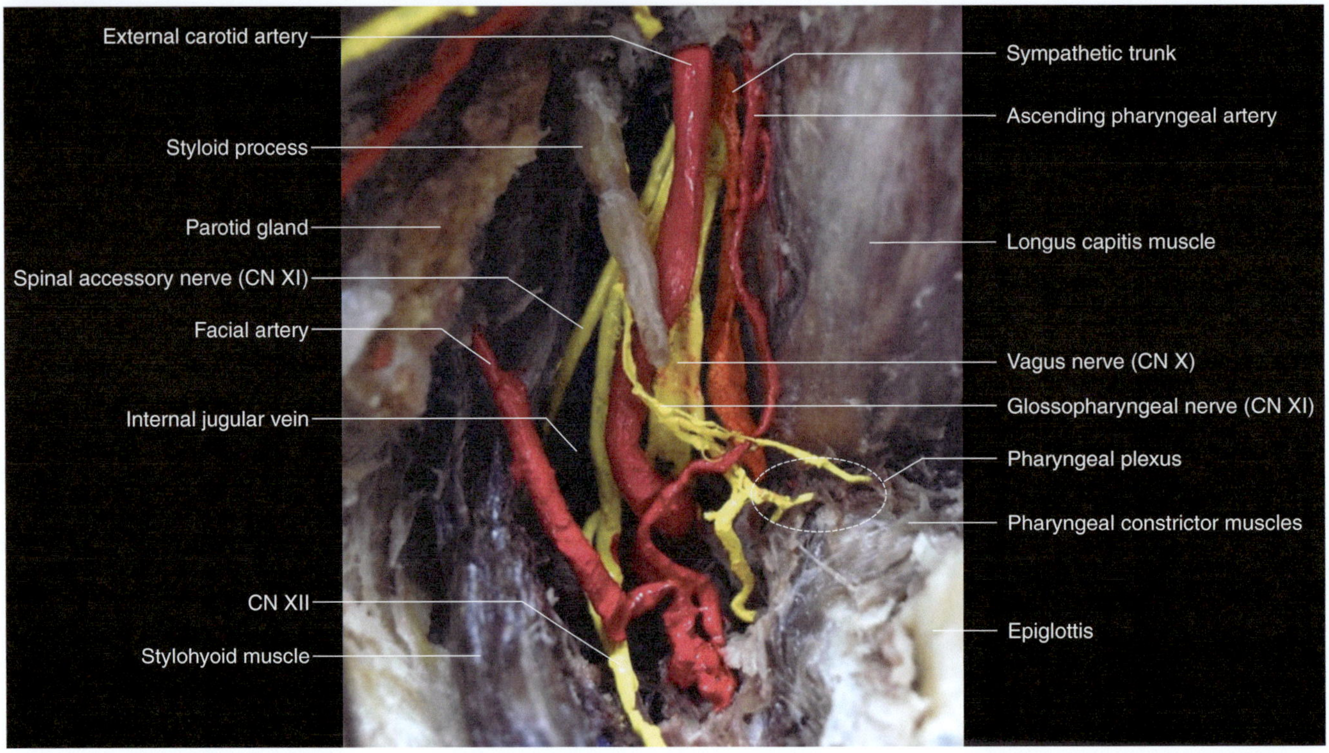

Fig. 4.65 Anterior view (transoral view) of the right parapharyngeal space

Fig. 4.66 Anterior view (transoral view) of the right parapharyngeal space. Most of the structures in the prestyloid (lateral styloid) space have been removed. Note Rouvière's lymph node lies on the surface of the lateral border of the longus capitis and medial to the internal carotid artery. Rouvière lymph node is located within the buccopharyngeal fascia at the C1 or C2 vertebral level near the opening of the carotid canal and drains into the jugulodigastric node

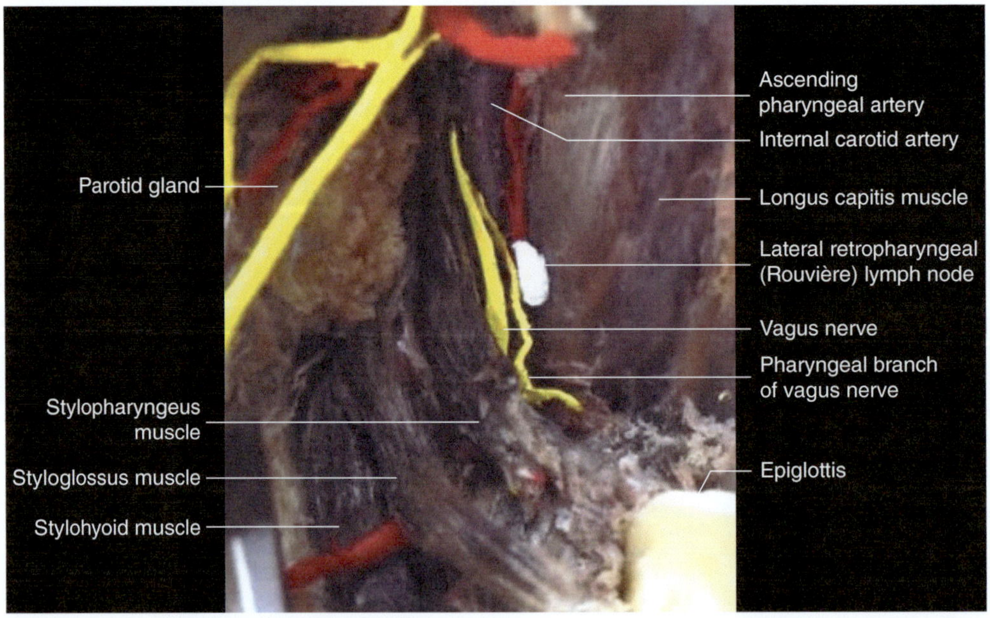

4.6 Larynx

Summary
The larynx is the airway that extends from the tongue to the trachea, which open into the laryngopharynx and forms the anterior wall of it. The larynx consists of five cartilages, i.e., epiglottic, thyroid, cricoid, corniculate, and arytenoid cartilages, and hyoid bone. Intrinsic muscles of the larynx are innervated by vagus nerve branches, either external branch of the superior laryngeal nerve or recurrent laryngeal nerve. Dysfunction of the intrinsic muscles can result in hoarseness or loss of tone. Internal branch of the superior laryngeal nerve supplies the sensory fibers to the larynx. The larynx is supplied by the superior thyroid branch of the external carotid artery superiorly and inferior thyroid branch of the thyrocervical trunk (branch of subclavian artery).

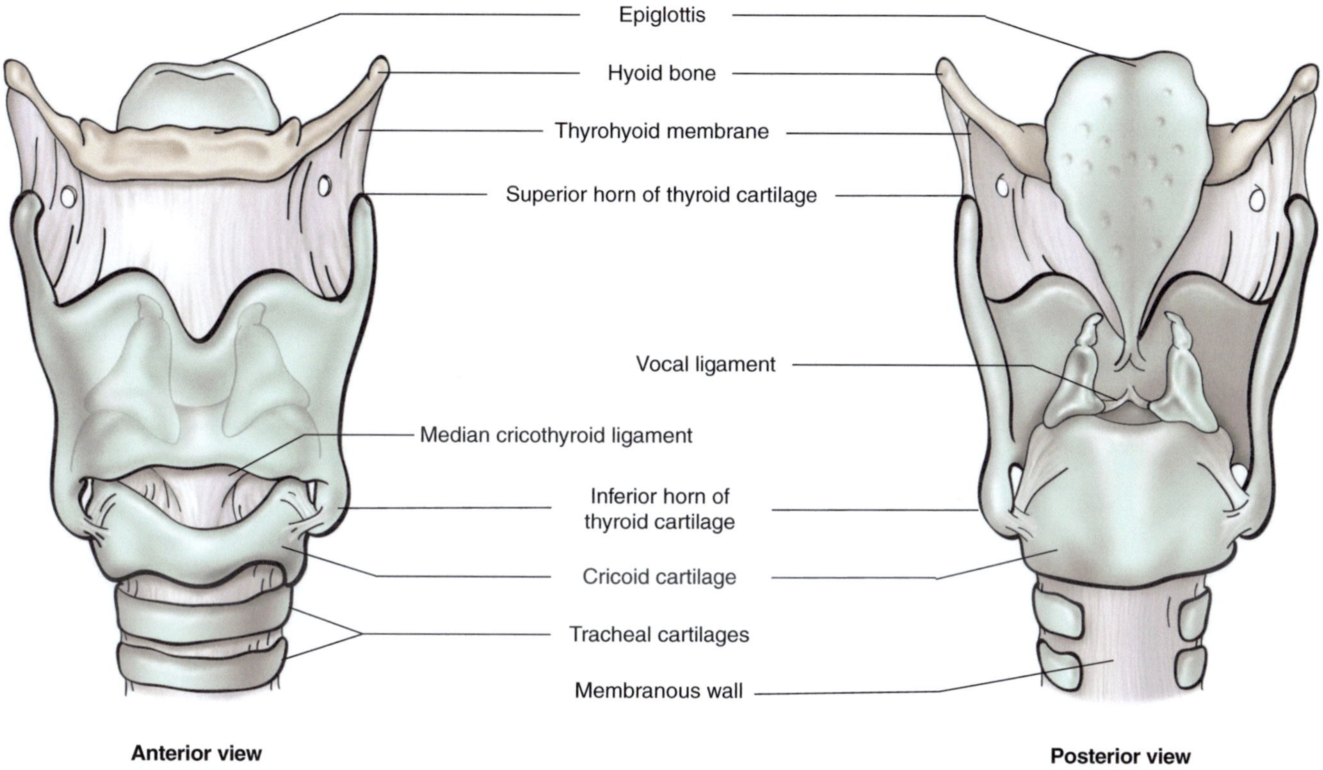

Fig. 4.67 Anterior and posterior views of larynx

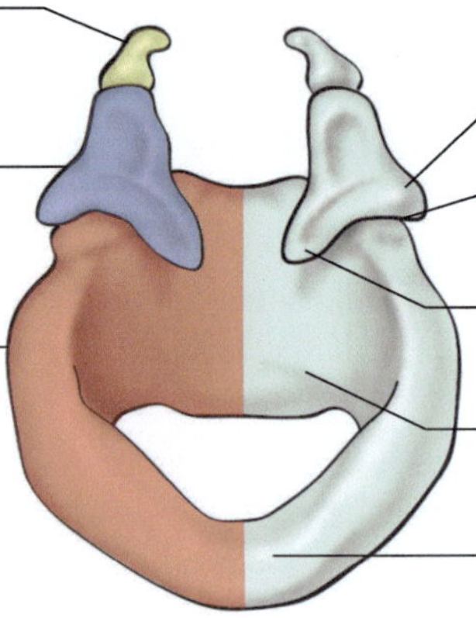

Fig. 4.68 Anterosuperior view of the cricoid, arytenoid, and corniculate cartilages

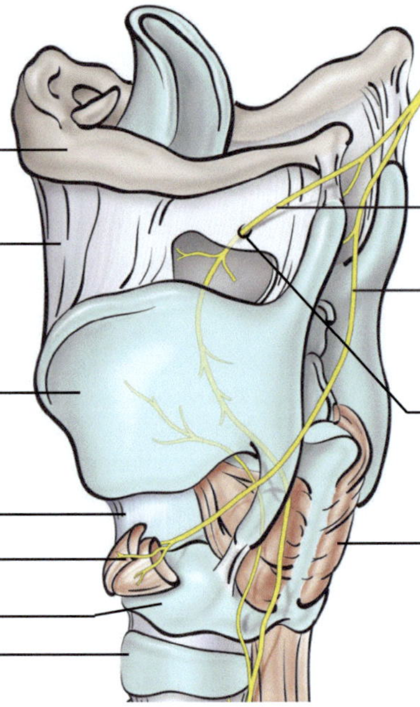

Fig. 4.69 Lateral view of the larynx. The external branch of the superior laryngeal nerve innervates the cricothyroid muscle that increases the tension of the vocal ligaments. Internal branch mainly consists of sensory fibers and it communicates with the anterior branch of the recurrent laryngeal nerve to form the nerve of Galen medial to the thyroid cartilage

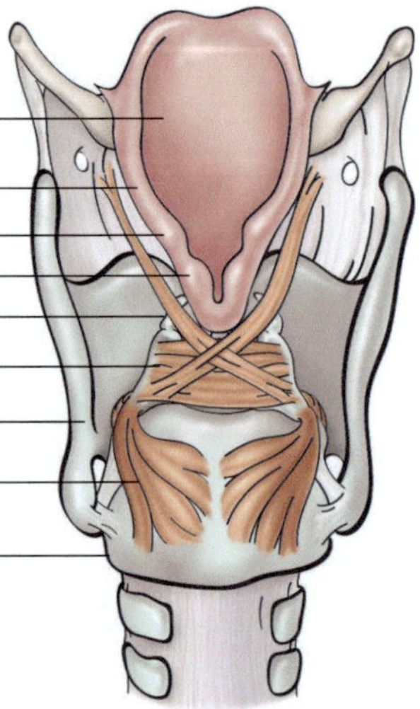

Fig. 4.70 Posterior view of the larynx

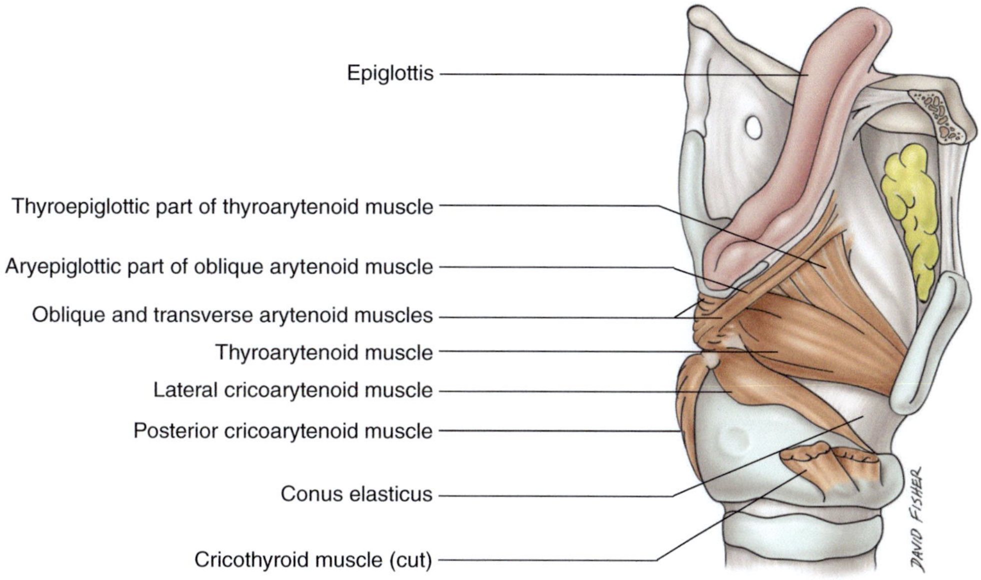

Fig. 4.71 Postrolateral view of the larynx. Right side of the thyroid cartilage has been removed

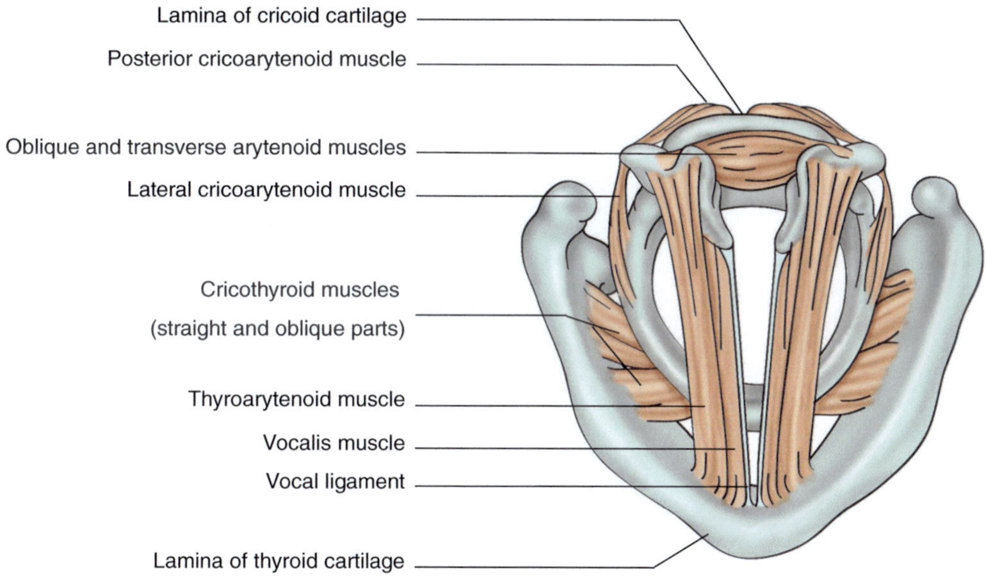

Fig. 4.72 Superior view of the larynx

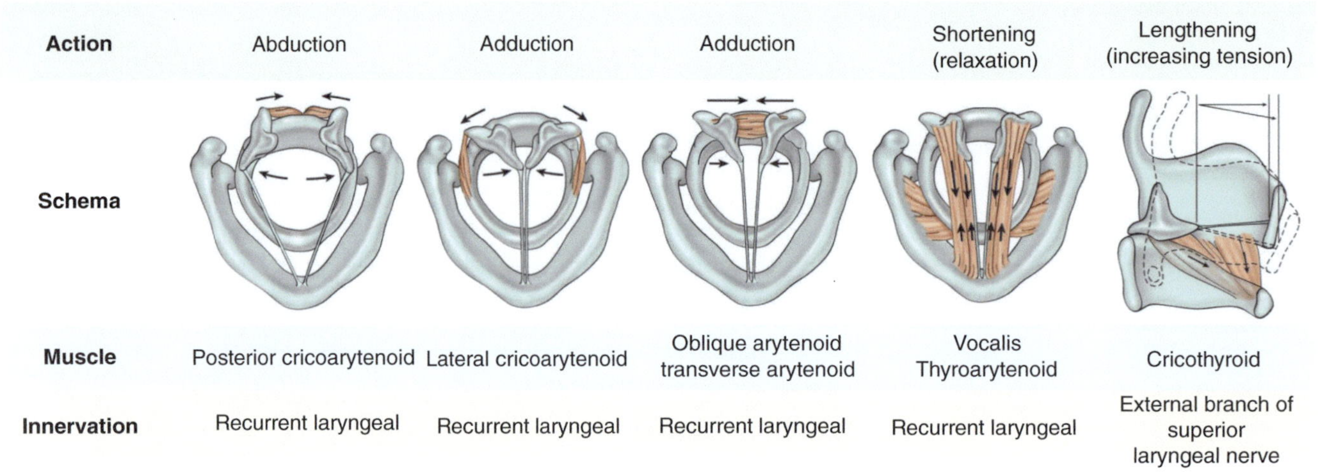

Fig. 4.73 Action of intrinsic muscles of the larynx to the vocal cord

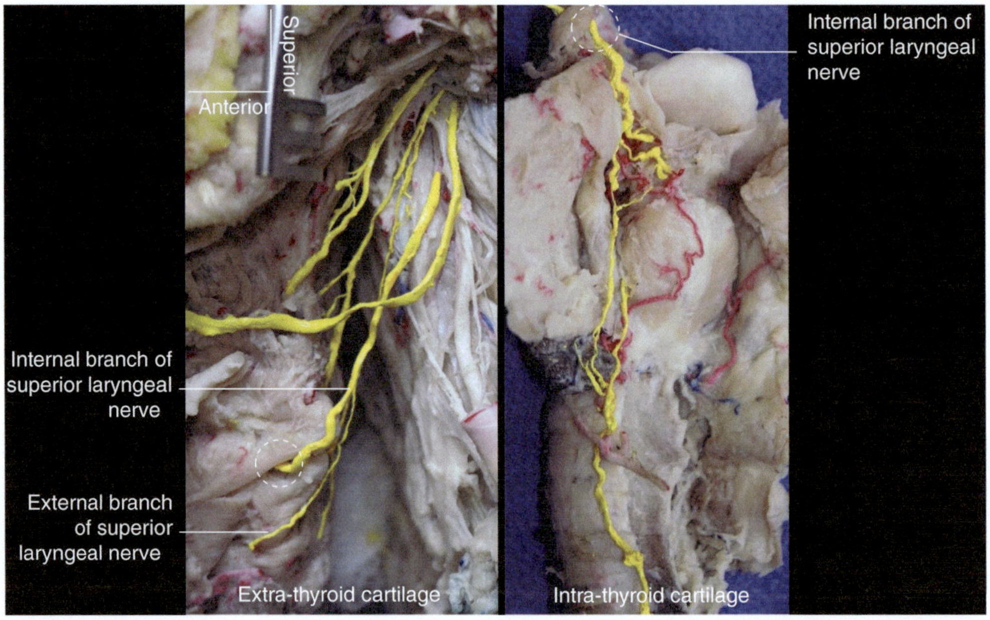

Fig. 4.74 The external branch of the superior laryngeal nerve innervates the cricothyroid muscle and cricopharyngeal part of the inferior pharyngeal constrictor (Sakamoto 2013; Standring 2020). The internal branch of the superior laryngeal nerve pierces the foramen for the superior laryngeal vessels and internal branch of the superior laryngeal nerve to provide sensory fibers to the larynx

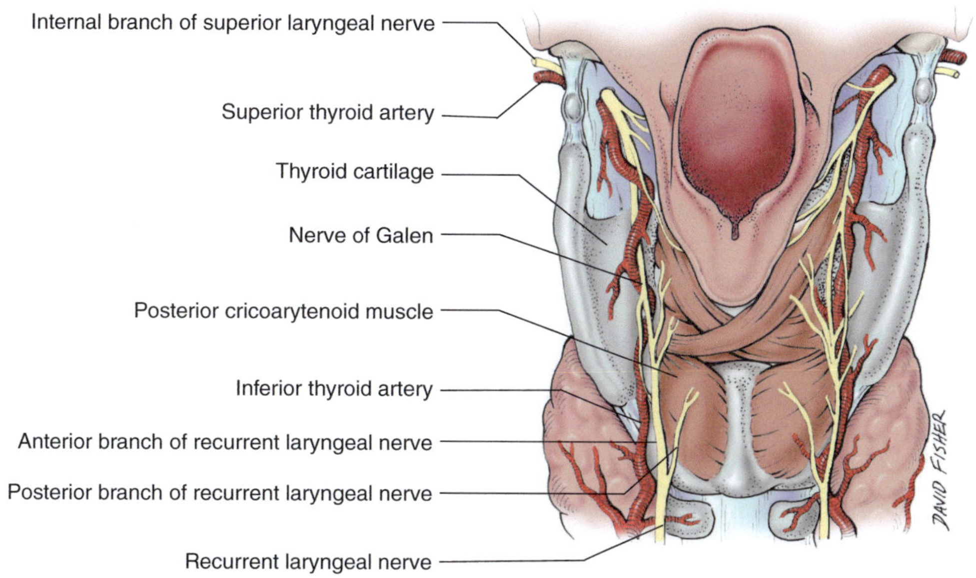

Fig. 4.75 The internal branch of the superior laryngeal nerve provides sensory branches to the larynx above the vocal cords and communicates with the anterior branch of the recurrent laryngeal nerve to form the nerve of Galen medial to the thyroid cartilage.

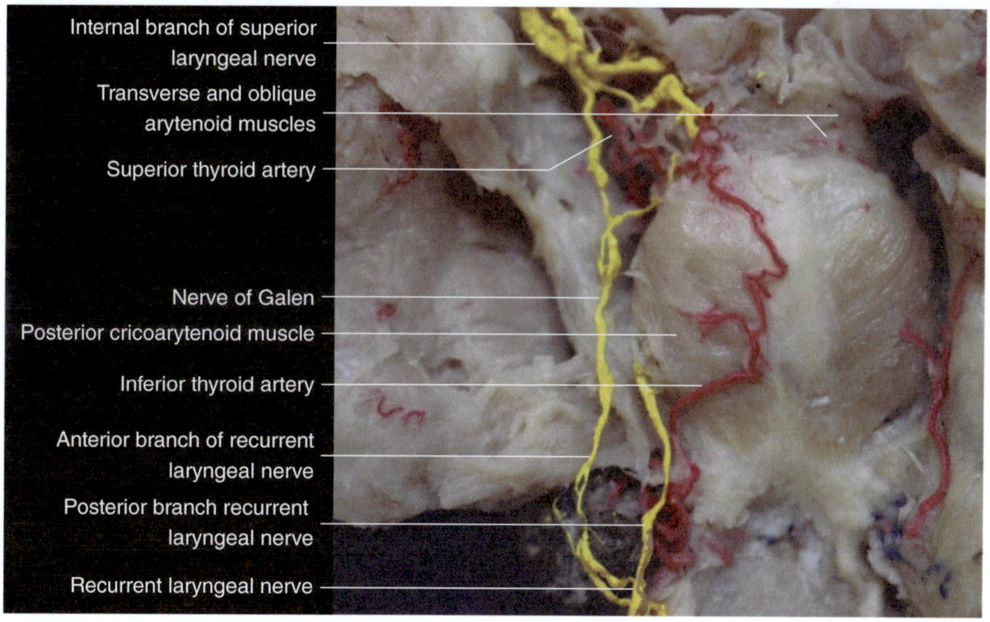

Fig. 4.76 The internal branch of the superior laryngeal nerve and anterior branch of the recurrent laryngeal nerve communicate to form the nerve of Galen medial to the thyroid cartilage. All the laryngeal muscles except the cricothyroid muscle are innervated by the recurrent laryngeal nerve

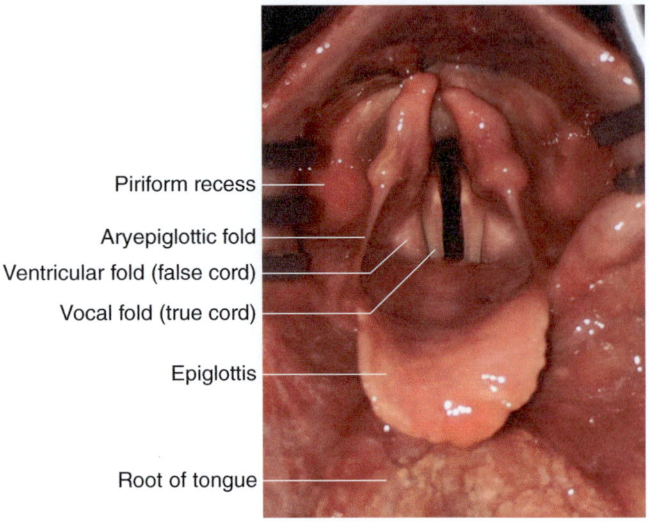

Fig. 4.77 Superior view of the larynx

4.7 Infratemporal and Pterygopalatine Fossae

Summary

The pterygopalatine fossa (PT fossa) is bounded by the greater wing of the sphenoid bone superiorly, pterygoid process posteriorly, and infratemporal surface of the maxilla anteriorly.

The infratemporal fossa (IT fossa) is situated medial and inferior to the zygomatic arch and is not fully bounded by bony structures. Its boundaries include the infratemporal crest of the sphenoid bone superiorly, infratemporal surface of the maxilla anteriorly, articular tubercle of the temporal bone posteriorly, lateral plate of the pterygoid process medially, medial pterygoid muscle inferiorly, and ramus of the mandible laterally.

The PT fossa is mainly related to V2 and its branches, and the IT fossa to V3 and its branches. Both fossae are supplied by the maxillary artery and its branches.

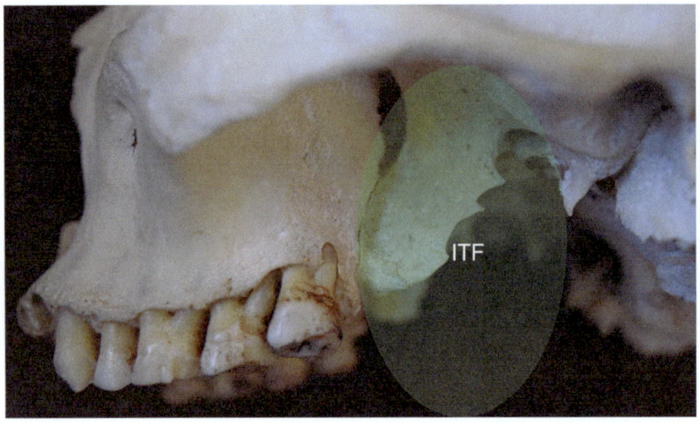

Fig. 4.78 Lateral view of the left infratemporal fossa (ITF)

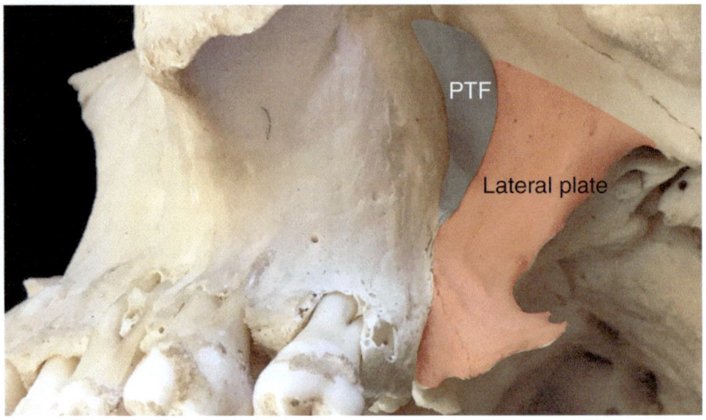

Fig. 4.79 Lateral view of the left ptyerygopalatine fossa (PTF)

Fig. 4.80 Lateral view of the left infratemporal and pterygopalatine fossae. The ramus of the mandible, lateral pterygoid muscle, posterior wall of the maxilla, infraorbital canal wall, foramen ovale (dashed line), and foramen rotundum (dashed line) are removed for clarity. Muscular branches are not shown. *BM* buccinator, *MPM* medial pterygoid muscle

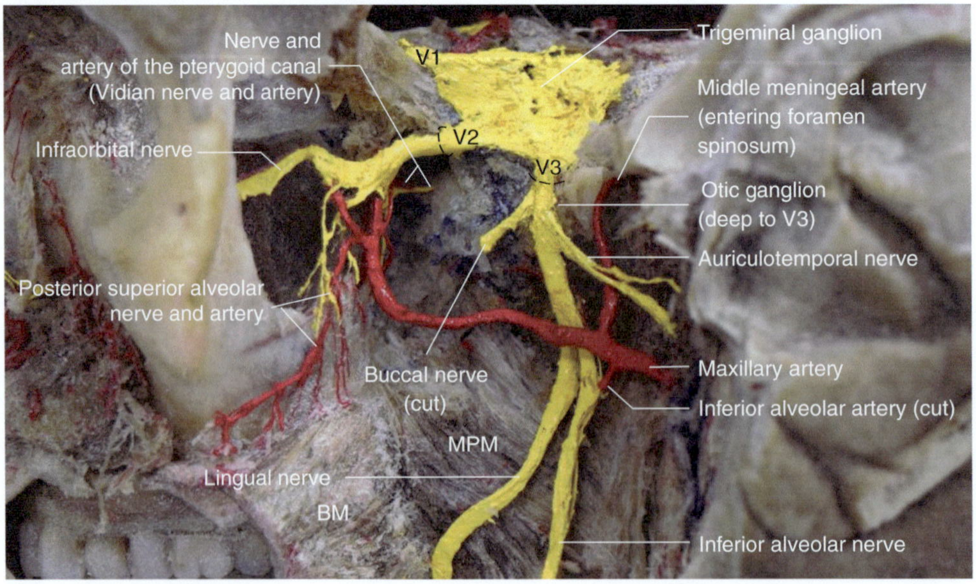

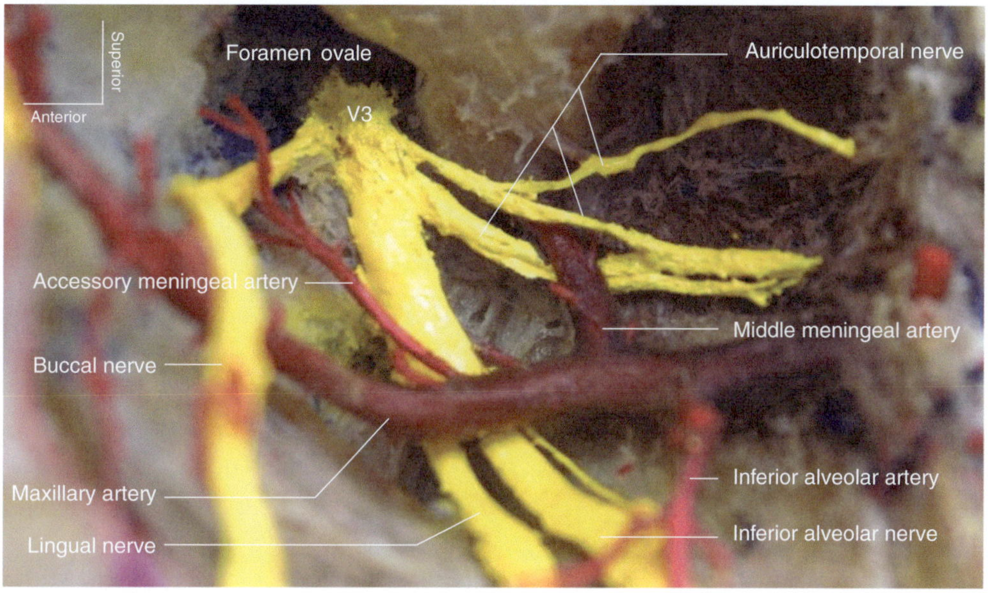

Fig. 4.81 Lateral magnified view of the left infratemporal fossa

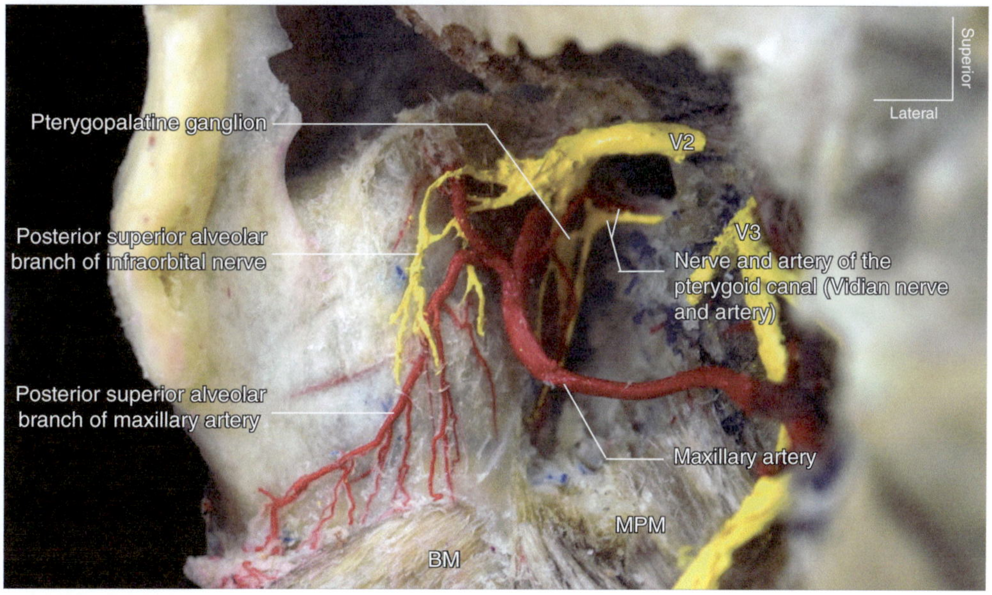

Fig. 4.82 Posterior view of the left pterygopalatine and infratemporal fossae. *BM* bucinator muscle, *MPM* medial pterygoid muscle

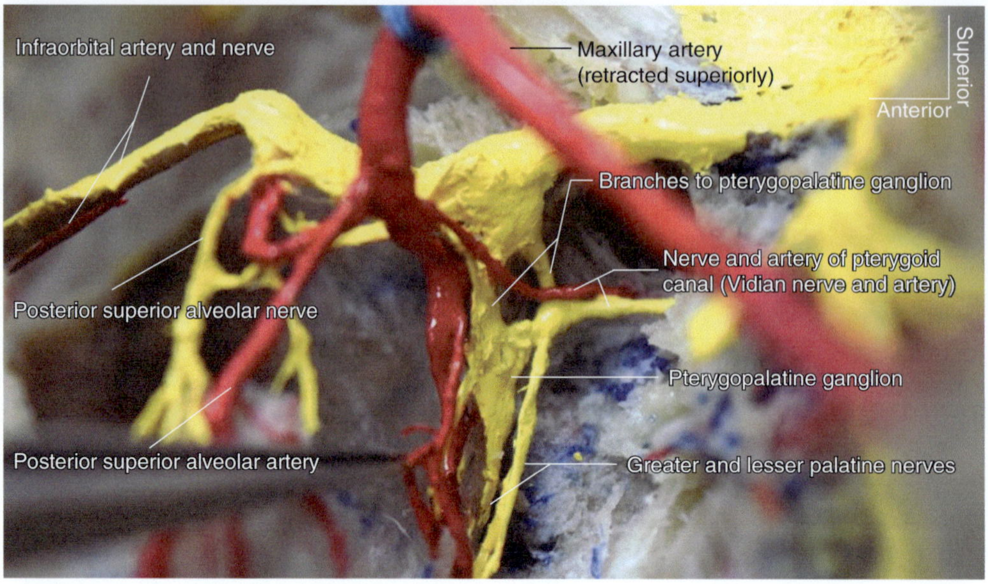

Fig. 4.83 Lateral magnified view of the left pterygopalatine fossa

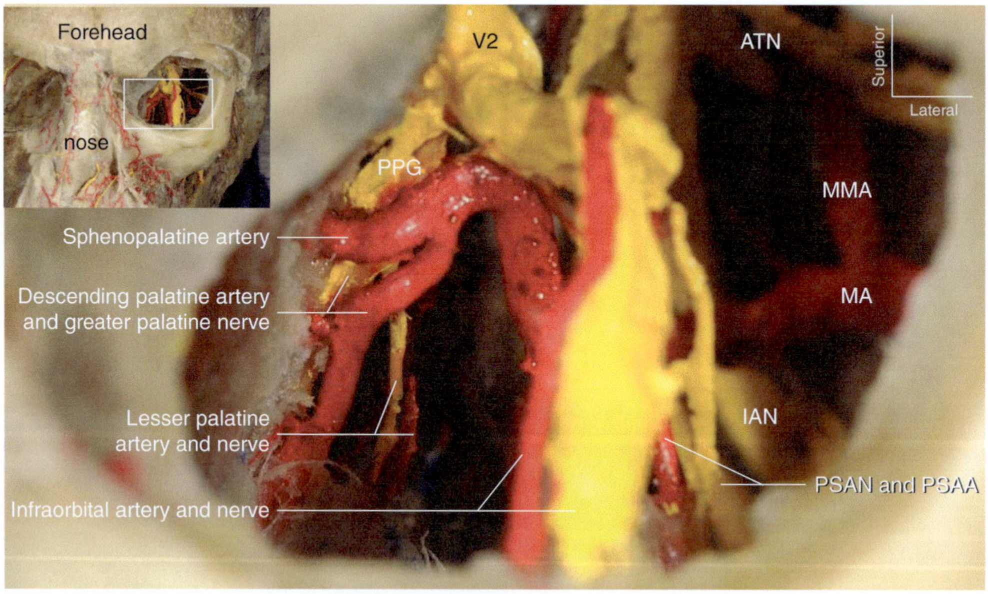

Fig. 4.84 Anterior magnified view (rectangular area in the left upper figure) of the left pterygopalatine fossa viewed through the orbit. The posterior wall of the maxilla and infraorbital canal have been removed. *ATN* auriculotemporal nerve, *IAN* inferior alveolar nerve, *MA* maxillary artery, *MMA* middle meningeal artery, *PPG* pterygopalatine fossa, *PSAA* posterior superior alveolar artery, *PSAN* posterior superior alveolar nerve

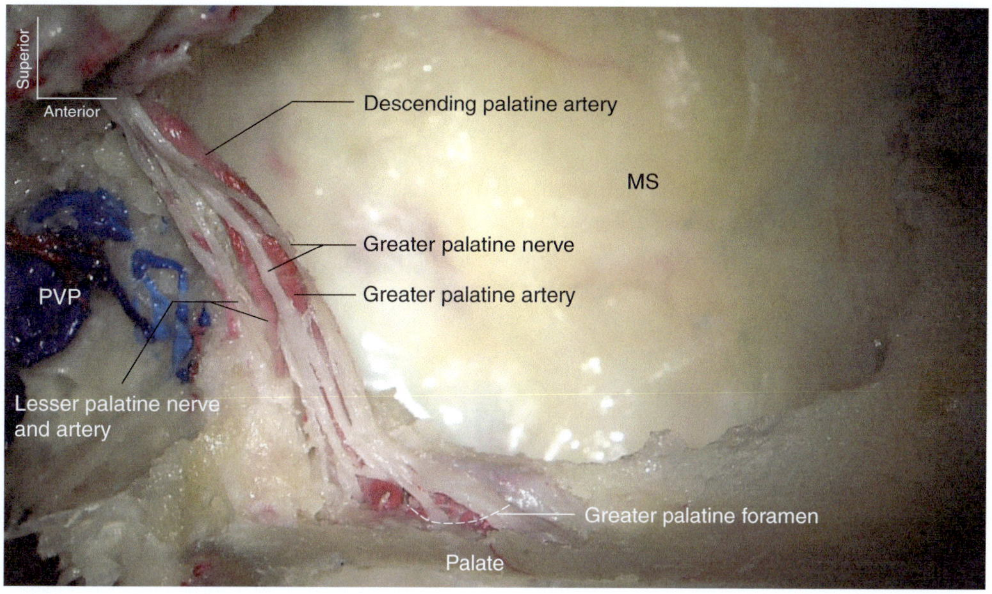

Fig. 4.85 Medial magnified view of the lower part of the left pterygopalatine fossa and greater palatine canal. The greater palatine canal has been removed. *MS* maxillary sinus, *PVP* pterygoid venous plexus

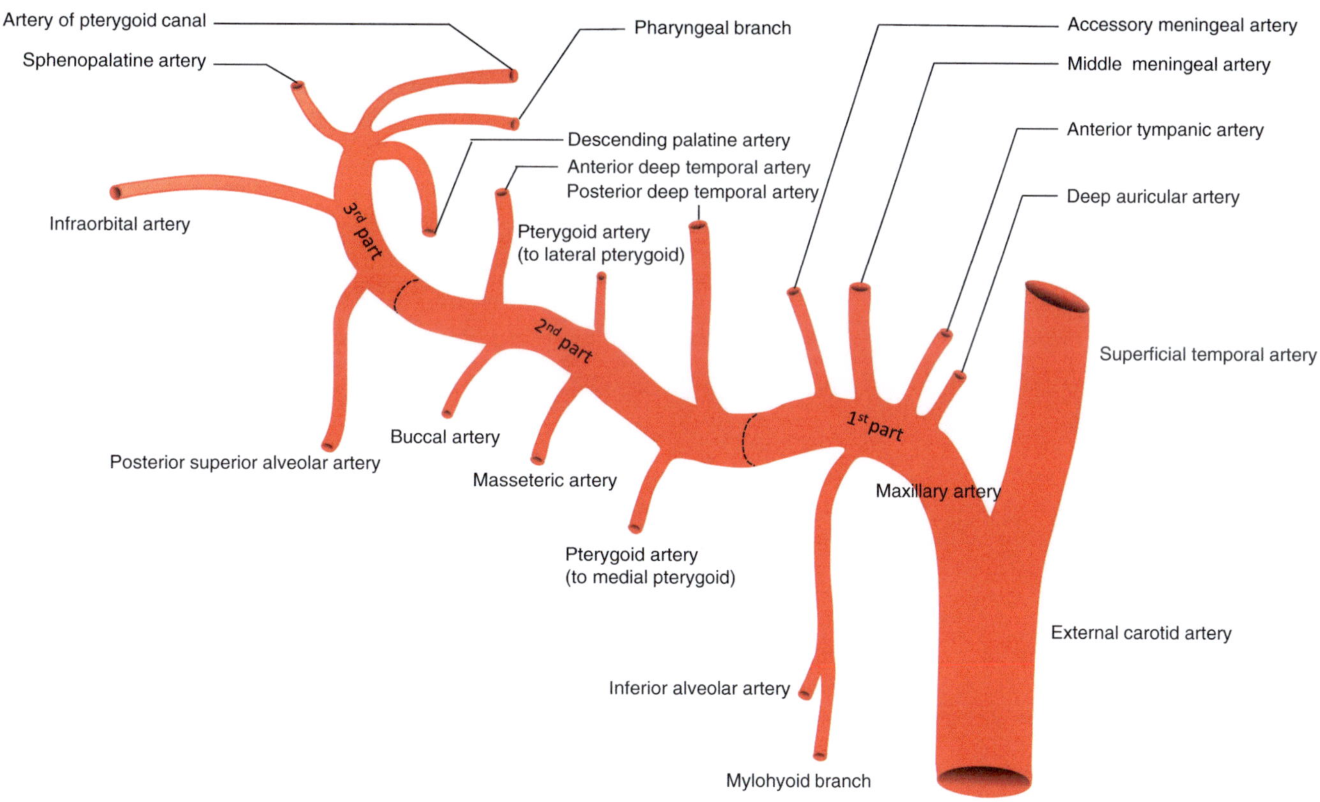

Fig. 4.86 Schematic drawing of the branches of the maxillary artery

4.8 Neck (Submental Space, Submandibular, etc.)

Summary

The anatomy of the neck can be considered to include the maxillofacial region, pharynx, and larynx. Given that surgeons incise/reflect the tissues of the neck layer by layer, it is better to understand the anatomical structures of the neck following the same order, from superficial to deep. A better understanding of the fasciae, spaces, triangles, and their boundaries helps the surgeon identify structures that they need to sacrifice or save. To avoid surgical complications, to operate safely and more effectively, knowledge of the anatomy of the neck is important. In this section, the anatomy of the neck, especially the lateral neck including the submandibular area will be reviewed.

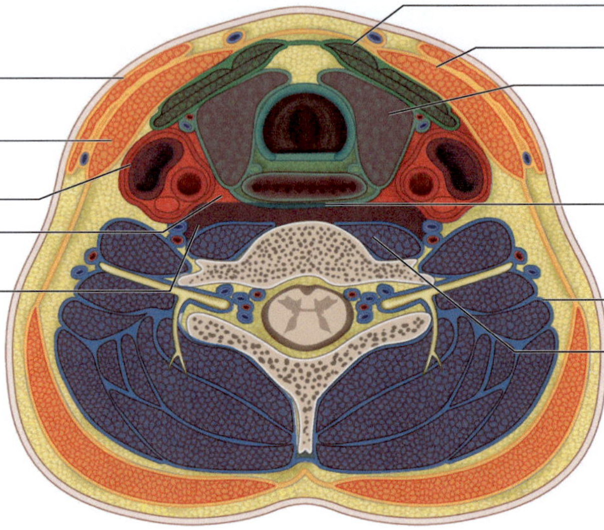

Fig. 4.87 Axial section of the neck (C6-7 vertebral level). The various fasciae of the neck are controversial. The superficial cervical fascia is currently considered to contain the platysma. The deep cervical fascia consists of investing, pretracheal, and prevertebral fasciae. The anatomical space posterior to the esophagus is divided into retropharyngeal and "danger" spaces by the alar fascia

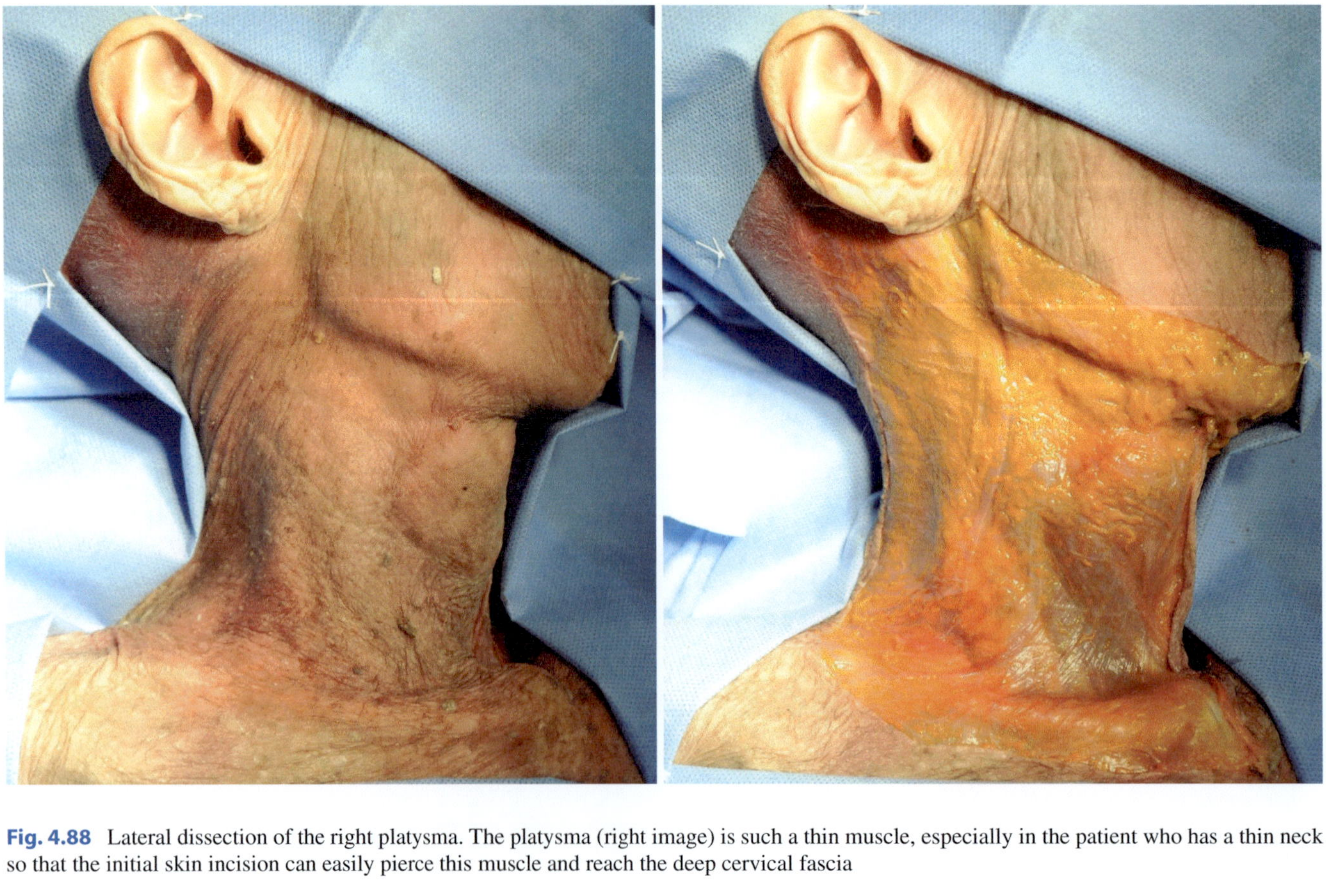

Fig. 4.88 Lateral dissection of the right platysma. The platysma (right image) is such a thin muscle, especially in the patient who has a thin neck so that the initial skin incision can easily pierce this muscle and reach the deep cervical fascia

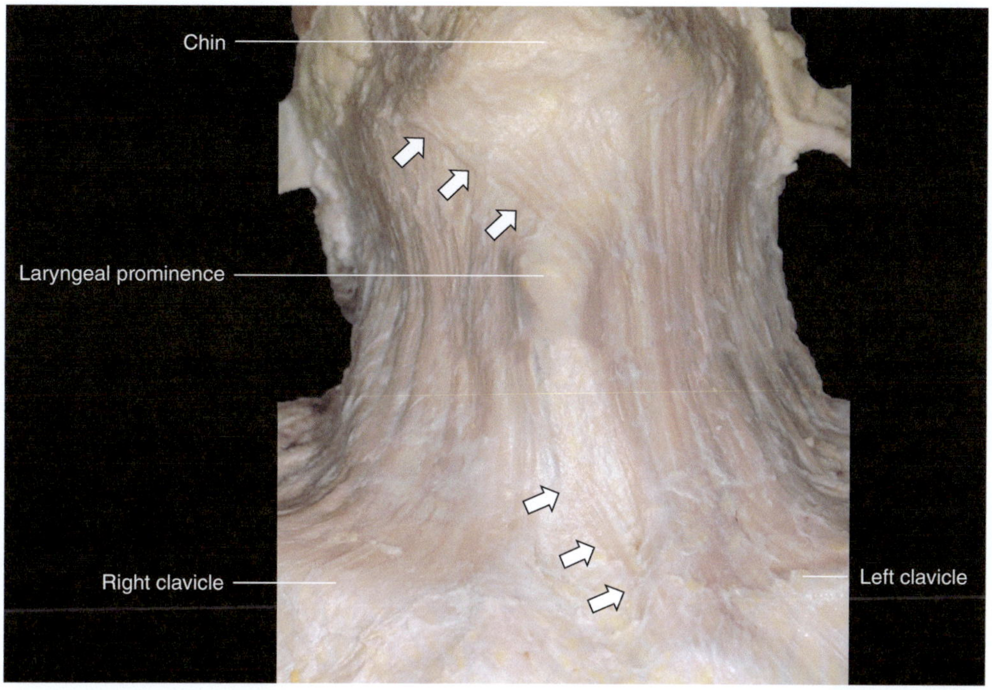

Fig. 4.89 Anterior dissection of the platysma. Note the muscle fibers of the left platysma joining the right. Both the ipsilateral and contralateral platysma often join the depressor anguli inferioris (normal variation). The platysma is innervated by the cervical branch of the facial nerve

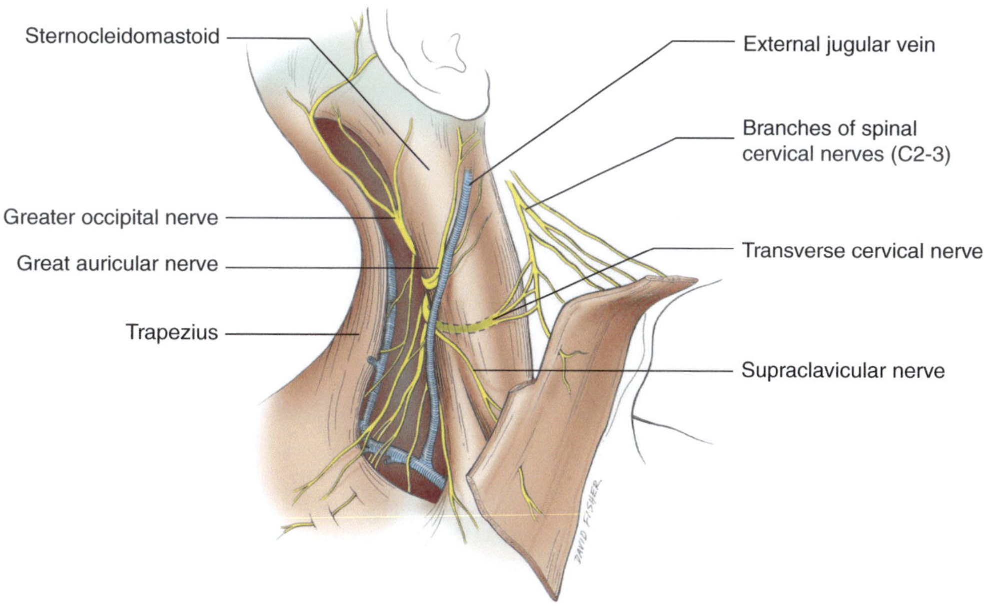

Fig. 4.90 Superficial structures of the left neck (deep to platysma). As anatomical landmarks, the mean distance from the GAN to the EJV, inferior border of the mastoid process, inferior border of the ear is 13.3, 27.7, and 31.0 mm, respectively (Altafulla et al. 2019). The trapezius is innervated by the spinal accessory nerve and cervical plexus (commonly C3-C4), and the sternocleidomastoid muscle is by the spinal accessory nerve and cervical plexus (commonly C2-3).

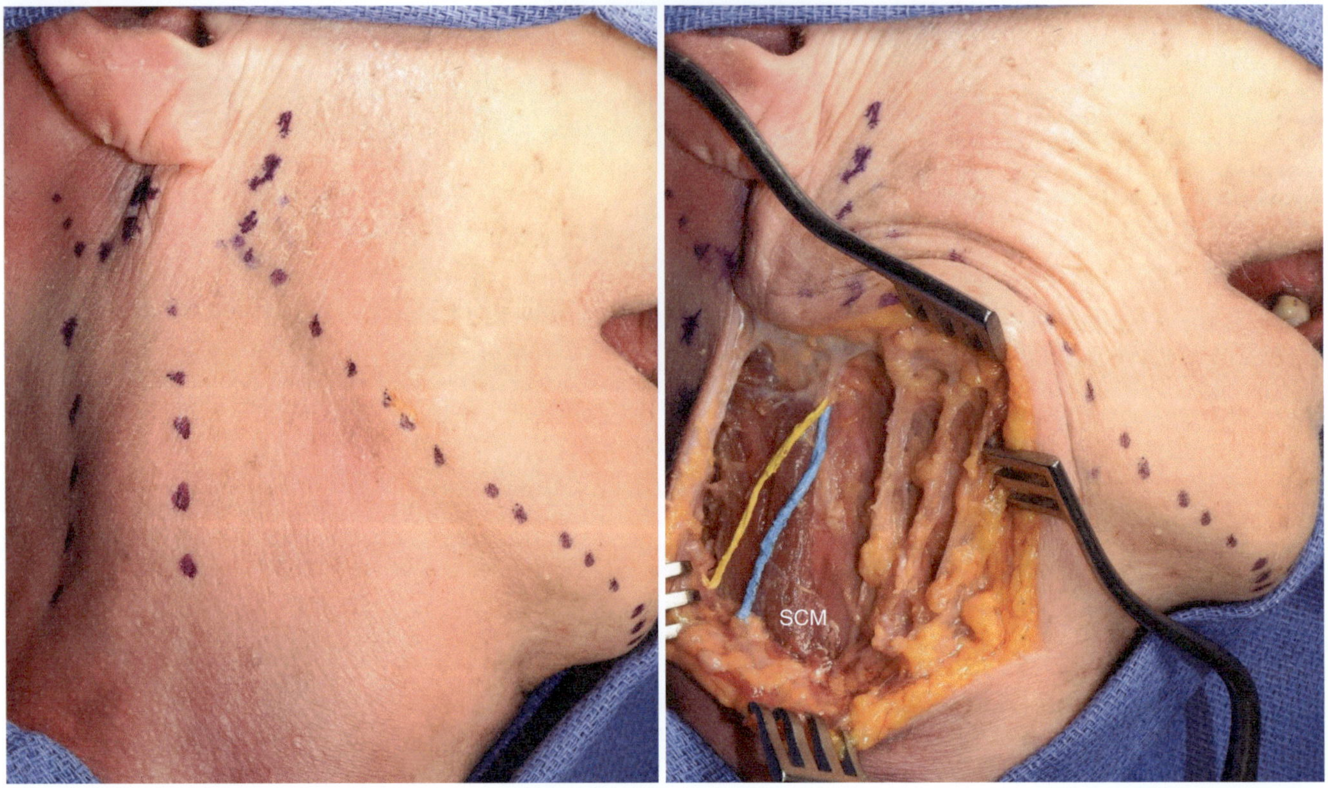

Fig. 4.91 Lateral dissection of the right neck. On the left, the edge of the mandible, sternocleidomastoid muscle (SCM), and mastoid process are outlined. On the right image, the platysma is excised and the SCM is seen deep to the great auricular nerve (yellow) and external jugular vein (blue)

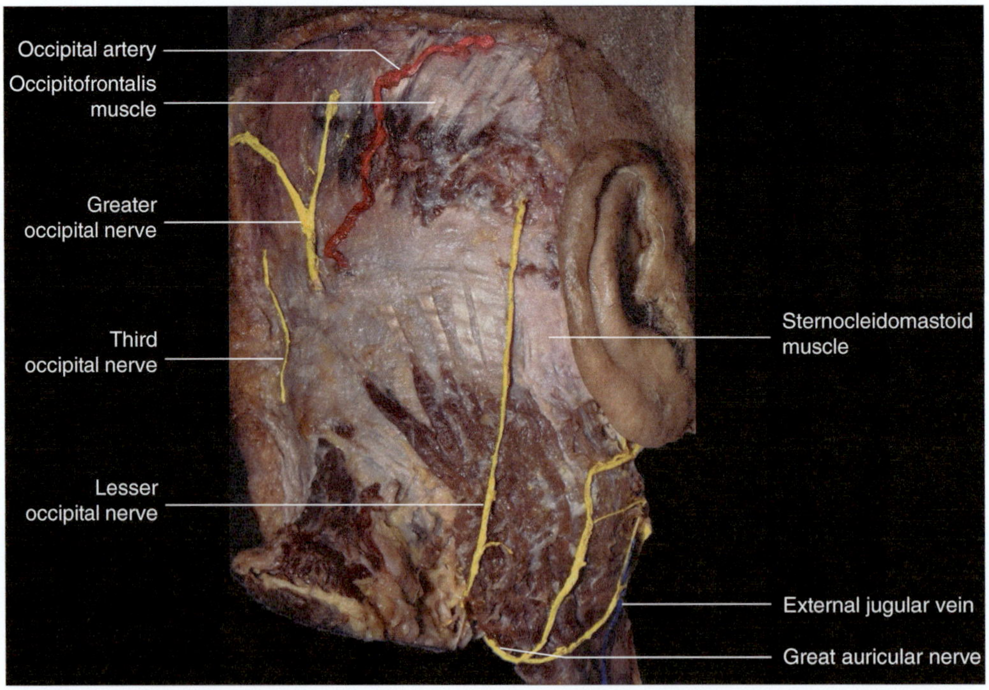

Fig. 4.92 Posterolateral dissection of the right neck

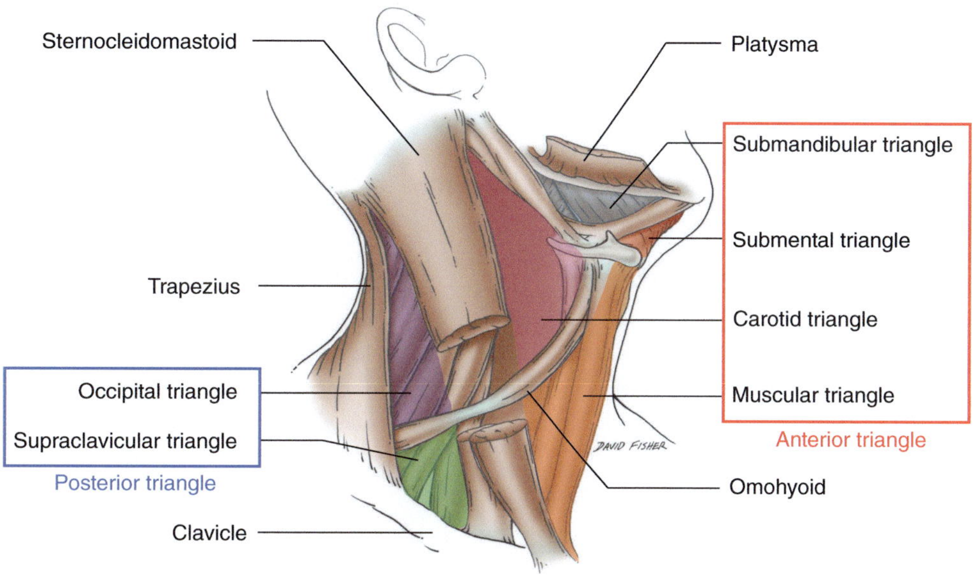

Fig. 4.93 Triangles of the neck. Multiple triangles are used as landmarks for identifying various anatomical structures. For example, the posterior triangle is where the spinal accessory nerve can be identified and the carotid arteries travel within the carotid triangle. In the submandibular triangle, the submandibular gland, facial artery and vein, and even the marginal mandibular branch of the facial nerve might be observed.

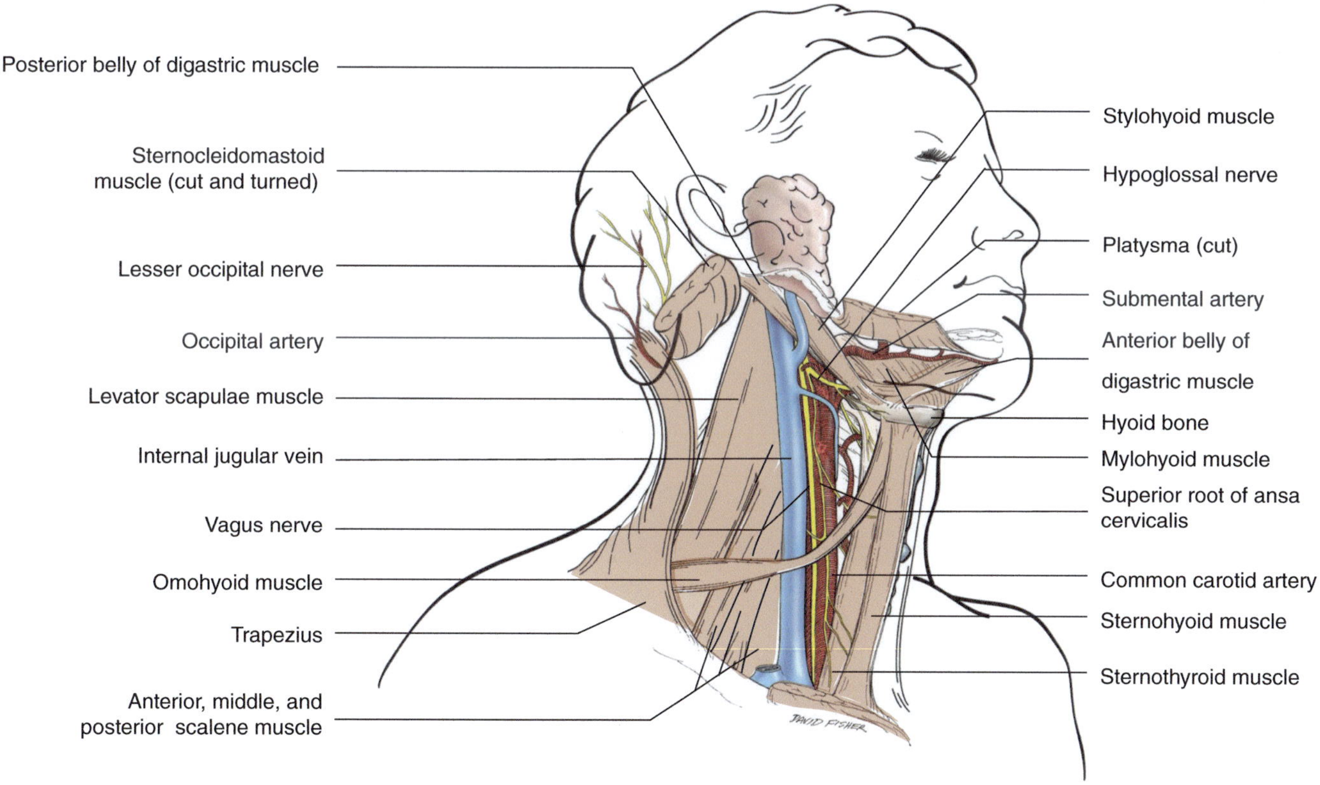

Fig. 4.94 Schematic drawing of the right neck deep to the sternocleidomastoid muscle

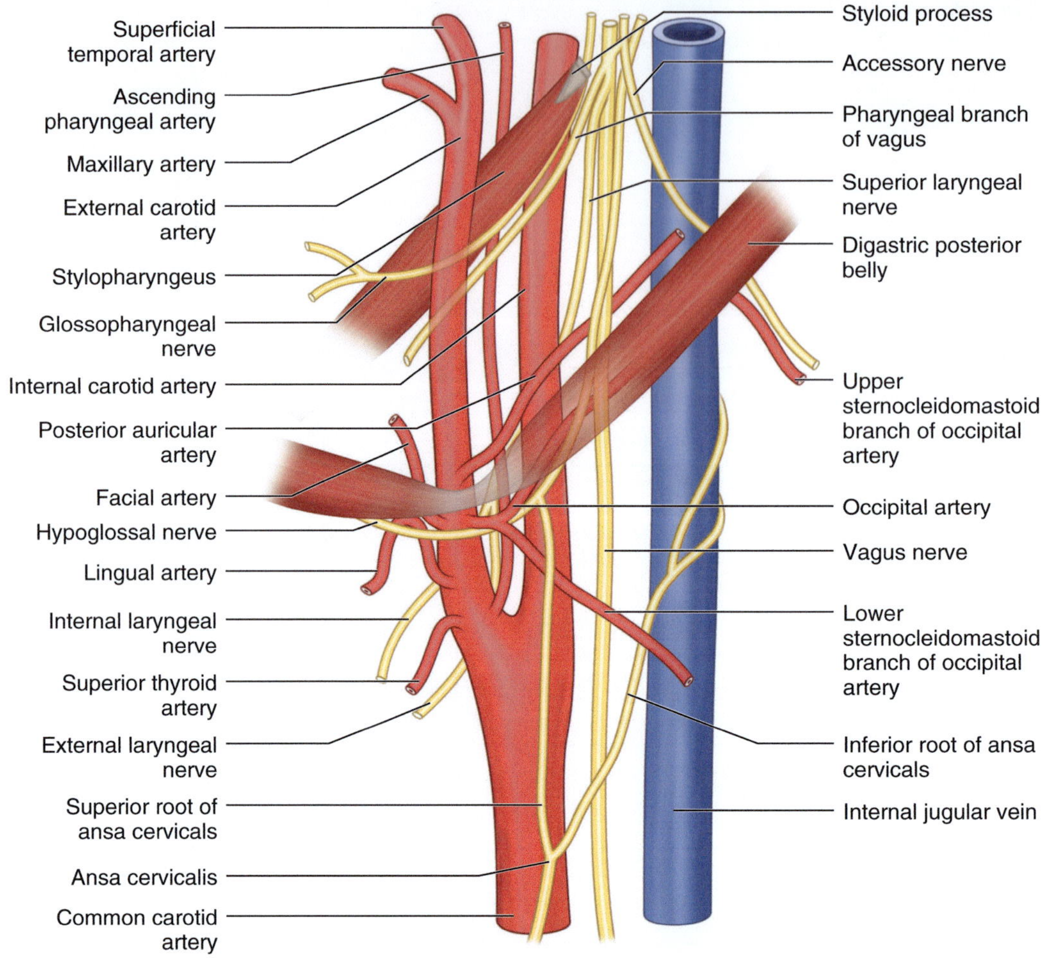

Fig. 4.95 Schematic drawing of the carotid arteries, internal jugular vein, and related structures

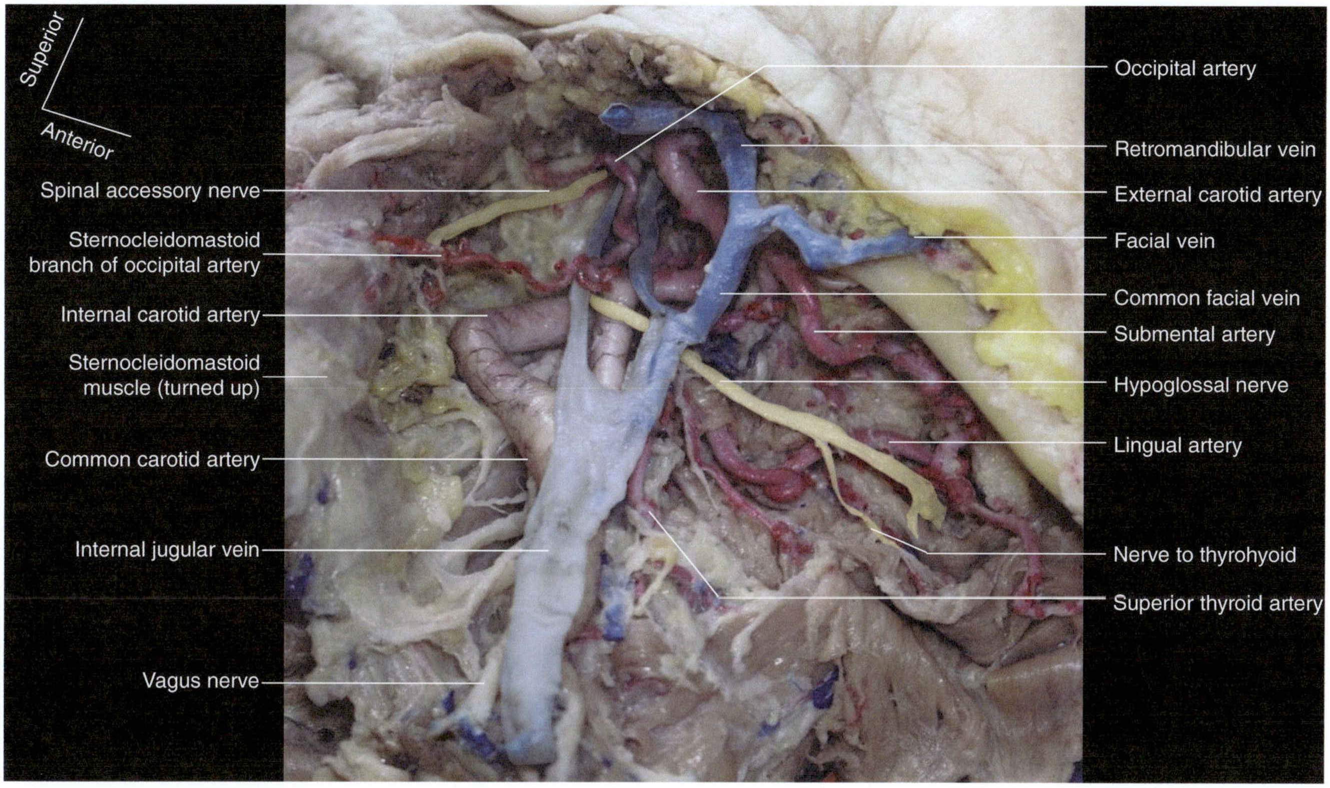

Fig. 4.96 Lateral dissection of the right neck

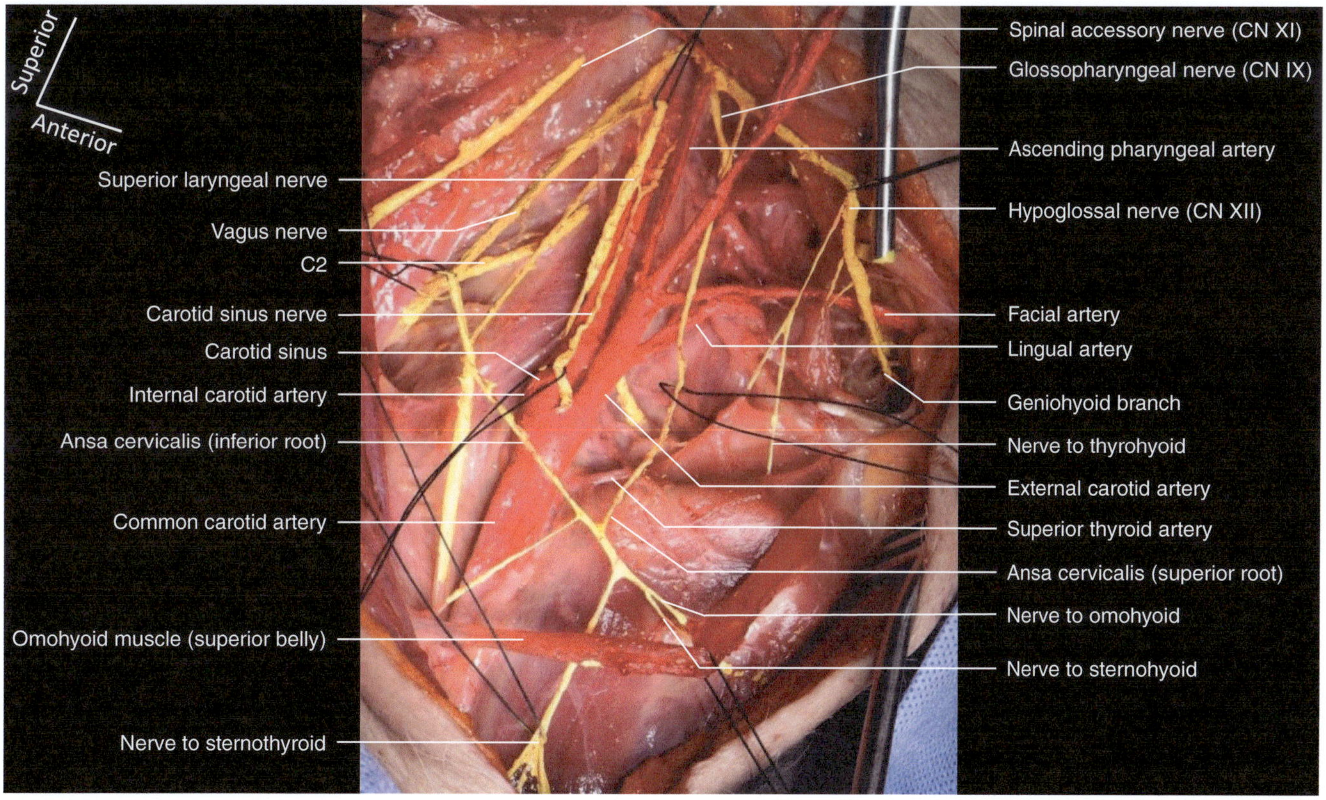

Fig. 4.97 Lateral dissection of the right neck. Note the ansa cervicalis gives branches to all the infrahyoid muscles (sternohyoid, sternothyroid, omohyoid, and thyrohyoid muscles)

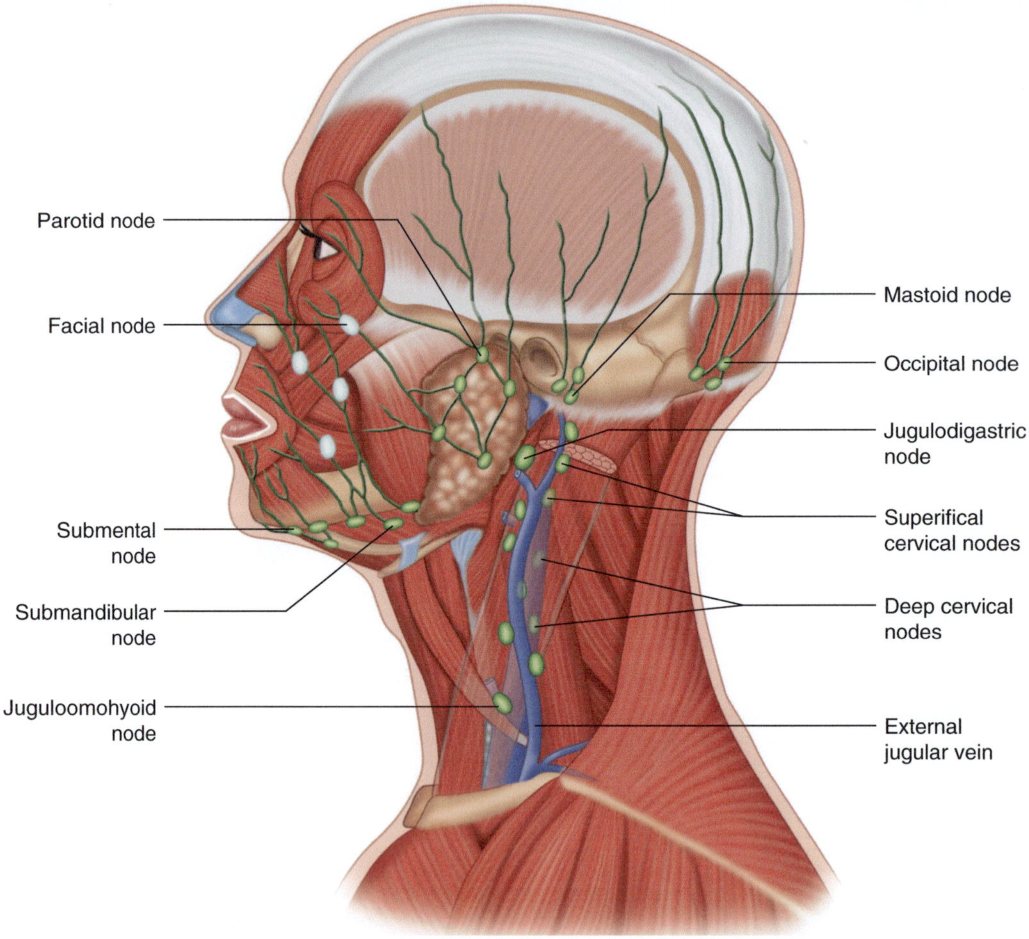

Fig. 4.98 Lymphatic system of the head and neck. The lymphatic vessels terminate into the venous angle via the thoracic duct on the left side

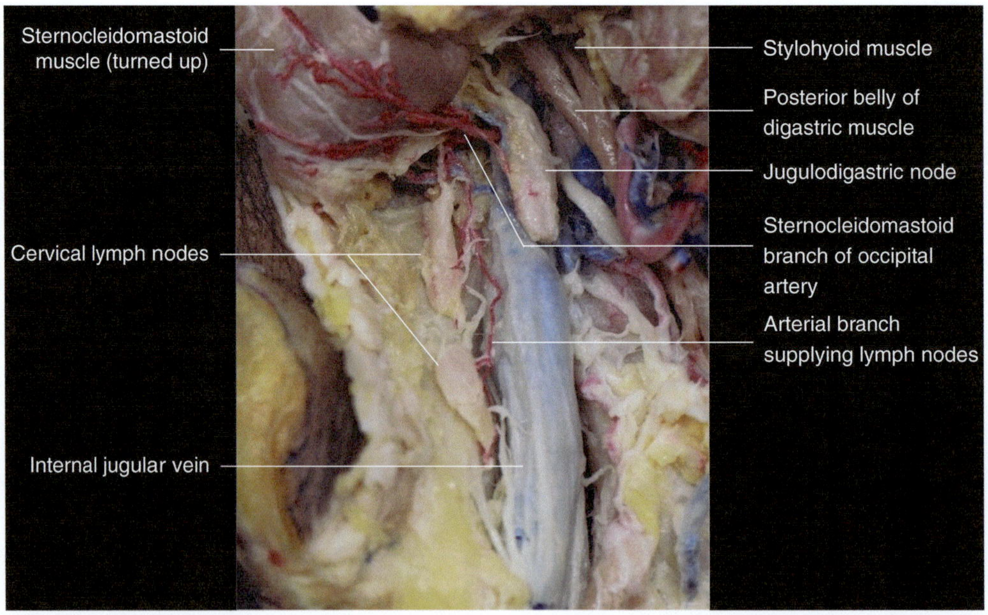

Fig. 4.99 Lateral dissection of the right neck. Note that the jugulodigastric node (JDN) is located inferior to the posterior belly of the digastric muscle. The JDN is the main node that receives lymphatic vessels from the oral and maxillofacial areas. Some cervical lymph nodes are supplied by the branches of the sternocleidomastoid branch of the occipital artery

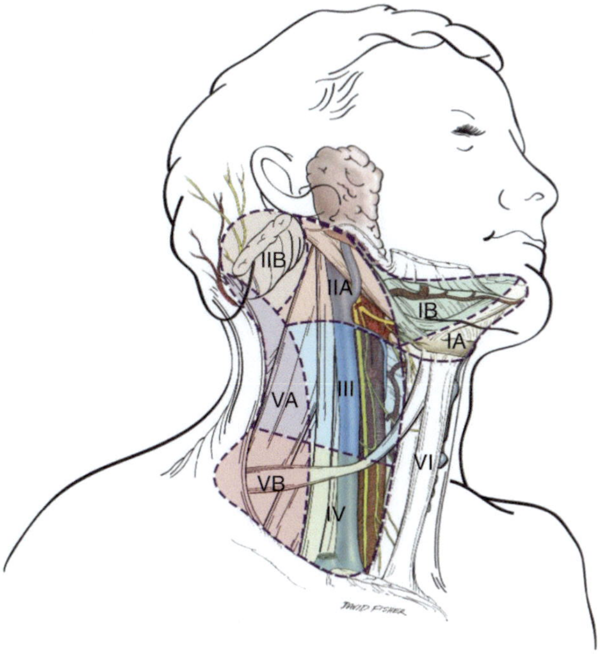

Fig. 4.100 Levels and sublevels of cervical lymph nodes for head and neck cancers and their metastases.

Level	Superior	Inferior	Anterior (medial)	Posterior (lateral)
IA	Symphysis of mandible	Body of hyoid	Anterior belly of contralateral digastric muscle	Anterior belly of ipsilateral digastric muscle
IB	Body of mandible	Posterior belly of digastric muscle	Anterior belly of contralateral digastric muscle	Stylohyoid muscle
IIA	Skull base	Horizontal plane defined by the inferior body of the hyoid bone	Stylohyoid muscle	Vertical plane defined by the spinal accessory nerve
IIB	Skull base	Horizontal plane defined by the inferior body of the hyoid bone	Vertical plane defined by the spinal accessory nerve	Lateral border of the sternohyoid muscle
III	Horizontal plane defined by inferior body of hyoid	Horizontal plane defined by the inferior border of the cricoid cartilage	Lateral border of the sternohyoid muscle	Lateral border of the sternocleidomastoid muscle or sensory branches of cervical plexus
IV	Horizontal plane defined by the inferior border of the cricoid cartilage	Clavicle	Lateral border of the sternohyoid muscle	Lateral border of the sternocleidomastoid muscle or sensory branches of cervical plexus
VA	Apex of the convergence of the sternocleidomastoid and trapezius muscles	Horizontal plane defined by the inferior border of the cricoid cartilage	Lateral border of the sternocleidomastoid muscle or sensory branches of cervical plexus	Anterior border of the trapezius muscle
VB	Horizontal plane defined by the lower border of the cricoid cartilage	Clavicle	Lateral border of the sternocleidomastoid muscle or sensory branches of cervical plexus	Anterior border of the trapezius muscle
VI	Hyoid bone	Suprasternal	Common carotid artery	Common carotid artery

After Robbins et al. (2002)

Fig. 4.101 Levels and sublevels of cervical lymph nodes with their anatomical boundaries. After Robbins et al. (2002)

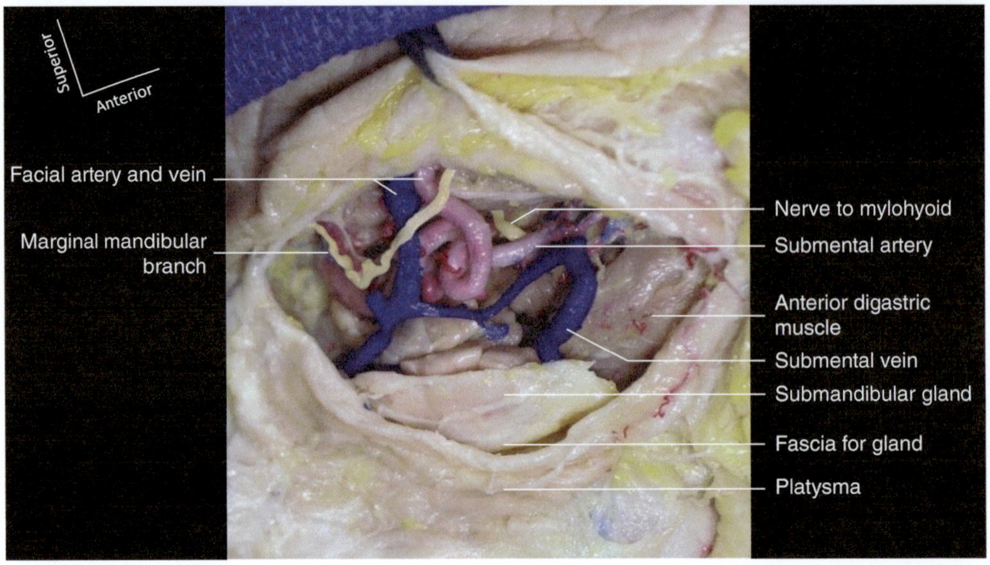

Fig. 4.102 Lateral view of the right submandibular area. A small transverse incision is made into the platysma to reach the submandibular space. The marginal mandibular branch (MMB) runs superficial to the submandibular gland so that the nerve is not damaged if the flap is elevated superiorly with the fascia for the submandibular gland. Note that the MMB is dissected within the elevated flap for better visualization in this photo

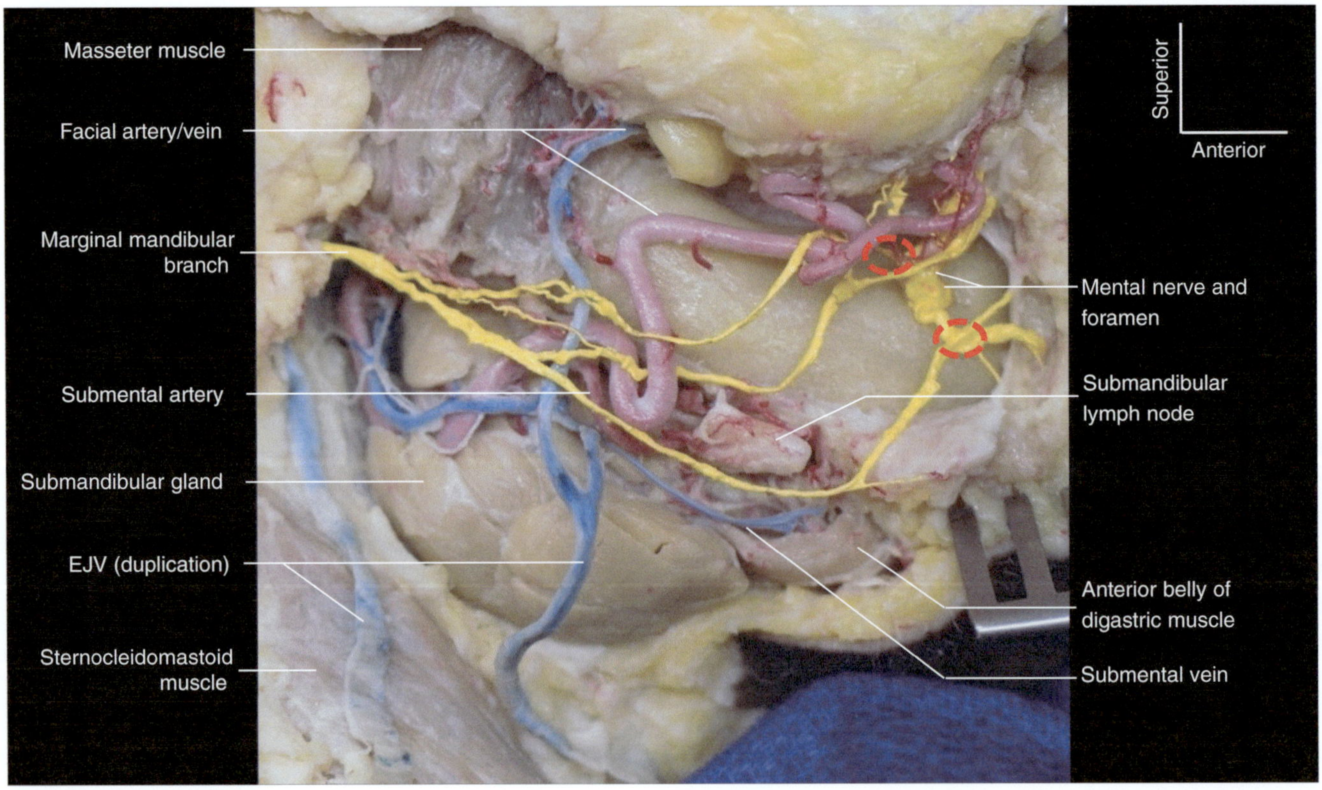

Fig. 4.103 Lateral view of the left submandibular area. The mental nerve and marginal mandibular branch of the facial nerve are seen to have communicating branches (red circles)

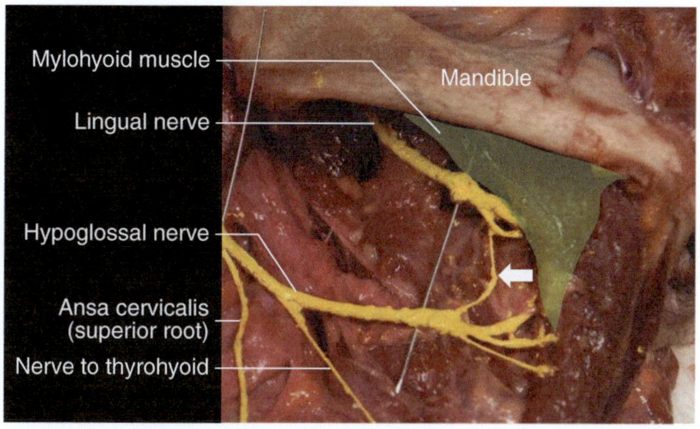

Fig. 4.104 Inferolateral view of the right submandibular area. The mental nerve and marginal mandibular branch of the facial nerve are seen to have a communicating branch (arrow)

Fig. 4.105 Triangles of the submandibular area. Lesser's and Pirogoff's triangles are useful for identifying the lingual artery, and Beclard's triangle is used for identifying both the lingual artery and hypoglossal nerve (Kikuta et al. 2019). © Fisher/Tubbs 2020. All Rights Reserved

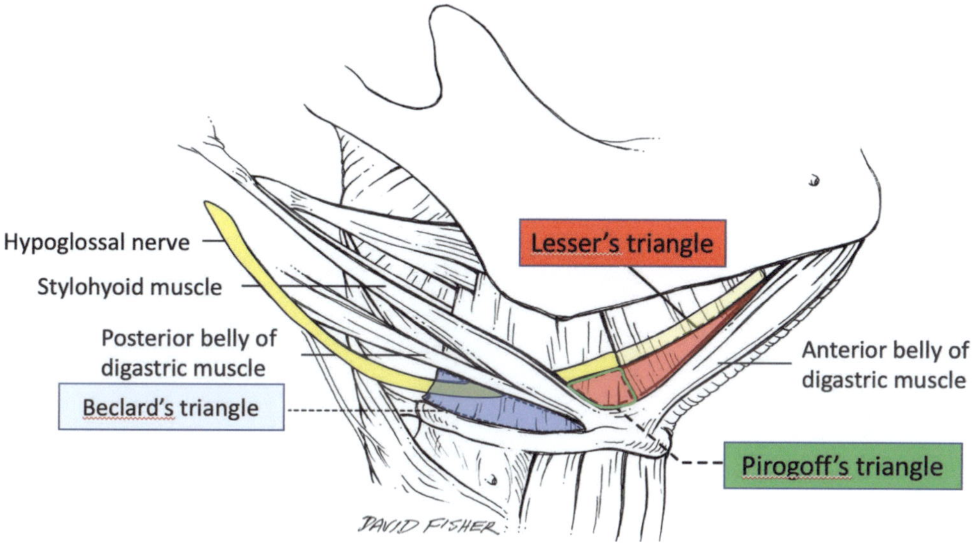

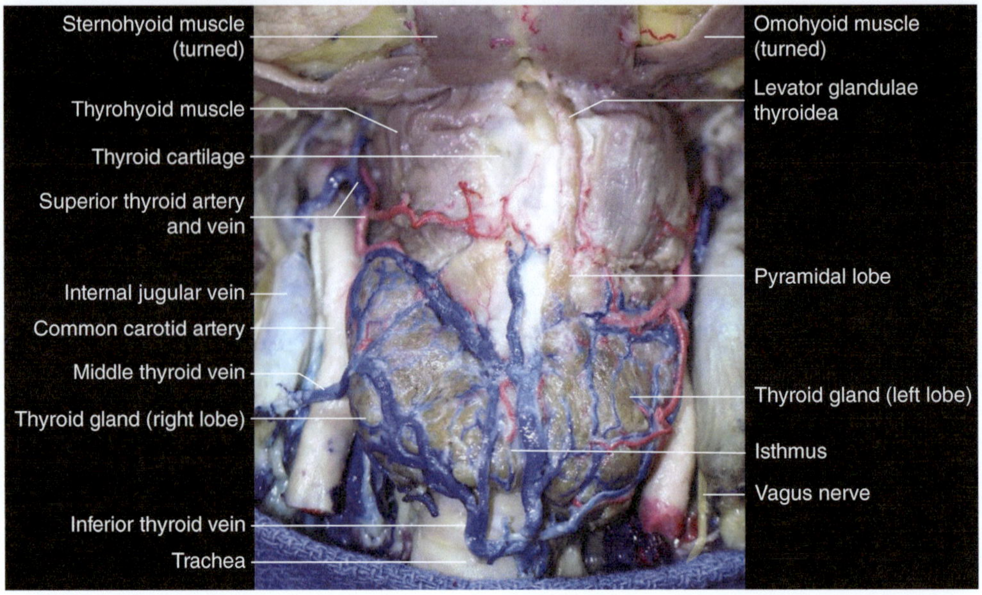

Fig. 4.106 Anterior view of the neck (infrahyoid level). The sternothyroid muscles are removed

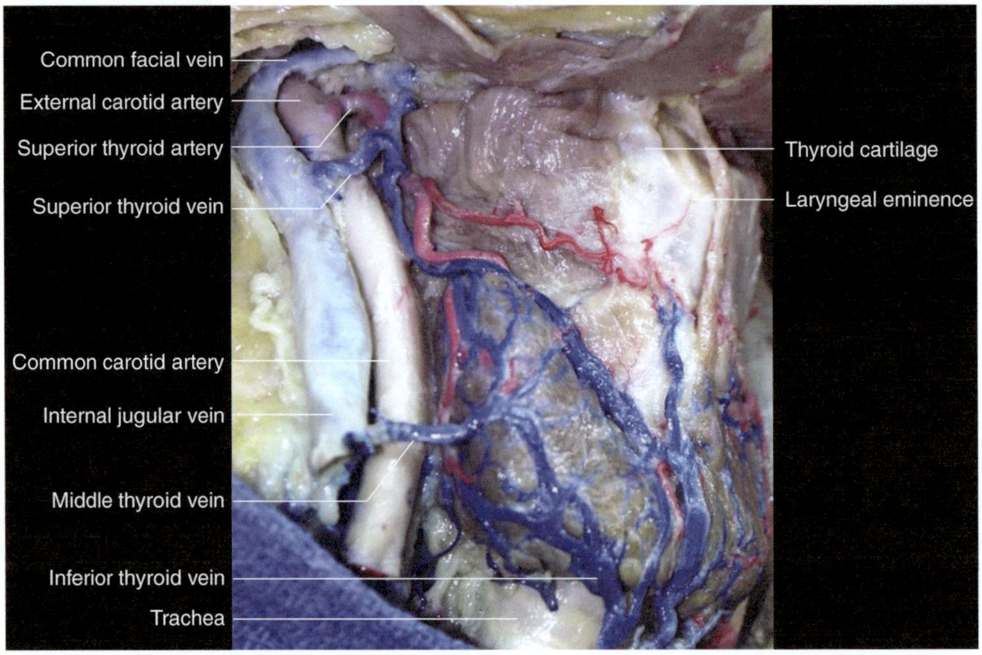

Fig. 4.107 Anterolateral view of the neck (infrahyoid level). The sternothyroid muscle is removed

4.9 Venous Drainage of the Oral and Maxillofacial Areas

Summary

The venous return of the head and neck region as well as the upper limbs terminates in the right atrium via the superior vena cava. The brachiocephalic vein on each side collects the venous blood from both the internal jugular and subclavian veins to drain into the superior vena cava. The subclavian veins drain blood from upper limbs and neck, and the external jugular and anterior jugular veins also drain blood from the neck. However, the majority of the venous drainage of the head and neck (including the brain) is collected into the internal jugular vein.

In this section, the venous drainage system of the head and neck will be shown.

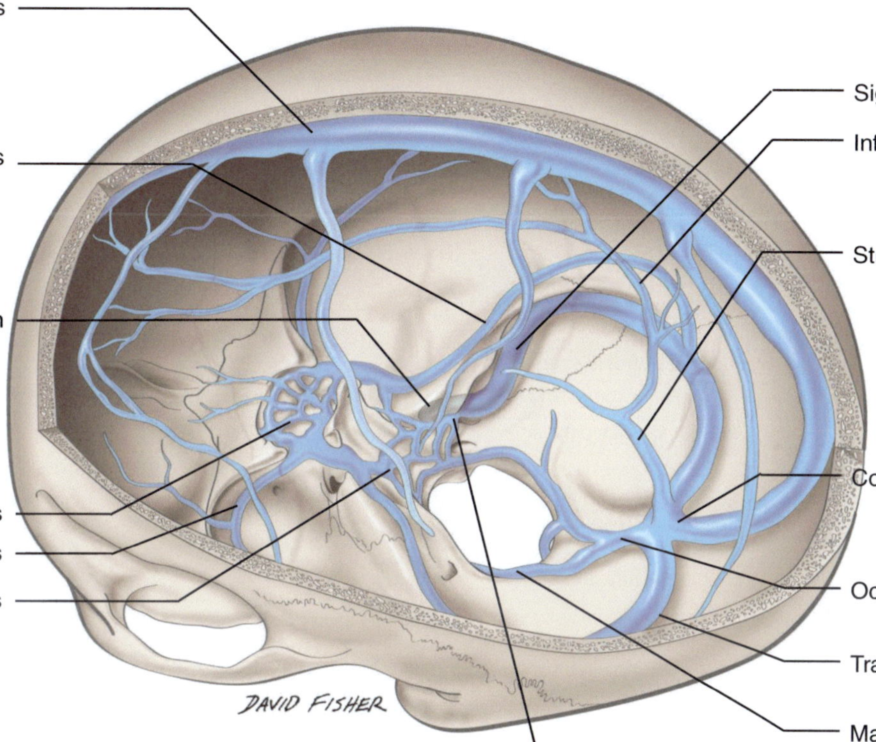

Fig. 4.108 Posterolateral view of the dural venous sinuses and superficial cerebral veins in the brain. The majority of the venous blood of the brain drains into the internal jugular vein via the sigmoid sinus or inferior petrosal sinus.

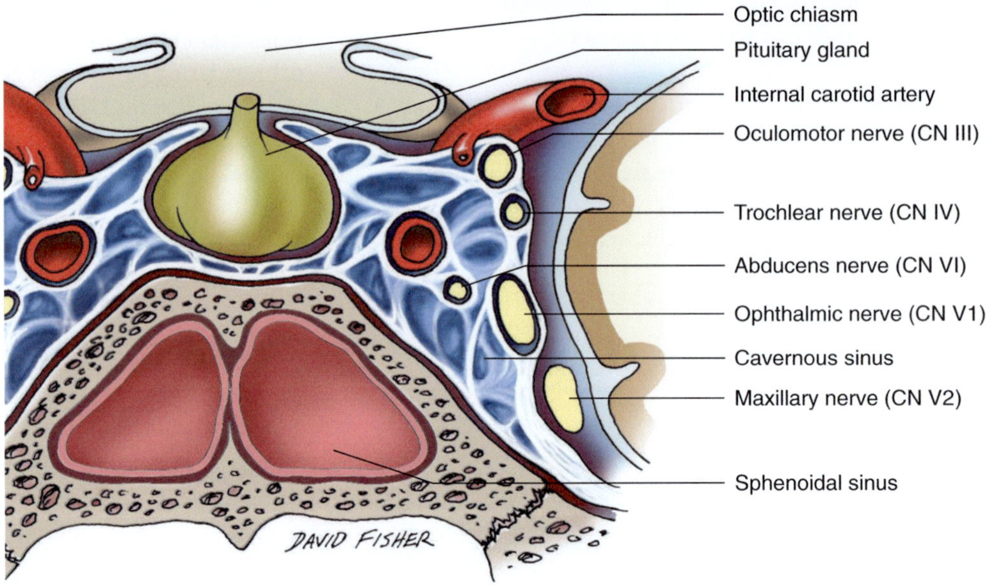

Fig. 4.109 Coronal image of the cavernous sinus. © Fisher/Tubbs 2020. All Rights Reserved

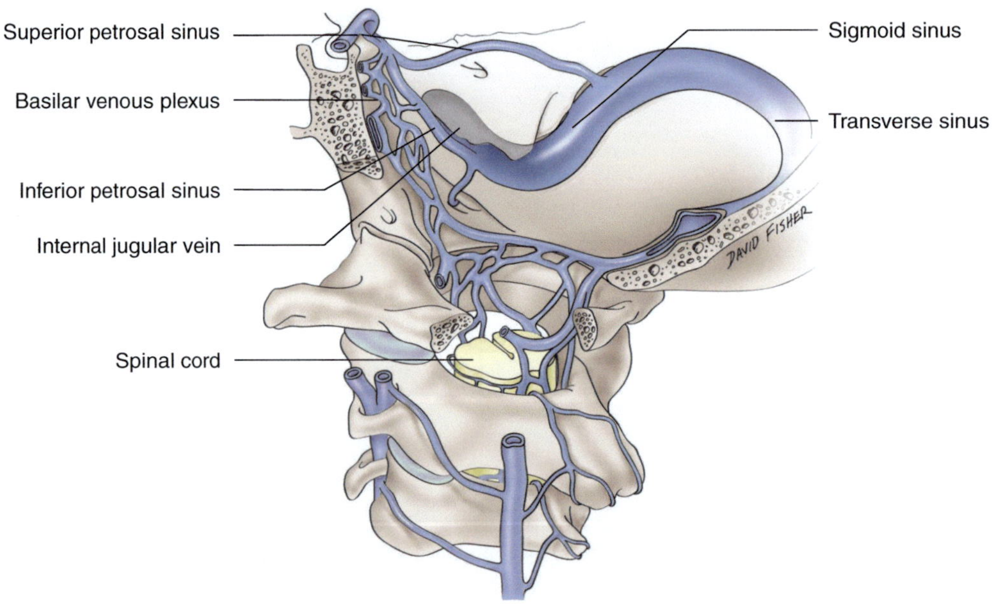

Fig. 4.110 Posterolateral view of the venous drainage of the posterior cranial fossa and craniocervical junction. © Fisher/Tubbs 2020. All Rights Reserved

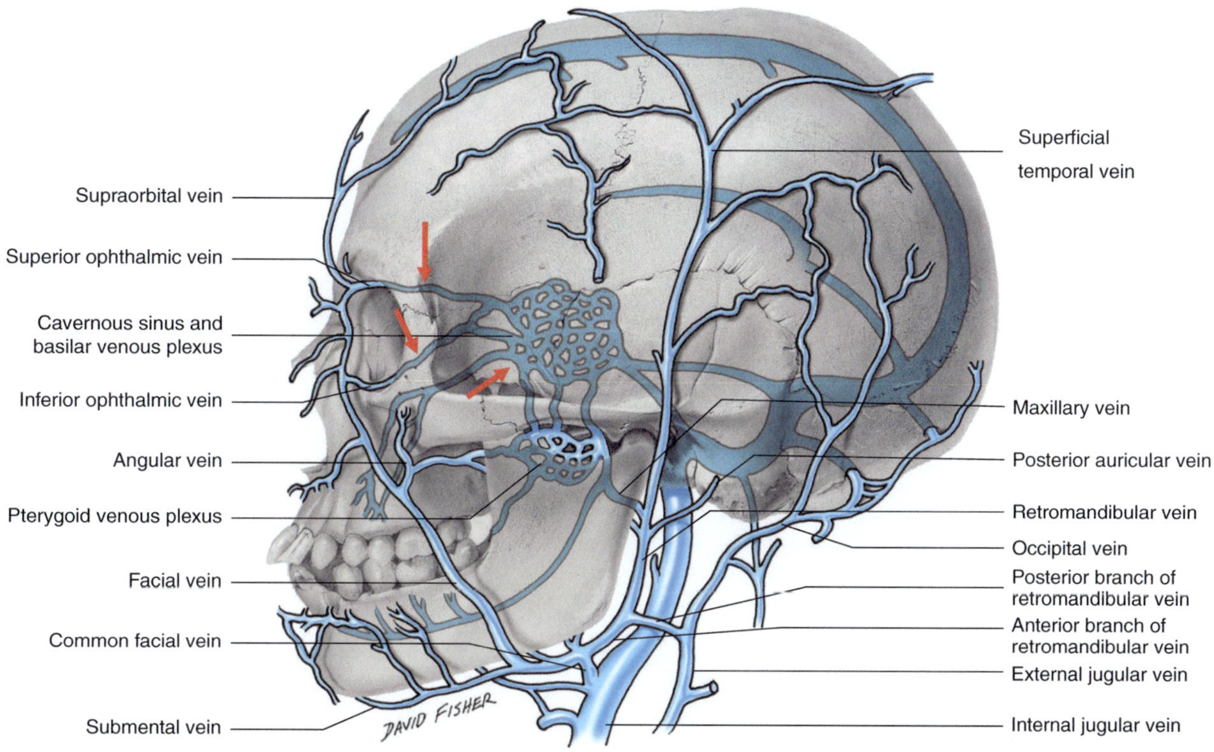

Fig. 4.111 Lateral view of the venous system of the head and neck region. The pterygoid venous plexus, and superior and inferior ophthalmic veins drain into the cavernous sinus (arrows). Unification of the internal jugular and subclavian veins forms the brachiocephalic vein on both sides which drains all the venous blood from the head, neck and upper limb into the superior vena cava

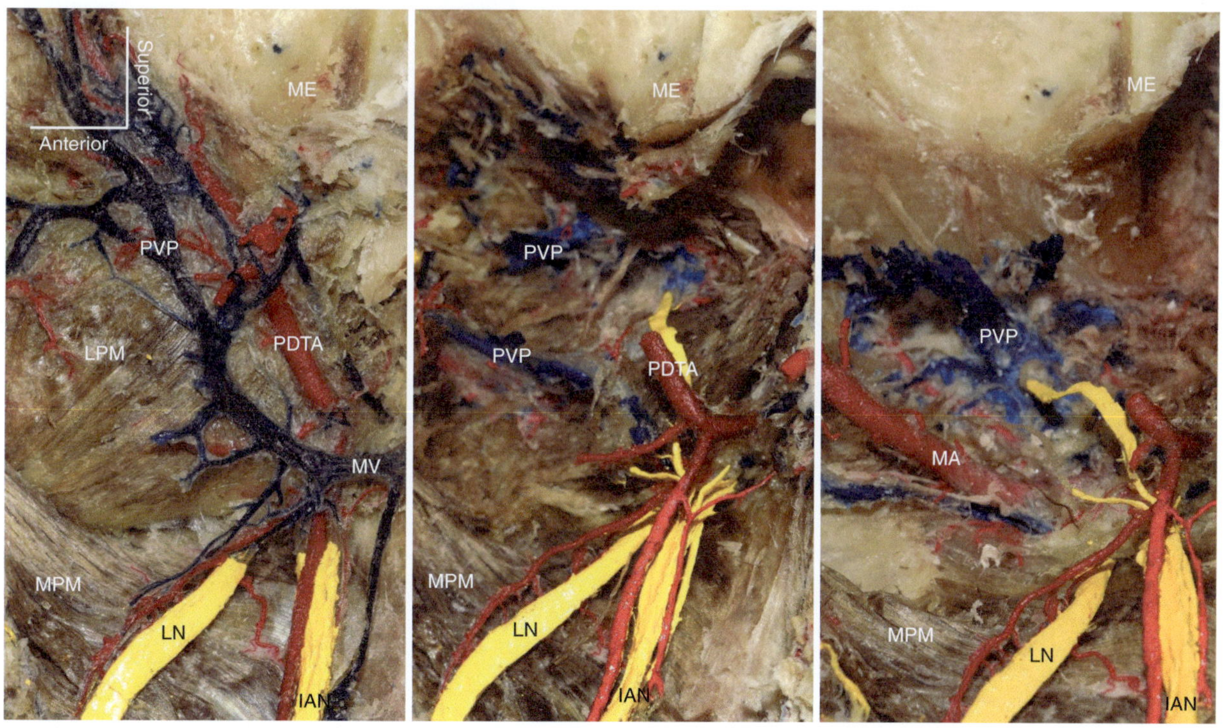

Fig. 4.112 Lateral view of the left infratemporal fossa. Note that the pterygoid venous plexus (PVP) is located lateral to (left image), inside (middle image), and medial to (right image) the lateral pterygoid muscle. *IAN* inferior alveolar nerve, *IAV* inferior alveolar vein, *LN* lingual nerve, *LPM* lateral pterygoid muscle, *MA* maxillary artery, *ME* mandibular eminence, *MPM* medial pterygoid muscle, *MV* maxillary vein, *PDTA* posterior deep temporal artery

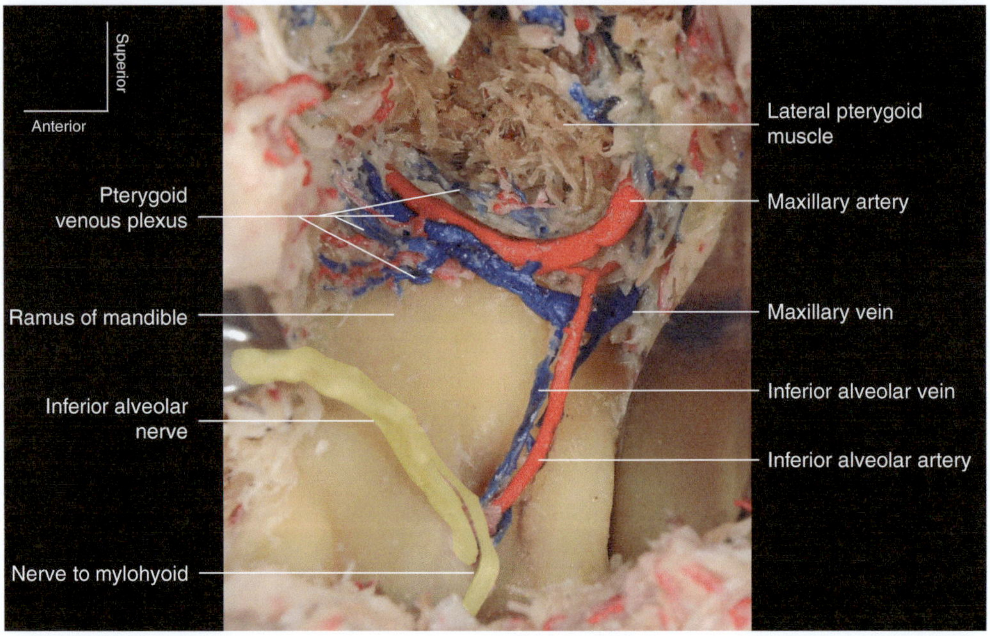

Fig. 4.113 Medial view of the right pterygomandibular space. The medial pterygoid muscle has been removed. The inferior alveolar nerve and nerve to the mylohyoid are reflected anteriorly. Note the pterygoid venous plexus draining into the maxillary vein

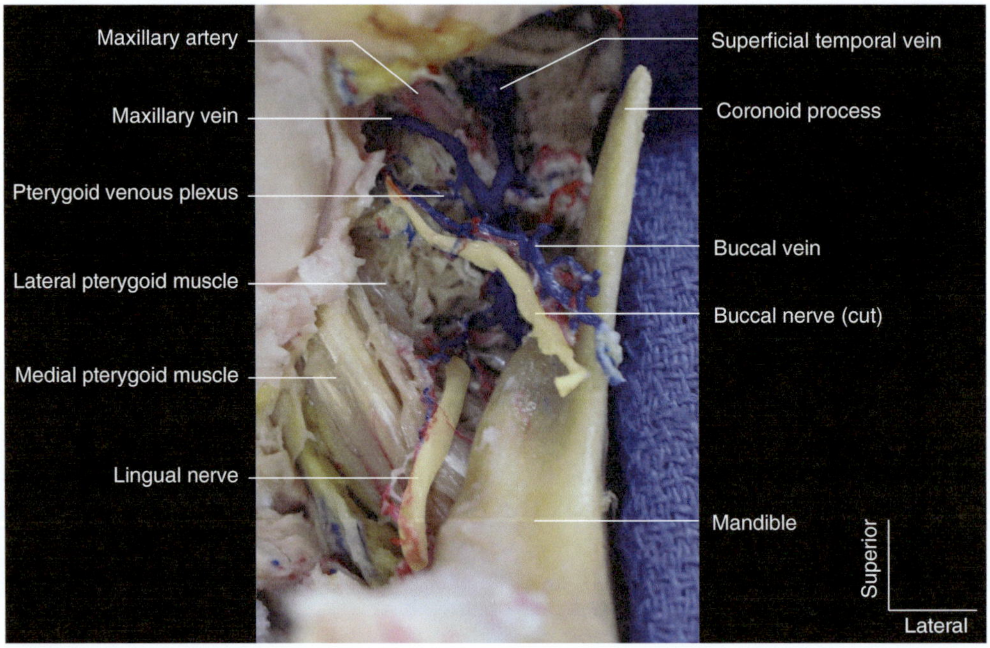

Fig. 4.114 Anterior view of the left pterygomandibular space. The medial pterygoid muscle has been removed. The inferior alveolar nerve and nerve to the mylohyoid are reflected anteriorly. Note the pterygoid venous plexus draining into the maxillary vein

References

Altafulla J, Iwanaga J, Lachkar S, Prickett J, Dupont G, Yilmaz E, Ishak B, Litvack Z, Tubbs RS. The great auricular nerve: anatomical study with application to nerve grafting procedures. World Neurosurg. 2019;125:e403–7. https://doi.org/10.1016/j.wneu.2019.01.087.

Farkas LG, Cheung G. Orbital measurements in the presence of epicanthi in healthy North American Caucasians. Ophthalmologica. 1979;179:309–15.

Iwanaga J, Kamura Y, Tanaka T, Watanabe K, Kusukawa J, Oskouian RJ, Tubbs RS. A new space of the face: the bucco-mandibular space. Clin Anat. 2017;30(7):958–62. https://doi.org/10.1002/ca.22964.

Kikuta S, Iwanaga J, Kusukawa J, Tubbs RS. Triangles of the neck: a review with clinical/surgical applications. Anat Cell Biol. 2019;52(2):120–7. https://doi.org/10.5115/acb.2019.52.2.120.

Lai C-S, Lai C-H, Wu Y-C, Chang K-P, Lee S-S, Lin S-D. Medial epicanthoplasty based on anatomic variations. J Plast Reconstr Aesthet Surg. 2012;65(9):1182–7.

Robbins KT, Clayman G, Levine PA, et al. Neck dissection classification update: revisions proposed by the American Head and Neck Society and the American Academy of Otolaryngology–Head and Neck Surgery. Arch Otolaryngol Head Neck Surg. 2002;128:751–8.

Sakamoto Y. Interrelationships between the innervations from the laryngeal nerves and the pharyngeal plexus to the inferior pharyngeal constrictor. Surg Radiol Anat. 2013;35(8):721–8. https://doi.org/10.1007/s00276-013-1102-8.

Standring S, editor. Gray's anatomy: the anatomical basis of clinical practice. London: Elsevier Health Sciences; 2020.

Cranial Nerves

5

5.1 Intracranial Course of the Cranial Nerves

Summary

There are 12 pairs of cranial nerves. The olfactory (CN I) and optic (CN II) nerves arise from the telencephalon and diencephalon, respectively, and the remaining cranial nerves originate from the brain stem with the spinal accessory nerve (CN XII) also arising partially from the cervical spinal cord. The trochlear nerve (CN IV) arises from the dorsal aspect of the midbrain and thus has the longest intracranial length of all cranial nerves. The oculomotor nerve (CN III) exits the midbrain in the crural cistern. The trigeminal nerve (CN V) arises from the pons and the abducens (VI), facial (VII), and vestibulocochlear (VIII) nerves arise from the pontomedullary junction. The glossopharyngeal nerve (CN IX), vagus nerve (CN X), cranial root of the accessory nerve (CN XI), and hypoglossal nerve (CN XII) originate from the medulla oblongata. In this section, the intracranial course of the cranial nerves will be shown.

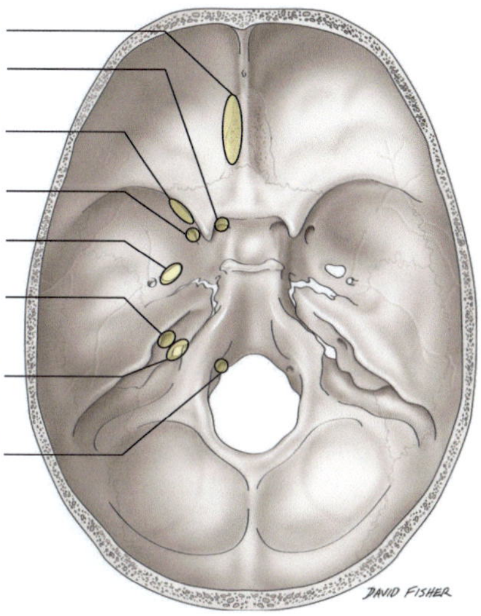

Fig. 5.1 Superior view of the intracranial pathway of the cranial nerves

J. Iwanaga, R. S. Tubbs, *Atlas of Oral and Maxillofacial Anatomy*, https://doi.org/10.1007/978-3-030-78327-3_5

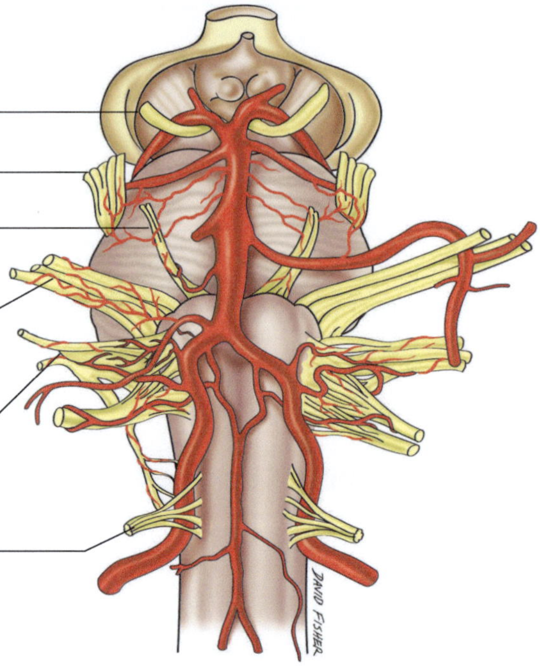

Fig. 5.2 Anterior view of the brainstem illustrating the origin of the cranial nerves, and related arteries. The olfactory nerve (CN I), optic nerve (CN II), and trochlear nerve (CN IV) are not shown

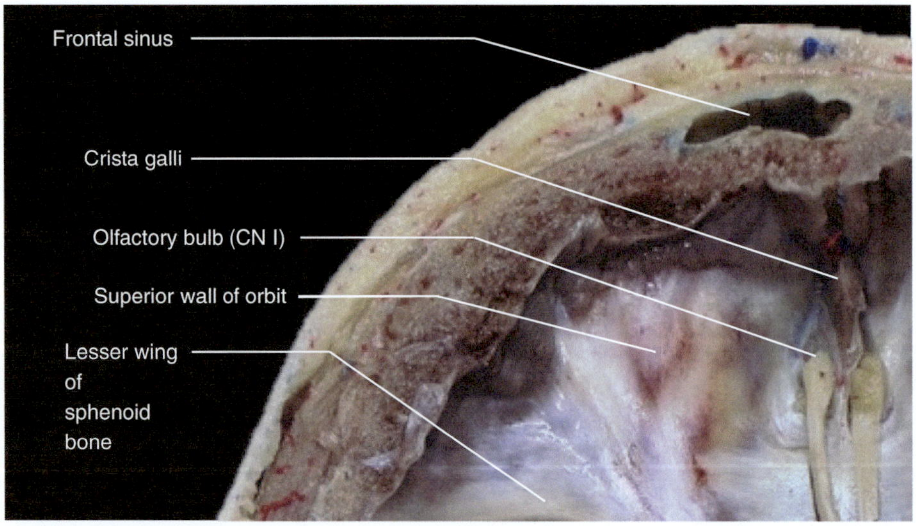

Fig. 5.3 Superior view of the anterior cranial fossa

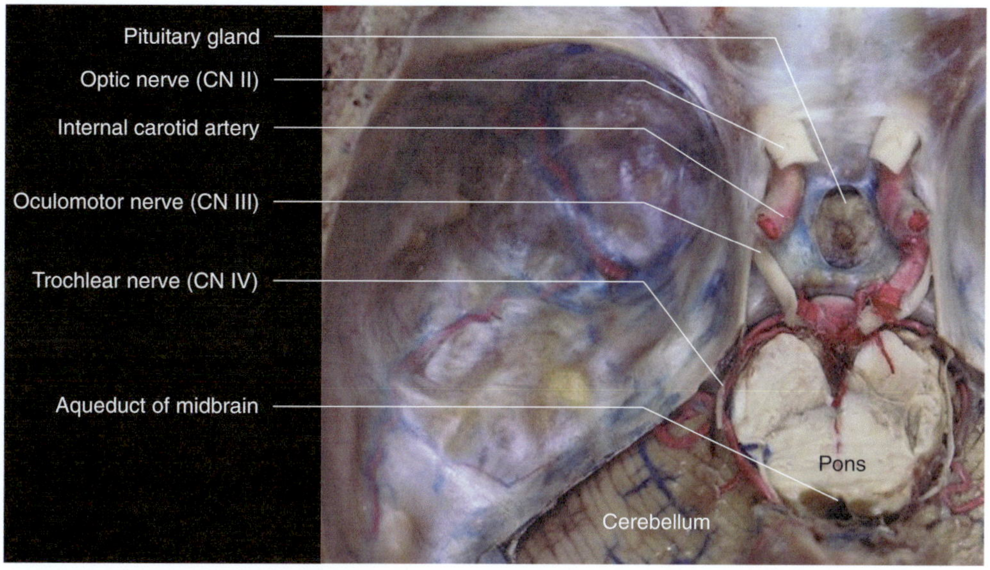

Fig. 5.4 Superior view of the middle and posterior cranial fossae showing cranial nerves II to IV. The tentorium cerebelli is removed

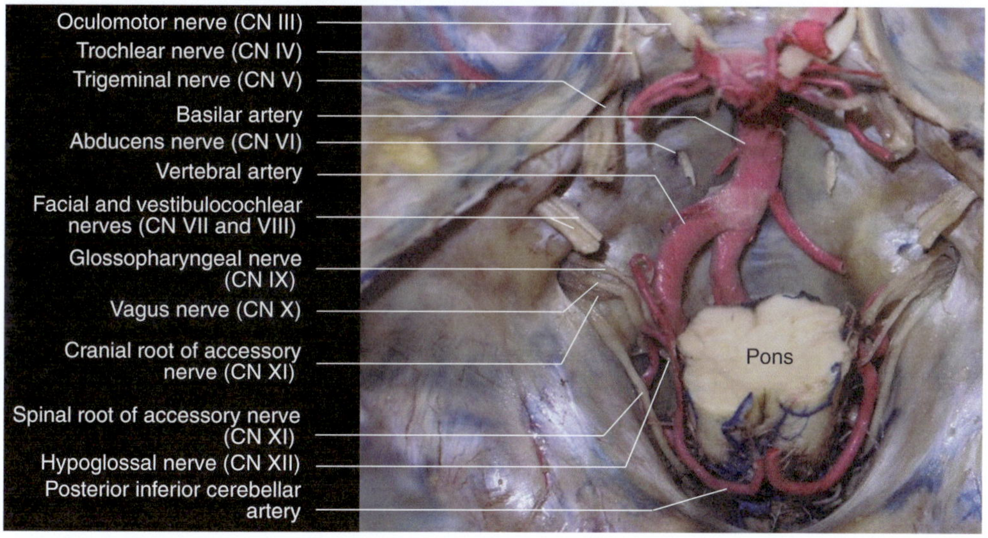

Fig. 5.5 Posterosuperior view of the posterior cranial fossa showing cranial nerves III to XII. The cerebellum and midbrain are removed

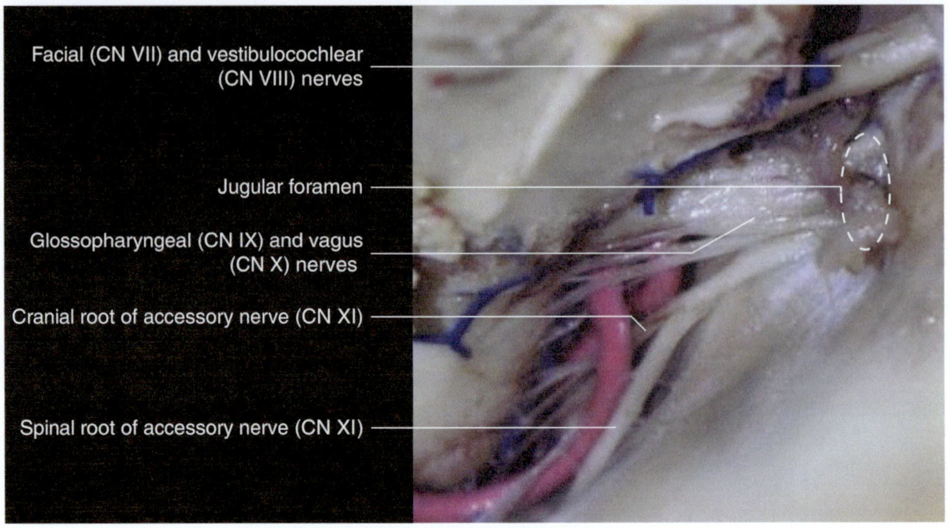

Fig. 5.6 Superior view of the right jugular foramen

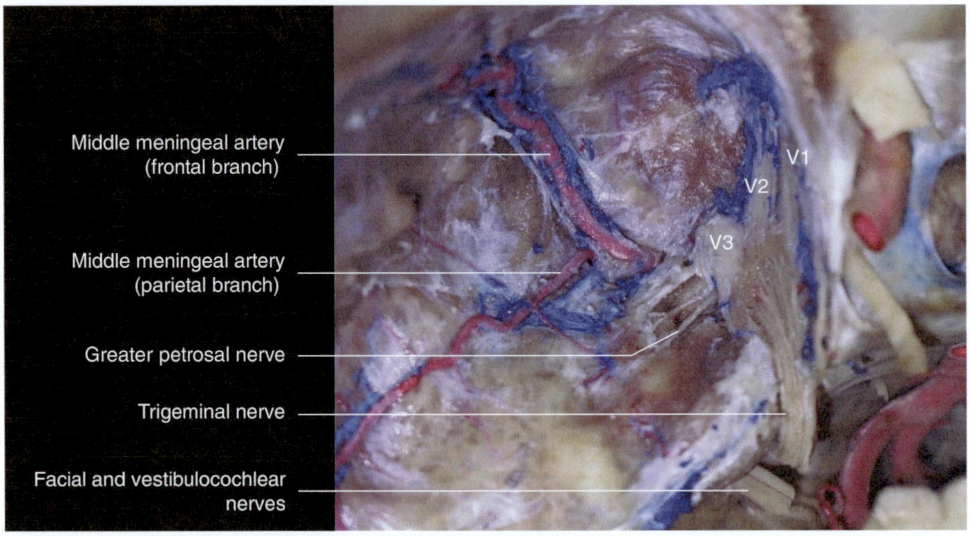

Fig. 5.7 Superior view of the left floor of the middle cranial fossa

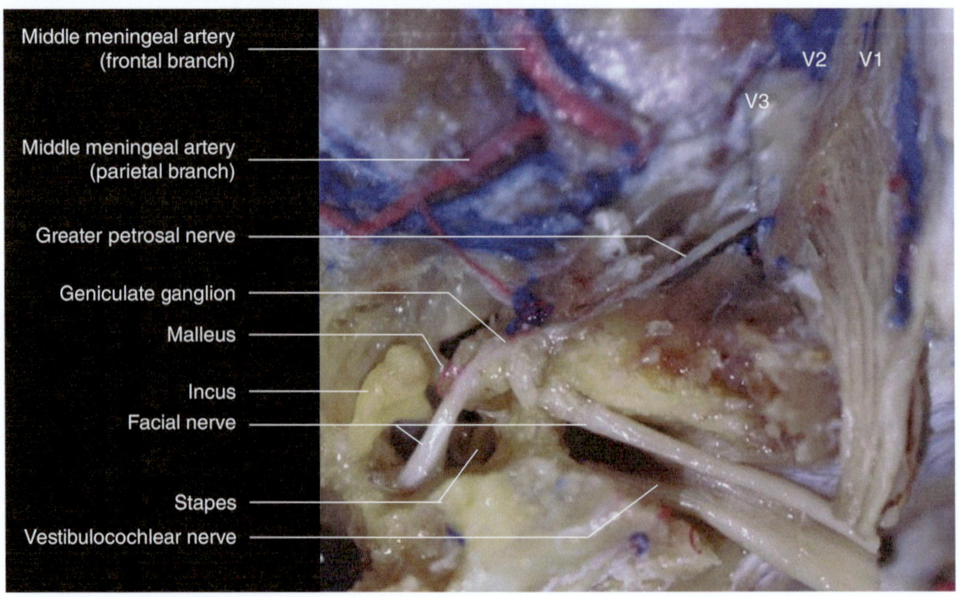

Fig. 5.8 Magnified superior view of the middle cranial fossa

MIX
Papier aus verantwortungsvollen Quellen
Paper from responsible sources
FSC® C105338

If you have any concerns about our products,
you can contact us on
ProductSafety@springernature.com

In case Publisher is established outside the EU,
the EU authorized representative is:
Springer Nature Customer Service Center GmbH
Europaplatz 3, 69115 Heidelberg, Germany

Printed by Libri Plureos GmbH
in Hamburg, Germany